Essentials of Human Genetics

Essentials of Human Genetics

Second Edition

Hema Purandarey MBBS MS
Medical and Reproductive Geneticist
Director and Consultant Medical Geneticist at
Centre for Genetic Health Care
Director Cytogenetics Division
Nicholas Piramal Group of Laboratories
Mumbai, India

Formerly
Associate Professor of Anatomy, Embryology and
Genetics, Grant Medical College
Mumbai, India

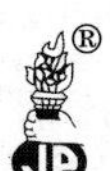

JAYPEE BROTHERS MEDICAL PUBLISHERS (P) LTD

New Delhi • Ahmedabad • Bengaluru • Chennai • Hyderabad • Kochi
Kolkata • Lucknow • Mumbai • Nagpur • St Louis (USA)

Published by

Jitendar P Vij
Jaypee Brothers Medical Publishers (P) Ltd
Corporate Office
4838/24 Ansari Road, Daryaganj, **New Delhi** - 110002, India, Phone: +91-11-43574357
Registered Office
B-3 EMCA House, 23/23B Ansari Road, Daryaganj, **New Delhi** - 110 002, India
Phones: +91-11-23272143, +91-11-23272703, +91-11-23282021
+91-11-23245672, Rel: +91-11-32558559, Fax: +91-11-23276490, +91-11-23245683
e-mail: jaypee@jaypeebrothers.com, Visit our website: www.jaypeebrothers.com

Branches

- 2/B, Akruti Society, Jodhpur Gam Road Satellite
  Ahmedabad 380 015, Phones: +91-79-26926233, Rel: +91-79-32988717
  Fax: +91-79-26927094, e-mail: ahmedabad@jaypeebrothers.com
- 202 Batavia Chambers, 8 Kumara Krupa Road, Kumara Park East
  Bengaluru 560 001, Phones: +91-80-22285971, +91-80-22382956, 91-80-22372664
  Rel: +91-80-32714073, Fax: +91-80-22281761 e-mail: bangalore@jaypeebrothers.com
- 282 IIIrd Floor, Khaleel Shirazi Estate, Fountain Plaza, Pantheon Road
  Chennai 600 008, Phones: +91-44-28193265, +91-44-28194897, Rel: +91-44-32972089
  Fax: +91-44-28193231 e-mail: chennai@jaypeebrothers.com
- 4-2-1067/1-3, 1st Floor, Balaji Building, Ramkote Cross Road,
  Hyderabad 500 095, Phones: +91-40-66610020, +91-40-24758498
  Rel:+91-40-32940929, Fax:+91-40-24758499 e-mail: hyderabad@jaypeebrothers.com
- No. 41/3098, B & B1, Kuruvi Building, St. Vincent Road
  Kochi 682 018, Kerala, Phones: +91-484-4036109, +91-484-2395739
  +91-484-2395740 e-mail: kochi@jaypeebrothers.com
- 1-A Indian Mirror Street, Wellington Square
  Kolkata 700 013, Phones: +91-33-22651926, +91-33-22276404
  +91-33-22276415, Rel: +91-33-32901926, Fax: +91-33-22656075
  e-mail: kolkata@jaypeebrothers.com
- Lekhraj Market III, B-2, Sector-4, Faizabad Road, Indira Nagar
  Lucknow 226 016 Phones: +91-522-3040553, +91-522-3040554
  e-mail: lucknow@jaypeebrothers.com
- 106 Amit Industrial Estate, 61 Dr SS Rao Road, Near MGM Hospital, Parel
  Mumbai 400 012, Phones: +91-22-24124863, +91-22-24104532,
  Rel: +91-22-32926896, Fax: +91-22-24160828
  e-mail: mumbai@jaypeebrothers.com
- "KAMALPUSHPA" 38, Reshimbag, Opp. Mohota Science College, Umred Road
  Nagpur 440 009 (MS), Phone: Rel: +91-712-3245220, Fax: +91-712-2704275
  e-mail: nagpur@jaypeebrothers.com

USA Office
1745, Pheasant Run Drive, Maryland Heights (Missouri), MO 63043, USA, Ph: 001-636-6279734
e-mail: jaypee@jaypeebrothers.com, anjulav@jaypeebrothers.com

Essentials of Human Genetics

First Edition: **2002**
Second Edition: **2009**

ISBN 978-81-8448-535-6

Typeset at JPBMP typesetting unit
Printed at Rajkamal Electric Press, B-35/9, G.T. Karnal Road, Delhi-33

To

My Granddaughter

Sree

Preface to the Second Edition

Medical genetics is one of the most rapidly advancing branch of medicine and is recognized as a clinical specialty which provides an insight into the functioning of the human body, in health and disease. Understanding the principles of human genetics is an important component in the diagnosis, management and prevention of several medical disorders.

To be a good medical practitioner, every medical student and professional needs to know the fundamentals of human genetics. The book is written with this view in mind and covers various basic aspects of the field. This is written after fifteen years of teaching experience in a medical college in the field of anatomy, embryology and genetics and twenty eight years of working experience in the clinical and laboratory aspects of medical genetics, and includes cases I have seen over the years.

Today, the treatment of genetic disorders is within reach due to advances in biotechnology. However, this is not available for most genetic disorders. As of now, the emphasis in medical genetics is on prenatal diagnosis, including presymptomatic testing and screening in pregnancy, the neonatal period and population screening.

Identification of genes responsible for human disease is a key factor in the progress in medical genetics. In February 2001, a major landmark was the mapping of 95% of the human genome, and the progress and benefits of this achievement are reviewed. Lastly but importantly, the ethical, legal and social issues concerning this field need to be understood and studied in context to the law of the land.

Self test is the best test to learn how much you know. Multiple-choice questions can quench this thirst. Most importantly, it is the work of other scientists and genetic professionals whose published works help us to substantiate our knowledge and help as reference.

I am confident that the basics given in the book will open minds of the readers to this exciting branch of new medicine. However, medicine is an everchanging science with continuous research and clinical experience altering the management. The efforts made in the making of this book, though are after the proper review to best of my ability, I disclaim all the responsibility of any errors or omissions and readers are therefore encouraged to confirm the same before putting into actual practice.

Hema Purandarey

Preface to the First Edition

Medical genetics is one of the most rapidly advancing branch of medicine and is recognised as a clinical speciality which provides an insight into the functioning of the human body, in health and disease. Understanding the principle of human genetics is an important component in the diagnosis, management and prevention of several disorders.

To be a good medical practitioner, every medical student and professional needs to know the fundamentals of human genetics. This book is written with this view in mind, and covers various basic aspects of the field. It was written after fifteen years of my teaching experience in a medical college and twenty years of working experience in the clinical and laboratory aspects of medical genetics, and includes cases I have seen over the years.

The initial chapters cover the brief history and burden of genetic diseases and factors predisposing to Mendelian and multifactorial diseases. The application of this knowledge in the diagnosis and prevention of genetic disease is also discussed. Chromosomes are the basic units of heredity and methods of their studies and types of abnormalities are discussed next. The disorders occurring due to these abnormalities are discussed later. The structure of DNA and factors altering DNA structure leading to various diseases, and methods of analysis are discussed next. The chapter on cancer genetics deals with constitutional and acquired genetic changes leading to malignant disorders.

Inborn errors of metabolism form an important group of disorders in pediatric practice and the chapter on biochemical genetics deals with the causes and classification of these disorders.

There are many congenital malformations which arise due to environmental insults or infections or teratogens, in addition to those occurring sporadically. These are described in the chapter on dysmorphology and congenital malformations.

Today the treatment of genetic disorders is within reach due to advances in biotechnology. However, this is not available for most genetic disorders. As of now, the emphasis in medical genetics is on prenatal diagnosis, including presymptomatic testing and screening in pregnancy, the neonatal period and population screening. These aspects are dealt with in the respective chapters.

An important chapter is that of genetic counseling as it is the first step in the patients medical history for arriving at a preliminary diagnosis and planning and discussing management options.

The chapter on population genetics deals with methods to study populations and statistical methods to estimate the incidence and recurrence of genetic diseases.

Identification of genes responsible for human diseases is a key factor in the progress in medical genetics. In February 2001, a major landmark was the mapping of 95% of the human genome, and the progress and benefits of this achievement are reviewed in the chapter on the human genome project. Lastly but importantly, the ethical, legal and social issues concerning this field are briefly discussed. Multiple-choice questions cover some important aspects of the field, and answers to the questions with the explanations have been provided.

This book covers the basics of medical genetics and references are provided at the end of the book for further reading. I hope this text provides something of interest to every reader; that it will be a basic introduction to those new to the field of medical genetics, and will provide a useful reference to those more experienced in the field of medical genetics.

Hema Purandarey

Acknowledgements

Dr Smita Purandare for so zealously going through and editing the entire manuscript and Dr Usha Desai, Dr Shilpa Purandare, Dr Anil Jalan, Dr Shrikant Purandare Dr Madan Naik for their inputs.

My staff, technicians and research students who have willingly helped me at all stages.

Contents

Fig. 3.10: Fish using whole chromosome paint probes (WCP) showing an 18;21 translocation by dual colour chromosome specific probes for chromosome 18 (red) and chromosome 21(green)

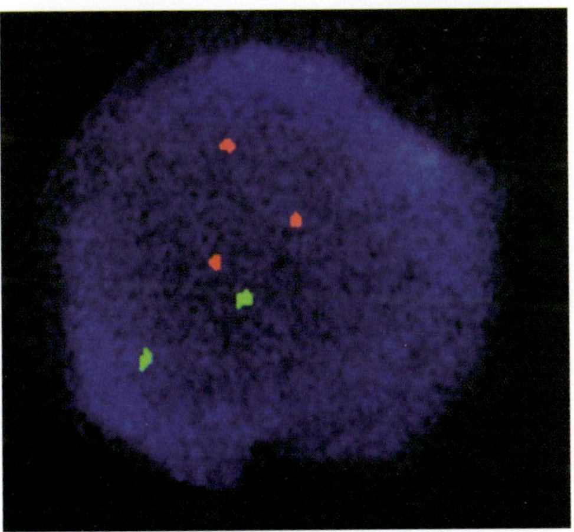

Fig. 3.11: Interphase FISH using locus specific identifier probes(LSI) Nuclear in situ hybridisation (NUCISH) performed with locus specific probes to detect chromosome 13(green), and chromosome 21(red). Three red signals indicating trisomy for chromosome 21

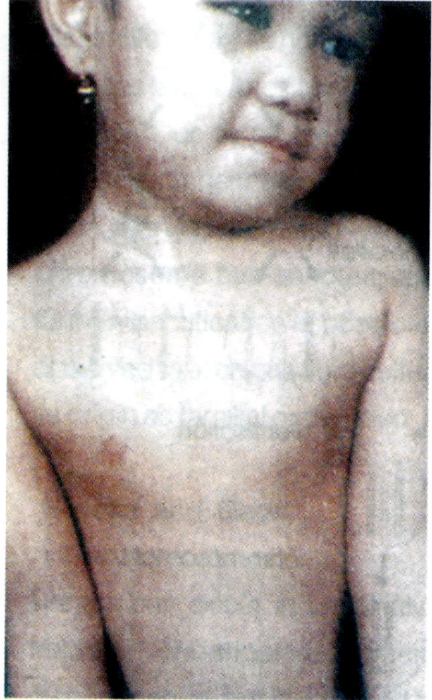

Fig. 3.20: Patterns of skin pigmentation on the body of a female child having mosaic cell line Metaphase spreads below.The skin conditions is called hypomelanosis of ITO

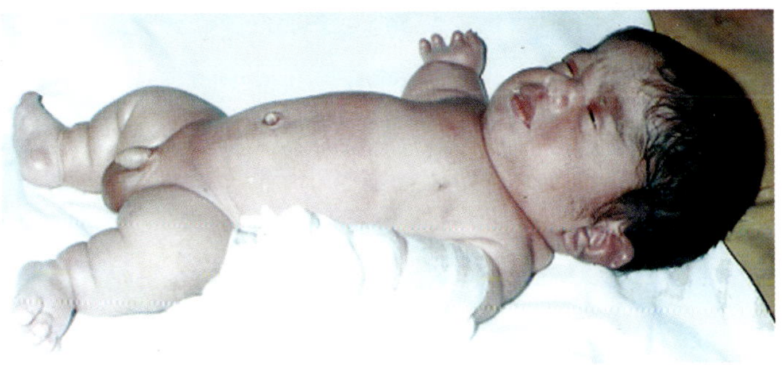

Fig. 6.5: Thanatophoric dysplasia

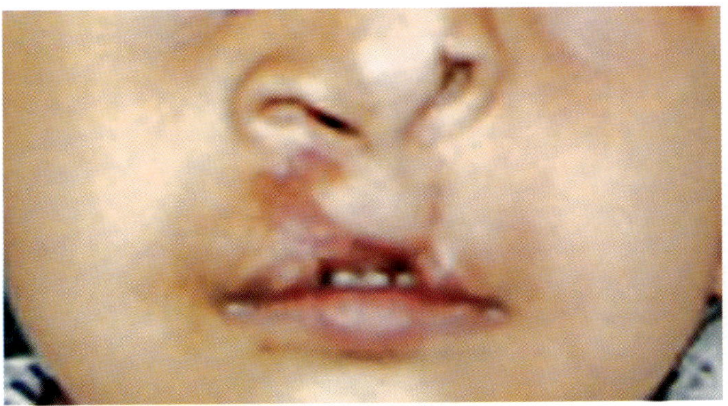

Fig. 9.2: Cleft lip with cleft palate

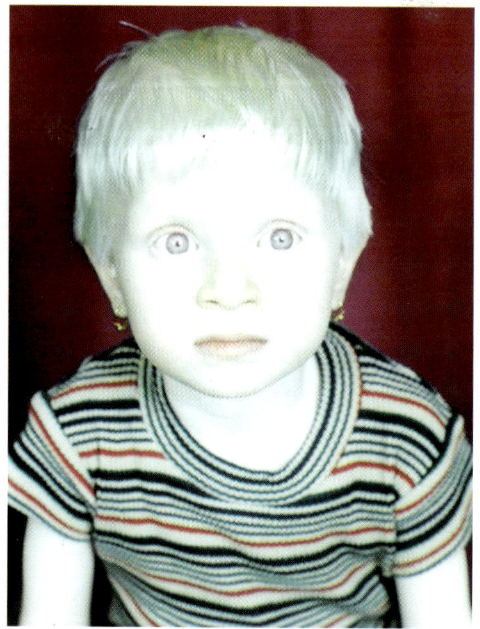

Fig. 10.2: Oculocutaneous albinism

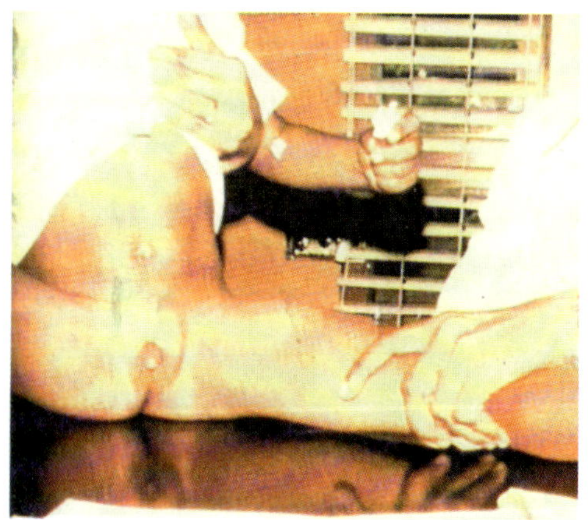

Fig. 10.3: Congenital adrenal hyperplasia

PLATE 5

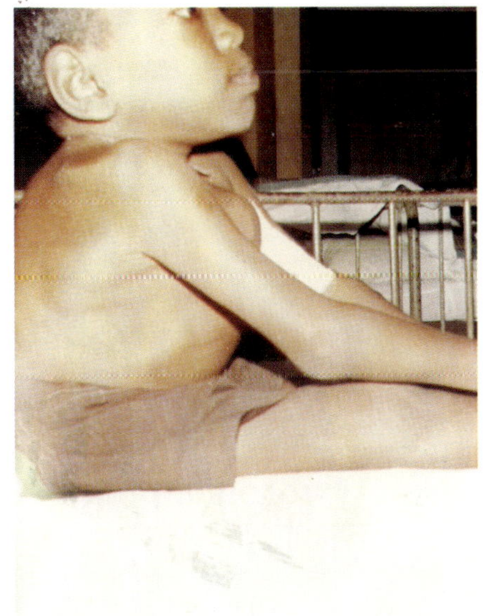

Fig. 10.5: Hunter's syndrome-(MPS II)

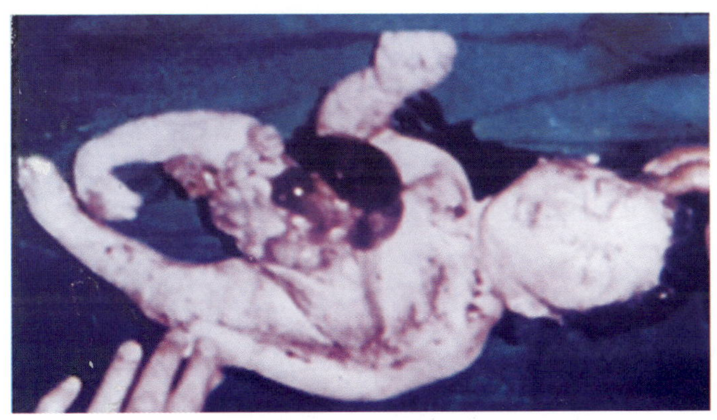

Fig. 18.2B: Exomphalos

CHAPTER 1

INTRODUCTION TO MEDICAL GENETICS

INTRODUCTION

Genetics is playing an increasingly important role in the practice of clinical medicine. Improved hygiene, better health care and awareness of good nutritional standards have resulted in an overall decrease in the incidence of infectious diseases. Additionally the role of genetic factors in the underlying pathology of disease is being better understood, the importance of genetics in medicine has increased.

The lifetime frequency of genetic disorders is estimated to be 7 per thousand, and this number includes cardiovascular diseases, which result from complex interactions of genes and environment and cancers, which result from accumulation of mutations in somatic cells. Genetic diseases are responsible for 10% of adult and 30-40% of pediatric hospital admissions. Congenital malformations when caused by genetic factors constitute a major cause of infant mortality.

Table 1.1 lists the burden of genetic diseases and their frequency in the general population. These figures necessitate today's physicians and health care professionals to understand the fundamentals and principles of genetic science in order to accurately counsel patients and their families. Patterns of genetic disorders vary in their occurrence, mode of inheritance and recurrence risk estimates. In addition, environmental factors also play a role in modifying both the risk factors and severity of the disease. Many birth defects caused by environmental

Table 1.1: Burden of genetic diseases

Burden of genetic disorders	*Frequency in population*
Oocyte aneuploidy	18%
Sperm aneuploidy	4%
1st trimester spontaneous abortion	50%
Perinatal deaths	30%
Stillbirths	5.6%
Chromosomal carriers	0.2%
Congenital malformation	3.6% (India)
Neonatal deaths	11.5%
Monogenic disorders	0.36%

factors and teratogens tend to mimic genetic disease, making it mandatory to take the role of these factors in human embryonic and adult development into consideration before making a final diagnosis.

WHY IS STUDY OF GENETIC DISORDERS IMPORTANT?

1. Mutations and pathological changes that result as a consequence of these mutations are established for generations and are irreversible.
2. Genetic disorders can manifest in many body systems and expression of the disease can occur any time during the life of individual.
3. Disease in any one individual in the family puts other members living or yet to be born at risk.
4. Genetic diseases have a major psychological and social impact.
5. Treatment for genetic disease is largely experimental and is only available at specialized centers.

Due to the recent advances in technology and increasing awareness of the patient population, physicians have an added responsibility in patient health care.

MENDEL'S LAWS

The principles of heredity and its understanding owes much to the pioneering work of an Austrian monk Gregor Mendel in 1865. Mendel studied clearly defined pairs of contrasting characters in the offspring of the garden pea (pisum sativum). However his work remained largely unnoticed until 1900. In his breeding experiments Mendel studied contrasting characters in garden peas e.g. tall pea plants were crossed with short pea plants (Fig. 1.1). All the plants in the first generation or F1 were tall. When the plants in this generation were subjected to interbreeding, the resulting plants were tall and short in a ratio of 3:1 [F2]. The characteristics in the F1 hide breeds are referred to as dominant, and those in the F2 are described as recessive. Mendel interpreted his findings suggesting that plant structure was controlled by factors one each from the parent. Wilhelm Johannsen coined these hereditary factors as genes. The first pure breed plants (tall and short) with identical genes used in the initial cross, are referred to as homozygous. The hybrid plants [F1], each of which inherit one gene for tallness and one for shortness are referred to as heterozygous. The combination of genetic material in the progeny is studied by constructing a square called Punnet's Square. On the basis of his experiments, the famous laws of Mendel were established. These are known as (1) Law of Unit inheritance, (2) Law of Segregation and (3) Law of Independent assortment.

1. *Unit Inheritance:* This law clearly states that blending of the characters of parents does not occur in the progeny.
2. *Segregation:* Two members of a gene pair (alleles) always segregate and pass to different gametes. However, if a

chromosomal pair fails to segregate, the offspring can inherit a severe abnormality.

3. *Independent assortment:* Gene pairs / characters assorted to a gamete are independent of each other. However, genes, which are closely linked on the same chromosome, do not assort independently but remain together from one generation to the other. This was not at that particular point of time recognized by Mendel.

Although Mendel presented and published his work in 1865, the significance of his discoveries was not realized until the early 1900 when three plant breeders De Vries, Correns and Tschermak confirmed his findings. It was around the same time that Charles Darwin's book on "The Origin of species" was published in 1859. Darwin emphasized the hereditary nature of the variability between members of a species, which is

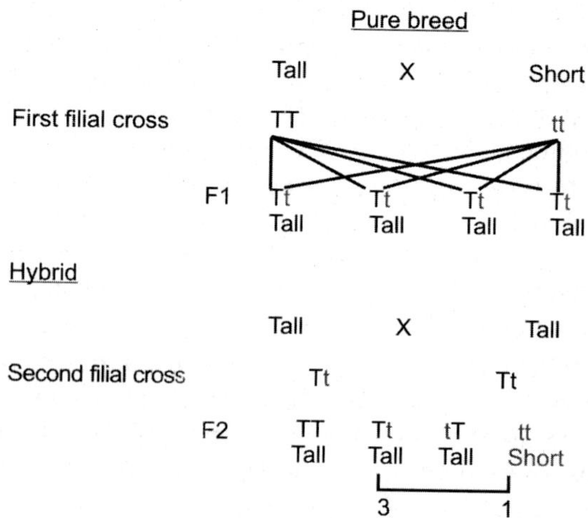

Fig. 1.1: Mendel's experiments

important in evolution. Heredity at the time was thought to involve blending of characters of both the parents. Archibald Garrod in 1902 proposed the idea that alkaptonuria was a recessive genetic disorder, and was the first to recognize the theory of a single gene. In collaboration with William Bateson, Garrod proposed that this was a Mendelian recessive trait with affected persons homozygous for the underactive gene. This was the first disease to be interpreted as a single gene trait. The urine of patients darkens on standing or on exposure to alkali. This is due to an inability on the part of the patient to metabolise homogentisic acid. Garrod also coined the term "Inborn error of metabolism". Several hundred such disorders have now been identified and this area is known as "Biochemical Genetics". In the 20th century the role of heredity became clearer and could explain different genetic mechanisms. Hereditary conditions are currently grouped as single gene disorders, chromosomal disorders and multifactorial disorders. Two other conditions now being considered are mitochondrial inheritance and somatic genetic diseases. As the understanding of the nature of biological structure and function of the living organism grew, the role of genes in life processes became increasingly recognized. In 1941, Beadle and Tatum formulated a hypothesis of one gene - one enzyme with the discovery that genes are composed of DNA. Since 1940, molecular analysis of genetic material has progressed rapidly. The intense interest in the composition of nucleic acids culminated in the discovery of the double helical structure for deoxyribonucleic acid (DNA) in 1953 by Watson and Crick for which they received the Nobel Prize in 1962.

HISTORY OF CHROMOSOMES AND CHROMOSOMAL TECHNIQUES

In order to understand and study the developmental process and expression of characters breeding experiments are to be performed. All breeding experiments are performed with looking at naturally existing genetic differences in a species. Mendel's experiments are well known and are described above. An ideal model for such experiments would be a model in which new generations are rapidly and easily maintained under laboratory conditions, and an organism that has variety in its physical characters with the chromosome number being minimum. In 1910, the American geneticist Thomas Hunt Morgan and his students, Sturtevant, Bridges and Muller, started experiments on a fruitfly, Drosophilia Meianogaster. Drosophilia produces new generation every 14 days, which is 25 times faster than the green pea.

The first mutant observed in the Drosophilia was colour of the eyes. Morgan once observed that in a culture bottle containing flies with red eyes, a male with white eyes was identified. This mutant male was crossed with red-eyed flies. In his experiment he crossed the white-eyed mutant male with red-eyed wild type female. In the F1 generation, both male and female were found to have red eyes. However in the F2 generation, half of the males were white eyed and other half of the males and females had red eyes. These experiments provided evidence that supported the hypothesis, that chromosomes are physical basis of inheritance.

By the late 1950's, human chromosome studies were developed and their role in sexual development, mental development and reproductive functions were understood. It was in 1956, Tjio and Levan established that normal diploid chromosome number in humans as 46. Various syndromes related to chromosomes were later identified. By 1970, with the combination of cytogenetics and molecular genetics, a new area of molecular cytogenetics emerged. Molecular cytogenetics techniques have opened a new vista in cytogenetic syndromes and many micro-deletion syndromes are now identified with the use of fluorescent in-situ hybridisation (FISH) technique.

SOME COMMONLY USED TERMS IN GENETICS

Human genetics—Human genetics is the scientific study of variation and heredity in human beings.

Medical genetics—Medical genetics is the application of the principles of human genetics to the practice of medicine. Medical genetics is the branch of medicine dealing with the inheritance, diagnosis and treatment of diseases caused by a single gene, chromosomal or multifactorial factors. This science also includes genetic counselling and screening.

Clinical genetics—The term Clinical Genetics is used in medical genetics and deals with the application of genetics to clinical problems in individual families.

Molecular genetics—Molecular genetics involves the interrelationship between DNA (deoxyribonucleic acid) and RNA (ribonucleic acid) and how these molecules are used to synthesize polypeptides, which are the basic component of all proteins.

Incidence—This refers to the rate of at which a disease occurs e.g., 1:1000 means in every 1000 individuals, one will have the disease.

Prevalence—Means proportion of a population affected at any one time. Prevalence of genetic disease is not as high as other disorders as the incidence and life expectancy is less, and the disorder may have a late age of onset.

Frequency-This is synonymous with incidence.

CLASSIFICATION OF GENETIC DISEASES

Genetic disorders may be classified into single gene, multifactorial, chromosomal, somatic genetic disorders and mitochondrial disorders. Detailed description of these disorders is provided in the chapters on Patterns of Inheritance and Polygenic and Multifactorial Inheritance.

Single Gene Disorders

Single gene disorders are due to deficiency or alteration in the structure of a single gene in an individual. Single gene disorders are further classified into autosomal dominant, autosomal recessive, X-linked traits.

Autosomal dominant traits—These traits are transmitted through the autosomes, and expressed when only a single copy of an abnormal gene is present. The transmission is vertical, from an affected individual to the progeny. Some examples of autosomal dominant disorders are Huntington's disease, Neurofibromatosis type-1, Marfan's syndrome, and Osteogenesis imperfecta. .

Autosomal recessive traits—These are transmitted through autosomes, but expressed only when both the copies of mutant gene are inherited. Some examples of autosomal recessive disorder are cystic fibrosis, Sickle cell anaemia, (3-thalassaemia, Galactosaemia, Phenylketonuria, Tay Sach's disease and Freidreich ataxia.

X-linked traits—These are transmitted due to mutant genes on the X chromosomes. The definition of dominant or recessive in these conditions is complicated by the inactivation of one of the X chromosomes in the cells of females during early development. Some examples of X-linked disorders are Duchenne Muscular Dystrophy, and Haemophilia A and B.

Multifactorial Disorders

There are many disorders, which have a familial clustering, but they do not follow any Mendelian pattern of inheritance. These disorders are due to an interaction between genes and environment.

Chromosomal Disorders

Mutations of genetic material sometimes involve large parts of the chromosome. When these are large enough to be visible under light microscopy these are termed as chromosomal aberrations. Chromosome aberrations affect 7.5% of conceptuses and have a live birth frequency of 0.6%. Abnormalities of the chromosomes may be classified as numerical aberrations, or structural aberrations. In numerical aberrations, somatic cells contain an abnormal number of normal chromosomes. Examples of these are aneuploidy and polyploidy. In structural aberrations, somatic cells contain one or more abnormal chromosomes. Examples of these include translocations, deletions, ring chromosomes, duplications, inversions and isochromosomes. Chromosomal abnormalities may occur in the sex chromosomes or the autosomes. They may occur in the germline of the parent or an ancestor, or may occur as the result of a somatic mutation, where only a proportion of cells are affected (see below).

Somatic Genetic Disorders

Genetic disorders may not originate at conception (in the germline) but can occur during the process of cell division (mitosis), which is a continuous process occurring throughout life for growth and repair of the body. During these mitotic divisions, there is a chance of error leading to single gene mutations or chromosomal aberrations. Such abnormalities can lead to malignancies thus giving rise to the term acquired or somatic genetic disease.

Mitochondrial Disorders

Disorders of mitochondrial function may involve genes encoded in the nuclear DNA or the mitochondrial DNA. Mitochondria are transmitted from a mother to all her offspring, while the sperm only contributes the nuclear DNA. Therefore mutations in the mitochondrial DNA are inherited maternally that is, females potentially pass the trait to all offspring and males do not transmit the trait. Some examples of these disorders include Leber hereditary optic neuropathy and mitochondrial myopathies.

CHAPTER 2

THE CELL AND CELL CYCLE

INTRODUCTION

The cell, the simplest living structure capable of independent existence, was first identified in 1663 by an English scientist Robert Hooke. It was not until 1838, that Schleiden and Schwann announced that the cell was the basic structural unit and functioned according to definite laws. The forms and functions of cells are diverse. They are controlled by genes, which lie on the chromosomes present in the cell nucleus. The chromosomes are involved in cell division as well as reproduction. To understand the basis of various genetic disorders, the study of cell structure and cell cycle is necessary. In unicellular organisms, a single cell carries out all the functions necessary for its survival. In higher organisms, however, cells associate to form colonies where different cells are allocated various functions, these being interdependent. The aggregates of cells, which have specialized functions, form different tissues, like blood, nervous tissue, bone and muscles. These tissues combine to form specialized organs such as the kidneys, heart and lungs. These in turn are grouped into functioning systems, like the urogenital, cardiovascular and respiratory systems.

COMPONENTS OF A CELL

Each cell has three basic components, (the cytoplasm, a cell membrane, which forms the cell wall, and a centrally placed body, the nucleus (Fig. 2.1).

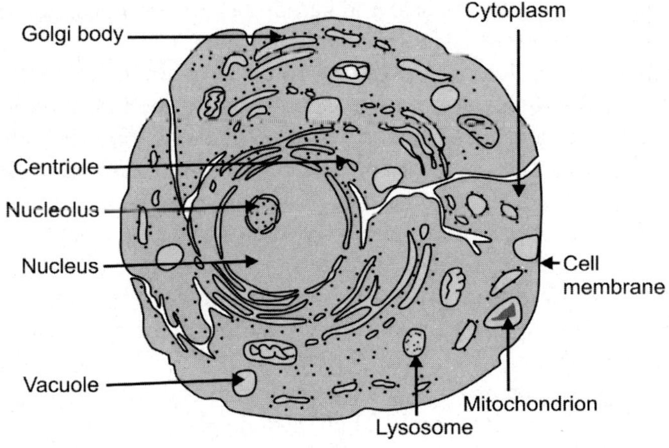

Fig 2.1: Components of a cell

Cytoplasm

The cytoplasm is a colloidal matrix composed of water and inorganic and organic compounds. Amongst the inorganic molecules are sodium, potassium, calcium, magnesium, bicarbonate and phosphates in trace amounts.

Organic molecules that impart colloidal property to the cytoplasm are monomers such as nucleotides, amino acids, monosaccharides and fatty acids along with their polymers, nucleic acids, proteins, polysaccharides and lipids. These constitute the macromolecules making up the major structural and functional units of the cell. The functions of each unit are different. Some proteins give structural support, like actin and myosin of the muscle and keratin of hair and nails. Some are involved in catalysis of metabolic reactions. Complex cellular reactions involve hormones, receptors and growth factors.

Nucleic acids are the repositories of genetic information and act as templates for the synthesis of proteins. Nucleic acids are of two types, deoxyribonucleic dcid (DNA) and ribonucleic acid (RNA). Purines and pyrimidines, are composed of a five-carbon sugar (pentose), a phosphate group, and a cyclic nitrogen compound. Purines are adenosine and guanine and pyrimidines are cytosine and thymine. Thymine is replaced by uracil in RNA. The sugar moiety in DNA is deoxyribose and that in RNA is ribose.

Lipids encompass a diverse group of compounds that are soluble in organic solvents. These include phospholipids in the cell membrane, sphingolipids in the nervous tissue, glycolipids in myelin sheath and steroids including male and female hormones, bile and adrenocortical hormones.

Cell Membrane

The cell membrane, also termed plasmalemma, defines the cellular boundary and acts as a physical barrier for cellular contents. It consists primarily of phospholipids and proteins. The membrane has selective permeability, which allows the to and fro passage of molecules. This is achieved by three mechanisms: passive diffusion, active transport and enclosure.

Passive diffusion is a term used to describe movement of substances from a region of high concentration to regions of lower concentration. Active transport requires energy and moves substances against a concentration gradient. Enclosure in vesicles that move substances into the cells is called endocytosis or pinocytosis, and out of cells is called exocytosis. Water moves freely across the membrane in both directions.

Glycoproteins are present on the protein lipid membrane surface. Their function is cell adhesion. Glycoproteins also have antigenic properties, and in red cells they determine blood groups.

Light microscopy has limitations in further identification of structures, which can be observed only by electron microscopy (EM). Some of these structures include the smooth endoplasmic reticulum, which functions in lipid metabolism. Rough ER, which has ribosomes attached to it, are the site of protein synthesis. Golgi apparatus is involved in the modifying, sorting and packing of molecules for secretion or delivery to other organelles. Lysosomes are vesicles containing digestive enzymes involved in the disposal of native or foreign waste products. Mitochondria are the powerhouses of cells, where oxidation of nutrients occurs to provide energy for synthesizing ATP. Structurally, mitochondria are small bodies with a double membrane. The inner membrane is folded into numerous projections called cristae, where oxidation of nutrients takes place. The other bodies in the cytoplasm are centrioles or basal bodies. Centrioles are responsible for the formation of spindle fibres, which separate chromosomes to respective daughter cells during cell division, and aid in the formation of cilia and flagella, which are needed for cell motility.

Nucleus

The nucleus carries the hereditary material, DNA, which determines specific functions and characteristics of a cell. The DNA lies in condensed form in linear arrays called chromosomes. Organisms with cells having a nucleus are called eukaryotes, and they are plants, animals and humans. Those without a proper nucleus are called prokaryotes, for example, bacteria. In prokaryotes the genetic material lies in the cytoplasm.

Cells lacking nuclei have limitations in their metabolic activity. When the cell goes through cell cycle, its appearance differs. The metaphase stage cell has its nucleus in a condensed spherical body and is darkly stained (heterochromatin). In interphase, two types of chromatin are seen.

The nucleus has an outer nuclear membrane and contains nucleoli and chromatin. The nuclear membrane or envelope is a double membrane with ribosomes attached to the outside. The membrane at many sites is continuous with the ER. When a cell divides, the nuclear membrane disappears. Within the nucleus, there is nucleolus and chromatin. The size and number of nucleoli vary with the cell type and the metabolic state of the cell. The nucleoli are larger in rapidly dividing cells and in cells with active protein synthesis. All the ribosomes in the cytoplasm originate in the nucleolus. Each nucleolus is formed along the nucleolar-organizing region of one or more specific chromosomes and is recognizable during cell division. The nucleolus is composed of RNA, protein and some amount of DNA.

The chromatin is composed of DNA, proteins (mainly histones), RNA and polysaccharides.

EUCHROMATIN AND HETEROCHROMATIN

During the cell cycle, chromosomes show a property of condensation (coiling) and decondensation. Maximum condensation occurs at metaphase. The staining intensity of the chromosomes varies owing to this property of condensation called heteropyknosis. More heavily stained parts of the chromosome are called areas of positive heteropyknosis and light areas are those of negative heteropyknosis. The chromatin in these variable regions is called heterochromatin and in the other regions in the cell it is called euchromatin. Heterochromatin is of two types, facultative and constitutive. The inactive X chromosome in the female gets condensed and is facultative heterochromatin while the other differentially staining areas of the chromosome seen in banding are constitutive heterochromatin.

X CHROMATIN AND Y CHROMATIN

X Chromatin

In 1949 Barr and Bertram in their experiments on cat nerve cells, observed a peculiar body, which they called as paranucleus (now called the Barr body), and this was present only in female cats. In 1961, Mary Lyon put forth a hypothesis that one of the X-chromosomes of females is inactivated and this chromosome could be of maternal or paternal origin. The inactivation is stable and occurs at embryogenesis. It was hypothesized that this was to compensate for the extra gene products produced in females who have two X-chromosomes and is called dosage compensation.

As a result of this random inactivation of X-chromosomes, females are always mosaic for the genes located on the X chromosome. The inactivated X is observed as a darkly stained body in the nucleus attached to the nuclear membrane (Fig. 2.2A). It is either triangular, oval or dumbbell shaped and is always one per each inactivated X chromosome. Males with XXY complement will show presence of one Barr body or females with XXX syndrome will have two Barr bodies. This test along with Y chromatin studies can be offered as a provisional diagnostic test in ambiguous genitalia. The inactivation centre is believed to reside on the Xq13 region on the long arm of the X chromosome.

Y Chromatin

In a normal male, the sex chromosomal pattern is XY The Y chromosome belongs to the G group of chromosomes and is easily distinguishable from chromosome 21 and 22. The

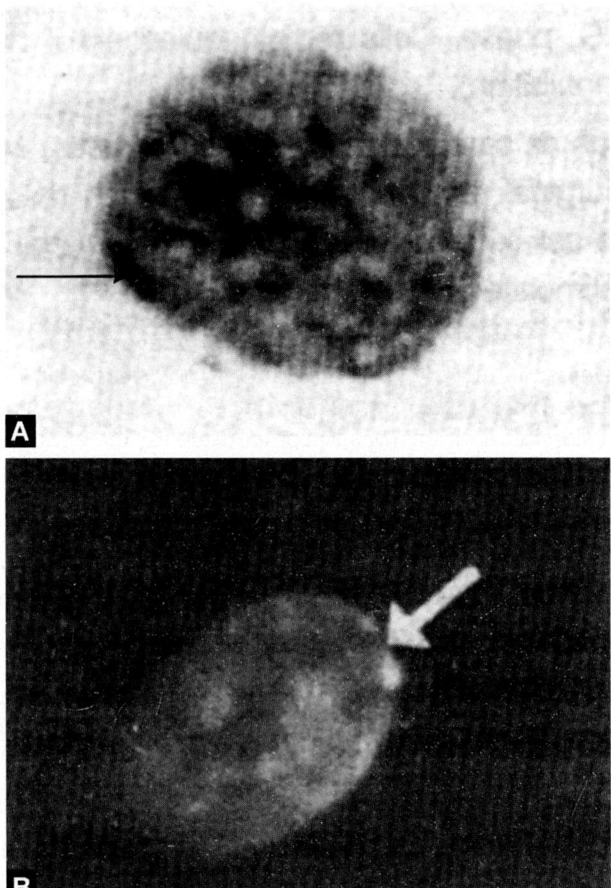

Figs 2.2A and B: Sex Chromatin in buccal mucosa. (A) X chromatin (B) Y chromatin

Y chromosome does not have a satellite and the long arms are straight. They do not diverge like long arms of chromosomes 21 and 22). The length of this segment varies. The Y chromosome is transmitted from father to son and the length of the Y can be studied as a family marker. When the buccal smears, peripheral blood smear or smears from seminal fluid are stained with a quinacrine dye, this fluorescent segment can be visualized in the interphase nuclei as a brightly fluorescent body called as Y chromatin (Fig. 2.2B).

The role of satellite DNA is becoming increasingly important in techniques like fluorescent *in situ* hybridisation (FISH). Repetitive DNA found in constitutive heterochromatin is called satellite DNA. Satellite DNA has highly repetitive sequences. A substantial portion of each fraction is made up of a single family of simple repeats. There are variations from mutations, sharing one to a few base pair differences. The alpha and beta satellite DNA is found at the centromere of all chromosomes. Satellite probes identify the centromeric regions of specific chromosomes and are used to identify aneuploidies or X and Y chromosomes in uncultured cells.

THE CELL CYCLE

For growth, cells need to multiply. In this process the cell mass increases, duplication of the genetic material occurs, and then cell division takes place. This assures that each newly formed daughter cell receives an equal component of genetic material. These orderly mannered stages of cell division are referred to as the cell cycle.

The cell cycle is divided into four phases (Fig. 2.3):

Mphase: This is a relatively brief phase in which mitosis and cell division occurs.

G1 phase: G1 phase follows mitosis. This is the gap phase, which covers the longest part of the cell cycle.

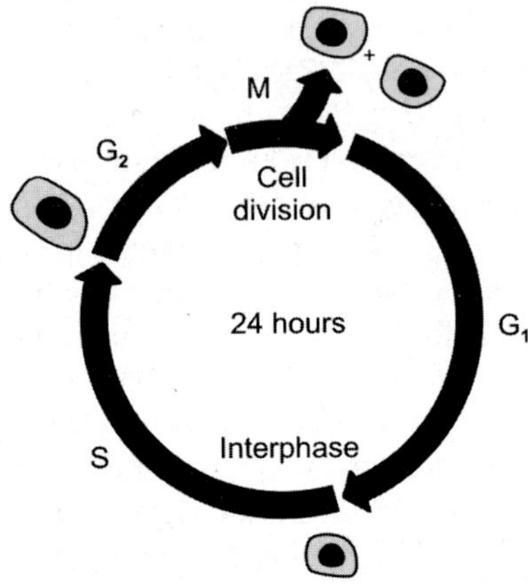

Fig. 2.3: Stages in cell cycle

S phase: This is the synthesis phase, which, in contrast to prokaryotes, is the only phase in which DNA is synthesized in eukaryotes.

G_2 phase: The cell, which has become tetraploid, now prepares itself for division. Two processes are involved in a cell division the first is called mitosis, where nuclear division occurs and the second cytokinesis, where changes occur in the cytoplasm, including division of the cell proper. G_2 is a relatively short phase. Once the cell enters the M phase, again a new round of cell division begins

Typically, cells in culture complete a cell cycle within 16-24 hr. This may vary from 8 hr to upto to 100 days or more for different types of cells. This variation usually occurs in the G_1 phase. Cells that have differentiated terminally never divide; they enter the G_0 phase also known as the quiescent phase. For a cell with a 24-hour cycle, G_1 phase requires 10 hours, S phase requires 9 hours, G_2 requires 4 hours and mitosis

1 hour. A cell's irreversible decision to proliferate is made during the G_1 phase. Cells remain quiescent if nutrients are inadequate or if they are in contact with each other (contact inhibition).

DNA synthesis may be induced by (i) various agents such as carcinogens or tumour viruses, which trigger uncontrolled cell proliferation (as seen in cancer) (ii) Surgical removal of a tissue which results in rapid regeneration (iii) mitogens which are proteins that bind to cell surface receptors and induce cell division (iv) certain cytoplasmic factors present in growing cells which stimulate DNA synthesis.

Mitosis

Mitosis is a continuous process, and is subdivided into 4 stages, prophase, metaphase, anaphase, and telophase. Between cell division, cells are said to be in interphase (Fig. 2.4). The type of tissue, temperature and nutritional health of cell determine the relative length of each stage.

Interphase: In late interphase, cells prepare to undergo mitosis. The nucleus assumes a reticulate appearance due to the maximally extended, uncoiled chromosomes. There is often a single nucleolus at this stage. A centrosome encompassed by astral rays and containing a medium centriole is seen at the surface of the nuclear envelope.

Prophase: Until prophase begins, it is usually not apparent that a cell is about to divide. Generally, the cell enlarges relative to the neighbouring cells.

Early prophase: During the early part of prophase divided chromosomes separate and take their positions at opposite poles. The chromosomes now coil into compact structures and appear shorter and thicker. The nucleoli disperse.

Late prophase: At the end of prophase, chromosomes become clearly visible and nucleoli disappear.

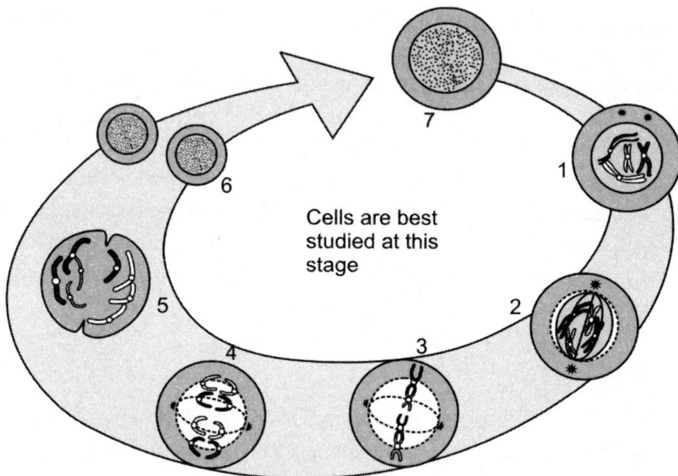

Fig. 2.4: Normal cell division stages in mitosis 1. Prophase 2. Prometaphase 3. Metaphase 4. Anaphase 5. Telophase 6. Interphase

Prometaphase: This is the portion of prophase immediately preceding metaphase. The chromosomes attain their maximum thickness and minimum length. Each chromosome that has split longitudinally for most of its length remains connected at a single point at the centromere. These separated chromosomes are called sister chromatids. The nuclear membrane begins to break down and chromosomes are left in the cytoplasm. A mitotic apparatus begins to assemble, and chromosomes start taking their positions at the equatorial plane after attachment of the centromeres of each chromosome to spindle fibres. The spindle apparatus seen now, consists of centromeres, their encompassing astral rays, a gelatinous spindle made up of fibres extending between centrosomes and traction fibres extending from each centrosome to the chromosomal centromere.

Metaphase: This is usually a very short stage. Chromosomes can be seen aligned equatorially in the mitotic apparatus and can be best studied and counted at this time.

Anaphase: During this phase the separation of chromosomes begins.

Early Anaphase: Each centromere divides longitudinally, thus converting two chromatids of the chromosomes into two daughter chromosomes. These daughter chromosomes disjoin and gradually move to opposite poles. This occurs due to pulling of the chromosomes by traction, in a process called karyokinesis. The longer chromosomes may still be adhered at their distal ends.

Late Anaphase: Chromosomes are pulled towards the pole and as they move away from the centre and the cell membrane starts invaginating. This process is called cytokinesis.

Telophase: This phase begins when sister chromatids reach the poles. The cell membrane invaginates from the area opposite the spindle equator. This process, which begins in late anaphase ends here. The nuclear membrane is formed around the chromosomes thus separating them from the centriole and the rest of the cytoplasm. Chromosomes become uncoiled again and spindle fibres and astral bodies disappear. The centriole divides as the centrosome prepares for the next mitosis.

The sequential and purposeful actions of mitosis focus on the movements of the chromosomes to ensure that they are distributed equally. It is essential that each chromosome of the parent cell have an identical counterpart in each of the daughter cells.

Meiosis

Union of two haploid germ cells or gametes, an egg from the mother and a sperm from the father form the diploid zygote.

These haploid cells cannot form by mitosis, as a reduction in the number of parental chromosomes to half is required. This occurs by a process termed meiosis involving two divisions. Reduction is affected because the two divisions involve only a single replication. There is orderly distribution of these replications in meiosis. In most organisms, meiotic cells are segregated in specialized organs generally termed gonads. (i) The female cells (containing abundant stored food to nourish the embryo in its early stages) are termed eggs or ova. This type of meiosis is called oogenesis and takes place in the ovary, (ii) In male, these are called spermatozoa and are produced by spermatogenesis in the testes.

The history of male and female gametes is different but the sequence is same. In males and females, there are two successive meiotic divisions. Meiosis I is known as reduction division since the chromosome number is reduced to haploid by pairing of homologous chromosomes in prophase and their segregation at anaphase in this division (Fig. 2.5A). The X and Y pair only at the tip of their short arms, as that is the homologous region.

Meiosis I

Prophase I: This is a complicated process, and differs from the mitotic prophase in a number of ways with important genetic consequences. It is long and critical, and is usually studied as five different stages, throughout which the chromosomes continually condense and become shorter and thicker. The stages of prophase I are described below.

Leptotene: Leptotene is characterized by the first appearance of 46 chromosomes. The chromosomes, which have already replicated during the S phase, become visible as thin threads that begin to condense. The sister chromatids are so closely aligned, that they cannot be distinguished as separate. Unlike mitotic chromosomes, meiotic chromosomes have alternating thicker and thinner regions. The pattern of thick regions (chromosomes) is characteristic for each chromosome.

Zygotene: In this stage, the chromosomes start pairing along their entire length. This pairing is also called synapsis and is very precise. Electron microscopy reveals the synaptonemal complex to be a ribbon like tripartite structure containing protein. This complex is essential for crossing over, which is the exchange of homologous segments between non-sister chromatids of a pair of homologous chromosomes. Crossing over, which occurs in the subsequent step, is biologically and clinically significant.

Pachytene: In this phase, the chromosomes become much more tightly coiled and mono pronounced. Synapsis is complete and structures called tetrads (as they contain four chromatids) are seen. Crossing over takes place at this stage.

Diplotene: The homologous chromosomes in each bivalent structure begin to repel each other. Here, their centromeres remain attached to each other and the chromosomes are held together only at points where the crossover takes place. These sites are termed chiasmata.

Diakinesis: When the prophase is nearing the end, the chromosomes move onto the spindle, and the tetrads become very contracted and densely stained. Terminalization is completed here.

Metaphase I: As in mitosis, the nuclear membrane disappears, and a spindle forms. The chromosomes align themselves on the equatorial plane. Their centromeres are oriented towards different poles.

Anaphase I: It is characterized by the separation of the chromosomes that had formerly formed the bivalents.

One of each pair moves to one pole of the spindle and the other member to the other pole. This is termed disjunction. This results in sorting of maternal and paternal chromosomes in random combinations. The possible number of combinations is 223. The process of crossing over imparts more variety. Anaphase I is the most error-prone step in meiosis.

Telophase I: The centromeres remain intact. Hence the 23 chromosomes at each pole remain double stranded and are called dyads. A nuclear membrane is formed around each group of 23 dyads.

Cytokinesis: The cell divides into two haploid daughter cells and enters interphase. Cytokinesis differs in spermatogenesis and oogenesis. In spermatogenesis, the cytoplasm is almost equally divided between two spermatocytes, but in oogenesis, one product (the secondary oocyte) receives almost all the cytoplasm, and the other becomes the first polar body. Here interphase is brief and there is no phase between the first and second meiotic divisions. After this phase, the chromosomes decondense again and meiosis II begins.

Meiosis II

This is the second meiotic division. This is similar to mitosis except that the chromosome number of the cell entering this phase is haploid (Fig. 2.5B). On completion of this division, four haploid cells, each containing 23 chromosomes is formed. Due to crossing over in meiosis I, the chromosomes of the daughter cells are not identical to those of the parent cell. Segregation of paternal and maternal forms of each gene takes place during either first or the second mitotic division, depending on whether they have been involved in a crossover event in meiosis I.

Chromosomal errors occur due to failure in the normal mitotic and meiotic divisions.

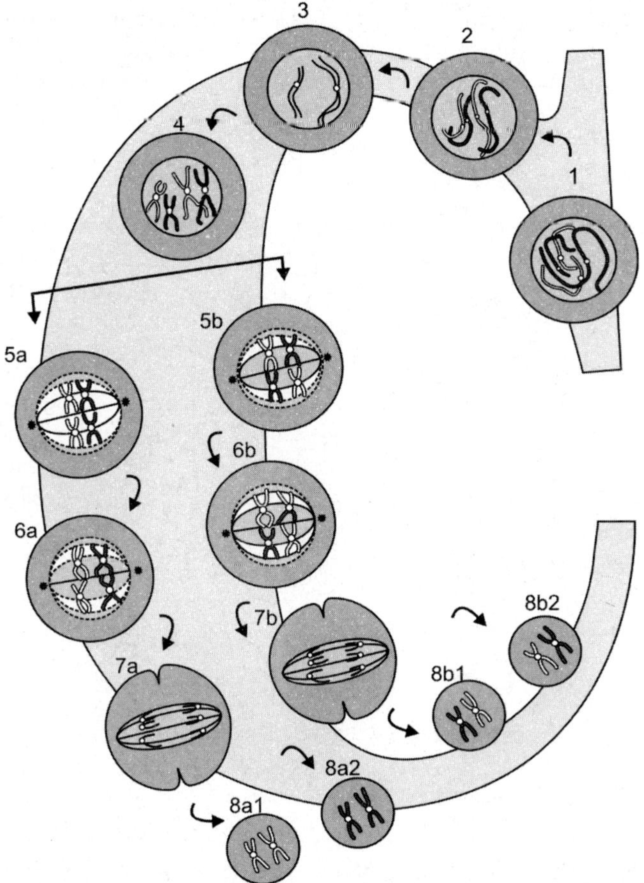

Fig. 2.5A: Stages of meiosis I. 1 through 4, stages of prophase I, 5a and b, metaphase I, 6a and 6b, anaphase I, 7a and 7b, telophase I and 8a1, 8a2, 8b1 and 8b2 represent the possible outcomes

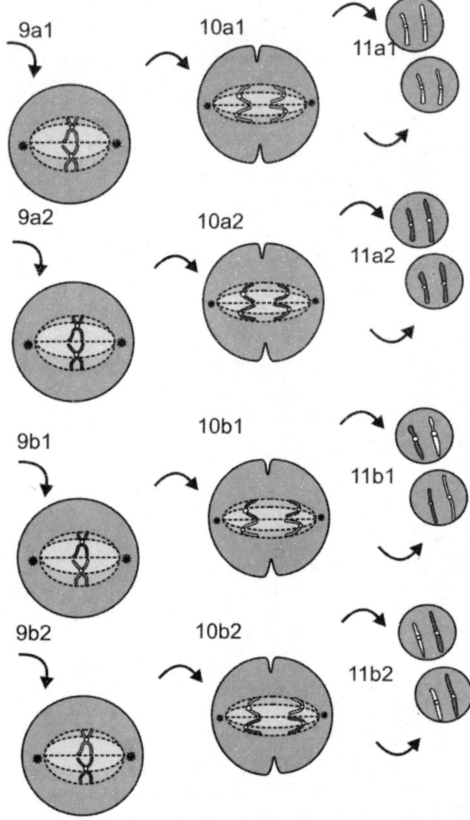

Fig. 2.5B: Stages of meiosis II, 9a1, 9a2, 9b1 and 9b2, anaphase II,10a1,10a2,10b1 and 10b2, stages of telophase II 11a1, 11a2,11b1,11b2 represent the possible outcomes

Gametogenesis

Male and female gametogenesis have a basic difference in the process, and various errors can occur in the genetic material leading to genetic variations or defects in the offspring (Fig. 2.6).

Oogenesis

Primordial germ cells give rise to oogonia by 20-30 mitotic divisions. This process occurs in the first few months of embryonic life. At the end of three months of embryogenesis, the oogonia mature into primary oocytes and meiosis starts. At birth these primary oocytes enter a phase of maturation arrest, dictyotene and the ovum is suspended in the prophase stage till meiosis I, which is completed at the time of ovulation. A single secondary oocyte is then formed, and the other cell is called polar body. The secondary oocyte receives most of the cytoplasm. The process of meiosis II commences during fertilization. Oogonia are present in embryonic life and at each menstrual cycle one egg matures and is released. In the reproductive life of a female, from first the onset of menstruation to menopause, approximately 300 ova are released. The others become atretic. The fact that many ova are available for maturation in every cycle is taken advantage of in assisted reproductive technology, where per cycle with hormonal induction about 20 to 25 mature ova can be made available for aspiration. As the process of oogenesis is a lengthy procedure, advanced maternal age plays a great role in chromosomal aneuploidy (numerical defects). There is always a chance that during this period a primary oocyte is exposed to intrinsic or extrinsic factors, which can damage spindle formation and the repair process, resulting in non-disjunction.

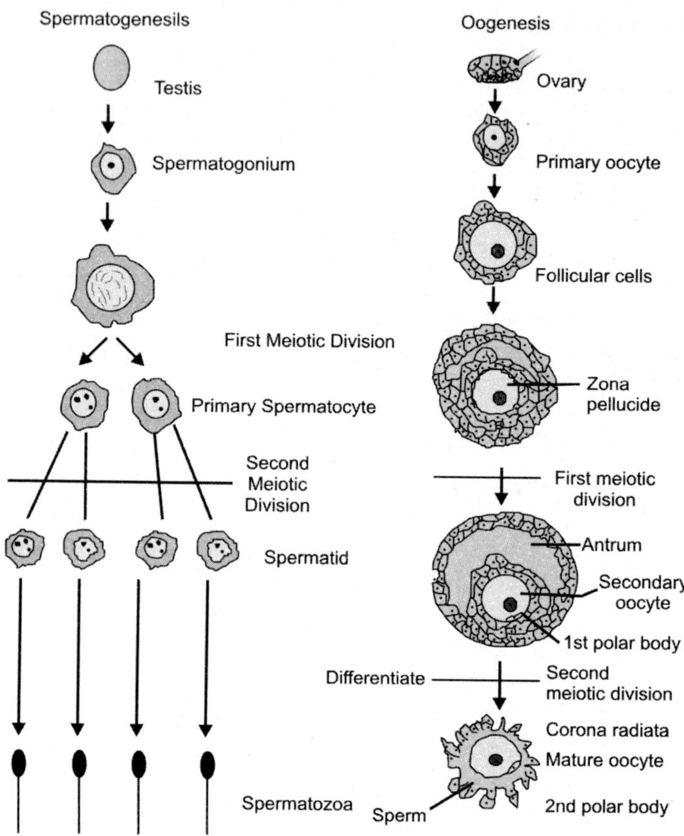

Fig. 2.6: Normal gametogenesis A. Spermatogenesis B. Oogenesis

Spermatogenesis

As compared to oogenesis, spermatogenesis is a quick process lasting for 60-65 days. Spermatogonia, which develop from the primordial ridge, undergo 30 mitotic divisions in embryonic life. At puberty they mature into primary spermatocytes, which enter a phase of meiosis I and are called secondary spermatocytes. These contain a haploid set of chromosomes called spermatocytes. These cells then undergo secondary meiotic division and spermatids are formed. These do not undergo any further cell division, and mature into spermatozoa. Each ejaculate contains about 100-200 million spermatozoa. The minimum requirement for fertility is 20 million spermatozoa with 50% motility, but with the advancement in IVF technology and intracytoplasmic sperm injection (ICSI), a single sperm can be utilized to achieve fertility. The process of spermatogenesis is continuous process. About 20-25 mitotic divisions occur per year. This means that a 50-years old man will have his sperm undergoing several mitotic divisions. Although paternal age is not associated with chromosomal defects in the foetus, some dominant mutations can arise due to DNA copy errors during the process of mitosis.

Chapter 3

CHROMOSOMES AND TYPES OF CHROMOSOMAL ABNORMALITIES

CHROMOSOMES

Chromosomes, composed of protein and DNA, are distinct dense bodies found in the nucleus of cells. The chromosomes are named for their ability to take up certain stains (Greek: *chromos* = coloured, *soma* = body). Genetic information is contained in the DNA of chromosomes in the form of linear sequences of bases (A, T, C, G). The DNA in an individual chromosome is one, long molecule which is highly coiled and condensed. The total number of bases in all the chromosomes of a human cell is approximately six billion and individual chromosomes range from 50 to 250 million bases. The DNA sequence for a single trait is called a gene. Each chromosome contains a few thousand genes, which range in size from a few thousand bases up to 2 million bases.

The number of chromosomes in human cells is 46, with 22 autosomal pairs (one of each type contributed by the mother and one of each type from the father) and 2 sex chromosomes – Two X chromosomes for females (one from father and one from mother) or an X and a Y chromosome for males (the X from the mother and the Y from the father). The normal chromosomal pattern in the females is 46, XX, and in the males, are 46, XY (Fig. 3.2). The gametes contain a single set of chromosomes, namely 22 autosomes and one sex chromosome. This single set of chromosomes is called haploid or 1n, in contrast to the chromosome set of a somatic cell, which is diploid, or 2n. At fertilization, each parent contributes a haploid set of chromosomes 1n to the foetus thus restoring the diploid set 2n. Since a male carries two different sex chromosomes X and Y it is clear that if he passes on his X chromosome to the foetus it will be a female foetus (as the contribution from the mother will always be X), and if a father passes on his Y chromosome the foetus will be a male.

Homologous chromosomes have genes at loci in the same sequence though slightly different forms may be present due to polymorphisms on the two different chromosomes. This alternative form of a gene found on the same homologous chromosome is called an allele.

CHROMOSOME MORPHOLOGY

Chromosomes can be visualized by light microscopy. During most of the cell cycle, interphase, the chromosomes are somewhat less condensed and are not visible as individual objects under the light microscope. However, during cell division, mitosis, the chromosomes become highly condensed and are then visible as dark distinct bodies within the nuclei of cells. The chromosomes are most easily seen and identified at the metaphase stage of cell division. The study of chromosomes is called cytogenetics. Various staining techniques have enabled identification of individual chromosomes. An arrangement of chromosomes is called karyotype (Figs 3.1 and 3.2).

During metaphase, chromosomes differ from each other in their morphology. Each chromosome is composed of two chromatids joined together at the primary constriction by a centromere. During cell division, the centromere is responsible for cell division. The centromere divides the chromosome into a short and long arm. The part of the chromosome above

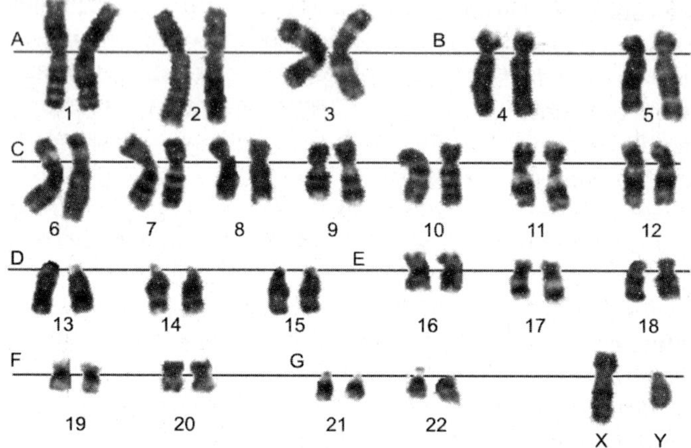

Fig. 3.1: GTG banded karyotype from peripheral blood of a normal male showing 22 pairs of autosomes and one pair of sex chromosomes, an X and a Y

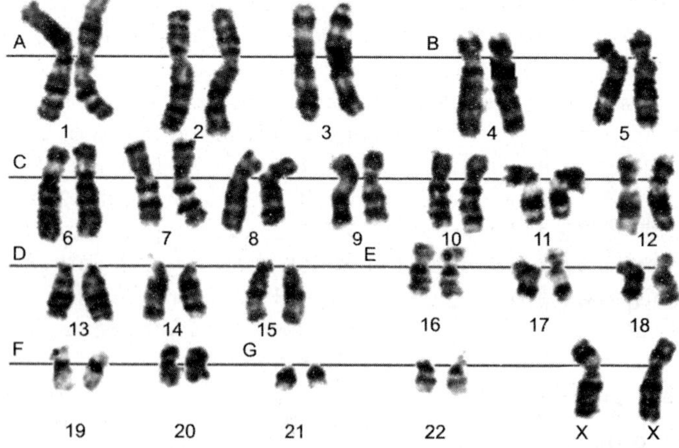

Fig. 3.2: GTG banded karyotype from peripheral blood of a normal female showing 22 pairs of autosomes and one pair of sex chromosomes, both chromosome X

the centromere is called short arm (p) and the part below is called long arm (q). The chromosomes are grouped from A to G on the basis of the length of the chromosome and position of the centromere Figure 3.3. The centromere is either in the middle of a chromosome i.e. metacentric where the short and long arms are equal or is above the centre i.e. sub-metacentric where the p arm is shorter than the q arm, or at the upper end of the chromosome when they are called acrocentric chromosomes. This group has a negligible p arm and a large q arm. The terminal end of a chromosome is called a telomere. Telomeres are specialized structures comprising DNA and protein, which cap the ends of eukaryotic chromosomes.

Besides primary constrictions at the centromere, some of the metaphase chromosomes have secondary constrictions. These secondary constrictions on the acrocentric chromosomes are the site for synthesis of ribosomal material in the interphase nucleus. These regions are termed the Nucleolus Organizer Regions (NORs).

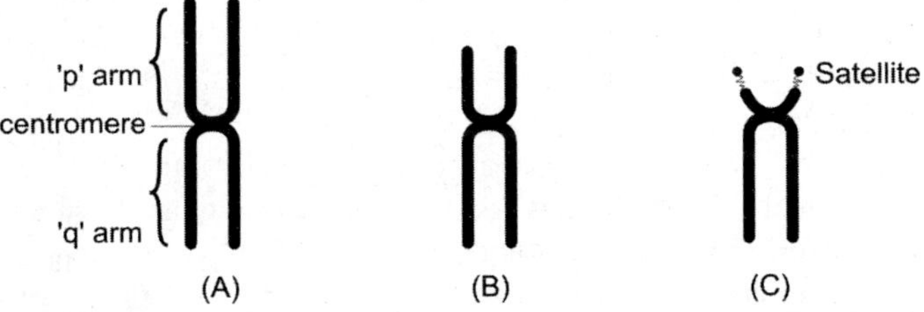

Figs 3.3A to C: Morphological chromosome classification according to centromere position, (A) Metacentric, (B) Submetacentric, (C) Acrocentric

METHODS OF CHROMOSOME STUDIES

Chromosome Preparation

Chromosomes can be studied from different tissues of the body. The basic principle involved in cytogenetic preparations is the same for all tissues, with slight modifications based on tissue physiology. Constitutional chromosomal patterns are best studied using peripheral blood, which is the most commonly used tissue for cytogenetic investigations. However, skin fibroblasts, and bone marrow are the other types of tissues used. For prenatal diagnosis, chorionic villi, amniotic fluid cells and foetal blood are the tissues that can be used.

Standard Procedures

The basic steps involved in cytogenetic preparation (Fig. 3.4) include growing the cells in tissue specific media, stimulating undivided cells (T lymphocytes) in blood by a mitogenic agent like phytohemagglutinin for 72 hours, and arresting the spindle formation in cell division by colchicine. In this step, the arrest occurs during metaphase. The chromosomes are in the condensed form in this phase of a cell cycle and the genes located on them cannot be transcribed. This is the most suitable stage for chromosome analysis. The next step is that of harvesting of the sample. In this stage, the cells are given hypotonic treatment so that they swell and chromosomes are released. These are then spread on a slide and can be stained with different staining techniques for visualization and analysis.

In certain acquired haematological malignancies where cells are in a state of spontaneous and continued division, karyotyping from unstimulated blood is also possible. Similarly foetal cord blood or blood from newborns also contain some dividing cells and can be directly karyotyped without stimulation. In prenatal foetal tissues, chorionic villi do not require stimulation as cells

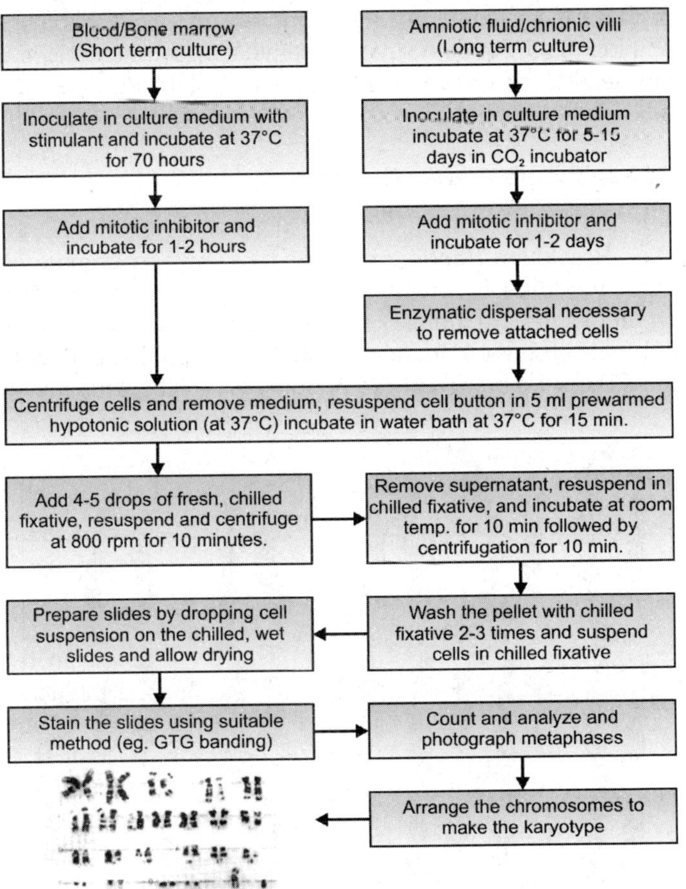

Fig. 3.4: Basic steps in cytogenetic preparations

of the villi are rapidly dividing and are mitotic. Cells from amniotic fluid also do not require stimulation by mitotic agents but need to be grown for at least ten days before they are ready for harvesting.

Chromosome Preparation for High Resolution Banding

High Resolution Banding involves banding and staining of chromosomes in prophase or prometaphase. As the chromosomes are more elongated in this phase, the number of bands observable increases to 800 as compared to 400 in the conventional metaphase banding (Fig. 3.5), thus minor

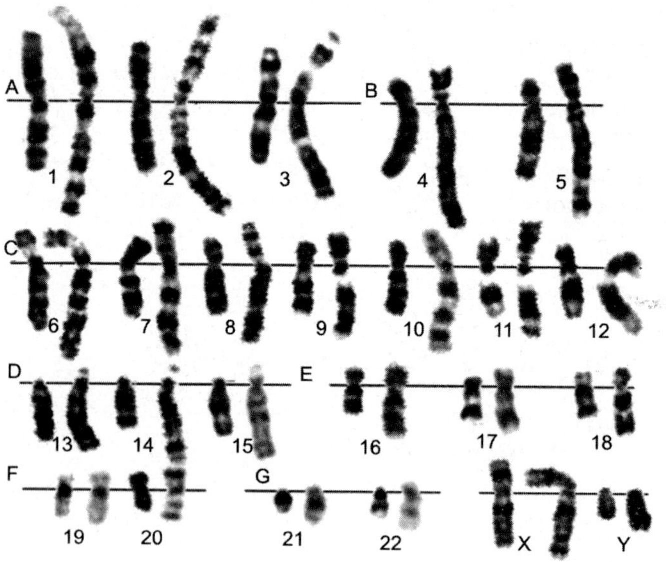

Fig. 3.5: Comparative karyotypes of routine GTG and high resolution banding

chromosomal aberrations are detectable. In this technique DNA synthesis in the cell is arrested in cell culture to synchronize the cells and release the block. The cultures are then harvested before they condense in late or early prometaphase.

Hereditary Fragile Sites

Several chromosomes have been seen to have fragile sites. They are often harmless on autosomes except for some syndromes and are of significance in chromosomal instability syndromes. The fragile site on the X chromosome at Xq27.3 (Fig. 3.6) is associated with the fragile X syndrome. This is the most common familial form of mental retardation, and is inherited as an X- linked disorder. This fragile site is rarely expressed in normal culture conditions, and it is expressed by either cultivating cells in folate-deficient medium, or treating the cells with thymidylate synthetase inhibitors such as fluorodeoxyuridine (FudR) in culture. The molecular basis of fragile-X syndrome is now known to be a triplet repeat expansion. DNA analysis of the size of the triplet repeat is now a more widely used method for diagnosis.

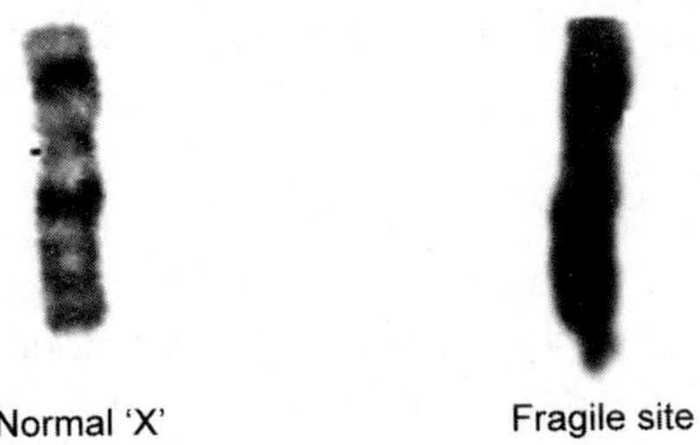

Fig. 3.6: Fragile site on the X chromosome at Xq27.3

ADVANTAGES OF USING PERIPHERAL BLOOD FOR CYTOGENETIC STUDIES

1. It represents the general constitutional chromosomal pattern of an individual. In rare situations, tissue mosaicism can be suspected if, with a classical clinical picture of a specific syndrome, a normal karyotype is seen. In such cases study from other tissues like skin fibroblasts can help to achieve a diagnosis.
2. Peripheral blood is obtained by simple, minimally invasive and safe technique of blood collection.
3. The culture period is short and gives a good yield.
4. In case of failure in culture growth, re-culturing is possible from the original sample after 4-5 days.
5. Cultures can grow even 48 hours postmortem.
6. A culture is possible in samples mailed by post.

CHROMOSOME STAINING

The most commonly used stains are Giemsa and Quinacrine. Giemsa is of two types:

1. Conventional Giemsa Stain,
2. Giemsa Trypsin Banding (GTG). The other banding techniques used are R-banding, C-banding and NOR-banding.

Conventional Giemsa Staining

Conventional Giemsa stain is of great value in studying chromosomal morphology (Fig. 3.7) which includes visualization of satellites, fragile sites, breaks and gaps and to study quadrilateral arrangements as seen in Bloom's Syndrome. The non-banded spreads are easier to count, and grouping is possible although individual chromosomes cannot be identified.

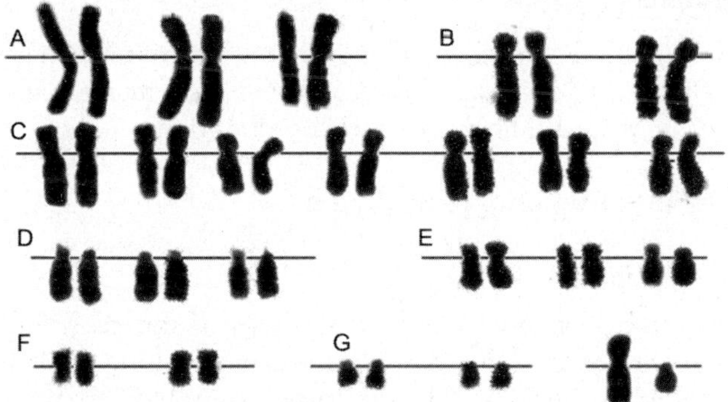

Fig. 3.7: Conventional Giemsa staining

Differential Staining Techniques

Giemsa Trypsin Banding (GTG)

In this method, trypsin is used to denature the chromosomal proteins, following which the slides are stained with Giemsa (Fig. 3.8A). Chromosomes stained by this method show definite patterns of light and dark bands.

Quinacrine Banding (QFQ)

Quinacrine banding is used in identification and structural rearrangement of Y chromosome (Fig. 3.8B), especially in ambiguous genitalia and in rapid analysis of chromosomal markers in haematological cancers and tumours. Quinacrine heteromorphism can sometimes be useful in identification of maternal v/s foetal cells, donor v/s recipient cells and inherited chromosomal variants.

R Banding

In this method chromosomes receive pre-treatment with heat. The light and dark bands thus produced show a reverse pattern of Giemsa and quinacrine banding (Fig. 3.8D).

Selective Staining Techniques

C Banding

This method allows selective staining of the constitutive heterochromatin. C-banding is done either by using alkali such as NaOH or $Ba(OH)_2$. Heteromorphisms in the C-bands are familial, and may be used as markers for certain cases. Unusual morphology in the heteromorphic C-bands, and translocations with a break point in C-banding regions can be identified by this method (Fig. 3.8C).

NOR Banding

NOR or nucleolar organizing regions are specific chromosomal regions that form and maintain the nucleoli in interphase nuclei. They consist of genes for the larger fraction (28S) of ribosomal RNA. These regions can be stained differentially in metaphase with Giemsa (N-banding) or by silver nitrate (Ag-NOR banding). The N-banding procedure reveals both inactive as well as active NORs, while the Ag-NOR reveals only active NORs. The pattern observed in Ag-NOR banding is consistent for an individual. They can be used in combination with Q-banding to identify paternal origin and the stages of meiotic non-disjunction in trisomies of acrocentrics. Ag-NOR staining has been important in examining the status of the NORs in determining the break points in Robertsonian as well as reciprocal translocations. Silver impregnation can be used to observe changes in activity of NORs in meiosis as well as in malignant cells.

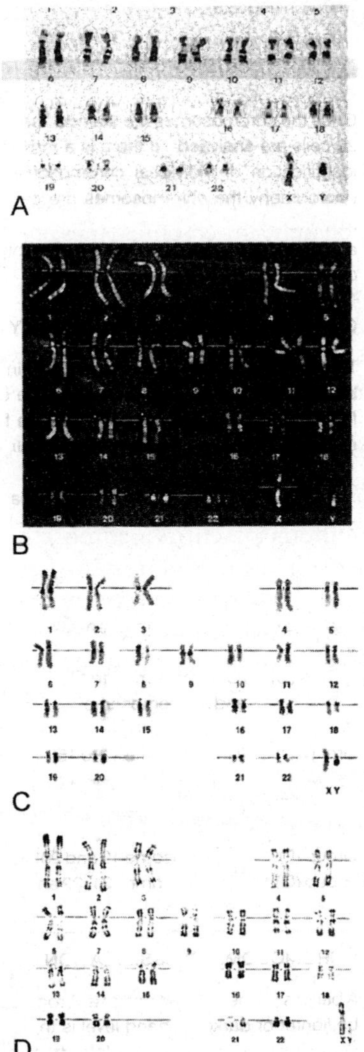

Figs 3.8A to D: Karyotypes using. (A) G-banding, (B) Q banding, (C) C-banding (D) R-banding

CHROMOSOME CLASSIFICATION AND ANALYSIS

Once the chromosomes are stained, they are ready for analysis. Numerical analysis is done first. A minimum of 20 cells are analysed. If there is a mosaic cell line, an additional 10,30 or 50 cells are analysed. Initially, the identification of individual chromosome is done under a microscope. Three fields are then chosen for photography the chromosomes are cut and pasted. This is called a karyotype. In the construction of the karyotype, the arrangement of the autosomes is done in decreasing order of length. The sex chromosomes X and Y are arranged at the end. The karyotyping by conventional photography is now slowly being replaced by computer image processing (Fig. 3.8).

CHROMOSOME CLASSIFICATION BY CONVENTIONAL GIEMSA STAIN

The earlier methods of chromosome staining allowed identification of chromosomes into seven groups on the basis of their length and position of the centromere (Fig. 3.1). The autosomes are arranged first in order followed by the sex chromosomes. The following table gives the method of classification of chromosomes stained by conventional solid Giemsa staining.

CHROMOSOME CLASSIFICATION BY CONVENTIONAL GIEMSA TRYPSIN BANDING

A band is defined as that part of a chromosome, which is clearly distinguishable from its adjacent segment. It can be lighter or darker. A band level is the total number of bands countable in a haploid state of chromosomes including sex chromosomes (Table 3.1). In order to attain a high band level that can detect minor chromosomal defects, long chromosomes are required. This is achieved by studying pro-metaphase

Table 3.1: Classification of unbanded chromosomes

Group (A)	(Chromosome 1 to 3)	Largest of the metacentric chromosomes. Number 1 is the longest metacentric, 2 long slightly sub-metacentric and 3 smaller metacentric
Group (B)	(Chromosome 4 and 5)	Large sub-metacentric chromosomes indistinguishable from each other.
Group (C)	(Chromosome 6 to 12) and X chromosome	Medium sized metacentric chromosomes, difficult to differentiate without banding. X chromosome belongs to this group.
Group (D)	(Chromosome 13 to 15)	Medium sized acrocentric chromosomes, which may or may not have satellites.
Group (E)	(Chromosome 16 to 18)	Short metacentric (number 16) and sub-metacentric chromosomes (17 and 18)
Group (F)	(Chromosome 19 and 20)	Short metacentric chromosomes
Group (G)	(Chromosomes 21, 22 and Y)	Short acrocentric with or without satellites. Y chromosome is without satellites.

chromosomes. A technique called high resolution banding is achieved by synchronization of culture followed by a short period of spindle blocking with colchicine, giving a high yield of pro-metaphase and prophase chromosomes.

Landmark bands, which were first demonstrated in a metaphase spread, were of a 250-band level. In earlier stages of metaphase, 400 band levels can be identified. In a routine

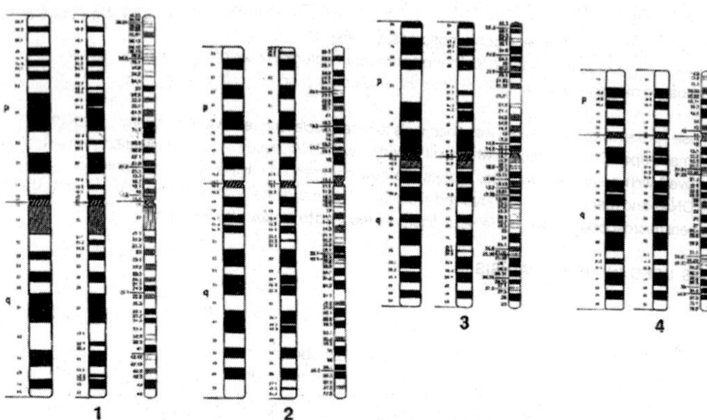

Fig. 3.9: G banded chromosomes arranged in increasing order from 500 to 900 bands. ISCN 1995 classification

cytogenetic laboratory, this band level is sufficient for peripheral blood methods and amniotic cell cultures.

In order to recognize small rearrangements 550 band levels is recommended (prophase or prometaphase stages). 850 band levels can be achieved in longer prophase and prometaphase chromosomes but is not required routinely. ISCN 1995 gives G-banded chromosomes arranged in increasing order of resolution from approximately 500 to 900 band stages (Fig. 3.9).

MOLECULAR CYTOGENETICS

Fluorescent In Situ Hybridization (FISH)

Conventional staining techniques have limitations in individual assessment of very minute chromosomal structural rearrangements or assessment of sub-microscopic deletions. Fluorescent *in situ* hybridisation (FISH) is one of the techniques in the field of cytogenetics since the first discovery of chromosomal banding. Denaturation of DNA sequences of metaphase chromosomes, hybridisation of DNA and RNA probes and identification of the target sequence of a chromosome with a probe is the principle of FISH. A fluorochrome tagged receptor molecule binds to DNA probes. A number of fluorochromes are used for this purpose. With the use of fluorescent microscope and special filters, signals are visualized.

In the technique of FISH, nucleic acid sequences of chromosomes (i.e. highly repeated satellite DNA / heterogeneous DNA sequences / specific gene loci sequence) are used as markers and hybridised to chromosomes in a metaphase spread. The technique allows one to detect chromosomal anomalies by specific probes that can be used in prenatal, postnatal or for preimplantation genetic diagnosis.

Diagnostic Applications of FISH

- Identification of specific chromosomes in interphase cells or metaphase spread.
- Identification of individual chromosomes and structural defects, especially microdeletions.
- Gene mapping.
- Identification of species-specific chromosomes by marker probes in hybrids.
- Assessment of radiation effects or damage on individual chromosomes or in metaphase spreads.
- Evaluation of chemical mutagenic effects in individual chromosomes or in metaphase spreads.

Metaphase spread slides are heated with chemicals to break nuclei and remove proteins from chromosomes in order to make open DNA molecules, which will hybridise with DNA probes. After hybridisation, marked probes are removed with a series of washes. Probes are now commercially available for all whole chromosomes, satellite DNAs and many specific loci involved in disease. These and other components can be supplied as kits. Fluorescent microscopes and a special set of filters are required to visualize the FISH results.

PROBES USED IN FISH ANALYSIS

Probes

DNA probes used for the FISH technique are direct-labelled probe and indirect labelled probe. A direct-labelled probe is pre-labelled with the fluorochrome. This probe attaches to the target of interest and allows a fluorescent signal to be bound to the target in the hybridisation stage. An indirect DNA probe is pre-labelled with a hapten. Once this is hybridised to the target sequence fluorochrome labelled antibodies to the hapten are used for probe detection. For this purpose digoxigenin or biotin / streptavidin conjugate is used. The length of the DNA probes used for FISH varies in the range of 20-22 nucleotides to 1Mbp. For detection of short ranges (20-25 nucleotides) synthetic oligomers are used while for tandemly repeated DNA sequences (1 mb) yeast artificial chromosome (YAC) clones are used. Other types of probes used include pools of cosmid contigs, P1 and P1 Derived Artificial Chromosomes (PACs), and Bacterial Artificial Chromosomes (BACs).

Chromosome Enumeration Probes (CEP)

CEP probes are made from chromosome specific sequences from highly repeated human satellite DNA sequences (Fig. 3.9). The metaphase target chromosome shows a compact, fluorescent spot where the CEP probe hybridises. These probes are useful in determining chromosome specific ploidy in preimplantation, prenatal, postnatal and haematological samples in cultured or uncultured specimens. They are also useful in detecting chromosome specific ploidy in tumour cells, especially in breast and myeloid cancers.

Whole Chromosome Paint Probes (WCP)

DNA probes, which are homologous to DNA sequences of the entire length of an individual chromosome, are called WCP probes. Any one WCP probe is a cocktail of probes for specific DNA sequences of a particular chromosome. These probes are made from chromosome specific recombinant DNA libraries obtained from flow sorted or microdissected, individual chromosomes. The target chromosome looks "painted" by WCP probes (Fig. 3.10). This helps to recognize an individual chromosome (marker) and identifies translocations, deletions and rearrangements of individual chromosomes in a metaphase spread. WCP probes may be used to detect chromosomal change due to chemical mutagens or radiation damages. It also helps in rapid identification of individual chromosomes in somatic cell hybrids.

Locus Specific Probes (LSI)

The DNA sequences of homologous chromosomes and positions of specific human gene loci can be identified by LSI probes (Fig. 3.11). The LSI probes are used in tumour, prenatal and postnatal samples.

Multiple Probe Co-hybridisation

Probes labelled with different colour fluoro probes can be mixed together and applied in a single hybridisation to allow simultaneous visualization of two different target sequences on the same nucleus or metaphase spread.

Fig. 3.10: Fish using whole chromosome paint probes (WCP) showing an 18;21 translocation by dual color chromosome specific probes for chromosome 18 (red) and chromosome 21(green) *(For color version see Plate 1)*

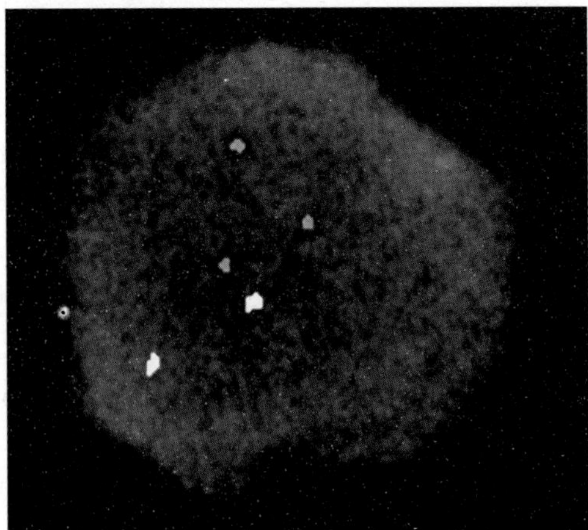

Fig. 3.11: Interphase FISH using locus specific identifier probes(LSI) Nuclear in situ hybridisation (NUCISH) performed with locus specific probes to detect chromosome 13(green), and chromosome 21(red). Three red signals indicating trisomy for chromosome 21 *(For color version see Plate 1)*

Probes for Telomeric Regions

Telomeric regions of chromosomes are lost due to deletions and unbalanced translocations.

Analysing FISH Results

FISH analysis requires an epi-illumination fluorescence microscope.

APPLICATION OF CHROMOSOMAL STUDIES

Chromosomal aberrations cannot be corrected, but they are of immense value in diagnosis, prognosis and management of genetic disorders. Some important applications are listed below:

1. To confirm the clinical diagnosis.
2. To identify carrier status of a couple and provide appropriate genetic counselling for prognosis, management and recurrence risk estimation.
3. To plan future prenatal diagnostic tests and consider available reproductive options.
4. In prenatal diagnosis to reassure the couple with normal results or in those with abnormal findings depending on the severity, offer possible options.
5. Karyotyping of products of conception in case of foetal loss may provide a clue to the type of genetic component involved.
6. Cytogenetic studies in malignant tissues especially haematological cancers, help in providing prognosis and assessing the drug response.
7. Chromosomal studies my help in assessment of environmental hazards in Bloom syndrome, Fanconi anaemia and ataxia telangiectasia (explained in the chapter on chromosomal syndromes)

CHROMOSOMAL ABNORMALITIES

Chromosome abnormalities are changes resulting in a visible alteration of chromosomes. An alternative definition of a chromosomal abnormality is an abnormality produced by specific chromosomal mechanisms. Most aberrations are produced by misrepair of broken chromosomes, improper recombination or improper segregation of chromosomes during mitosis or meiosis. Chromosome abnormalities are an important cause of mortality and morbidity and nearly 50 to 60% of foetal wastage.

A chromosomal abnormality may be present in all cells of the body (constitutional abnormality) or may be present only in certain cells or tissues (somatic abnormality). Chromosomal abnormalities, whether constitutional or somatic, fall into two categories, numerical and structural abnormalities (Table 3.2).

Various types of abnormal chromosomal patterns and rearrangements result into classical and non-classical syndromes. These are described in the chapter on chromosomal syndromes. The following pages describe the types of chromosomal abnormalities.

NUMERICAL CHROMOSOMAL ABNORMALITIES

Numerical abnormalities occur when the normal human chromosomal complement of 46 gets addition or loss of one or more chromosomes in the diploid number (2N). This is termed as aneuploidy. If a chromosomal complement has multiples of haploid number (1N) it is termed as polyploidy.

Polyploidy

Cell lines that contain multiples of the haploid number other than diploid are called polyploid. Triploidy (3n) 69 and tetraploidy (4n) 92 (Fig. 3.12) are the two most commonly

Table 3.2: Types of chromosomal abnormalities

Numerical	
• Aneuploidy	Monosomy
	Trisomy
	Tetrasomy
• Polyploidy	Triploidy
	Tetrploidy
Structural	
• Involving single chromosome	Deletion
	Insertion
	Inversion pericentric
	Paracentric
	Isochromosome
	Rings
• Involving more than one chromosome	
• Translocation	Reciprocal translocation
• More than one cell line	Mosaicism chimera

seen forms of polyploidy. Triploidy may be due to failure of the ovum or the sperm to divide at maturation. This may also be the result of fertilization of the ovum by two sperm, or fertilization of an ovum that has not expelled the first polar body. The phenotypic expression varies with the source of the extra set of chromosomes. When this extra set is of paternal origin, the foetuses have an abnormal placenta and are classified as hydatidiform moles. Those with an extra complement of maternal origin are aborted spontaneously.

Three sex types have been observed in triploidy, these being 69,XXX, 69,XXY and 69,XYY. Triploidy can result in abortions or in some cases live births that die at or shortly after birth. Tetraploidy may be seen as an artefact of tissue culture. True tetraploidy is very rare. All live born non-mosaics of polyploidy have died within a few hours of birth. Tetraploids are usually 92,XXXX or 92,XXYY. This is an indication that the cause of tetraploidy is the failure of completion of an early cleavage

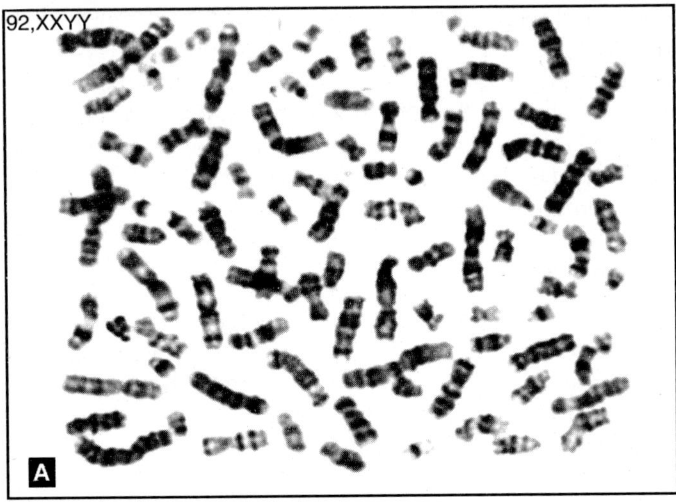

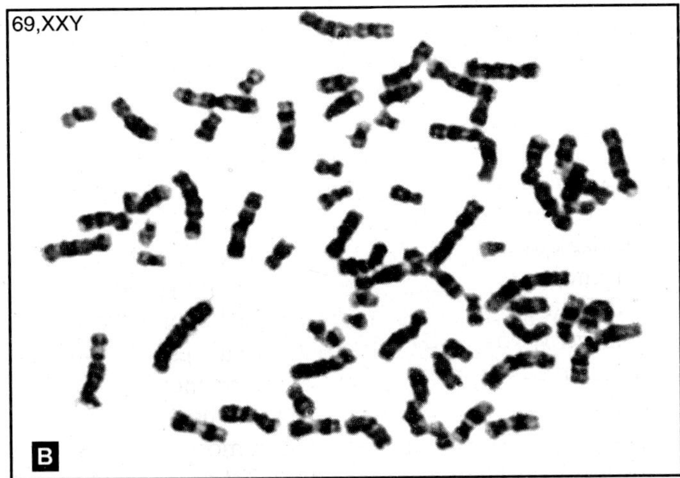

Figs 3.12A and B: Metaphase spreads showing (A) Teraploidy and (B) Triploidy

division of the zygote. Endoreduplication arises from failure of the centromeres to separate during anaphase; and this may be observed in tissue culture. The chromatids undergo the DNA synthesis phase for a second time and appear as four chromatids fastened at the centromere. This is a rare occurrence *in vivo*. Tumour cells may show a polyploid complement as a result of endoreduplication.

Aneuploidy

When a single chromosome is added to the normal chromosomal complement it is called trisomy. When two chromosomes are added it is called tetrasomy. When there is a loss of a single chromosome from the normal chromosomal complement it is called monosomy.

Numerous chromosomal abnormalities involving the loss or gain of an entire chromosome have been reported, many being seen only in spontaneously aborted foetuses. These are briefly mentioned below and discussed in chapter on Chromosomal disorders.

Trisomy

However, there are three well-defined chromosomal disorders that are compatible with postnatal survival. The 3 well recognized trisomies for an autosome are trisomy 21 (Down syndrome), trisomy 18 (Edward syndrome), and trisomy 13 (Fig. 3.13) (Patau syndrome). Each of these autosomal trisomies is seen to be associated with growth retardation, mental retardation and multiple systemic anomalies. Though each has a distinctive phenotype, there can be variation in expression or in severity and involvement of systems. Trisomies other than these usually result in pregnancy loss. Trisomy 16 is a common trisomy of the autosome seen in first trimester foetal losses. The commonly known syndromes are 47, XXY

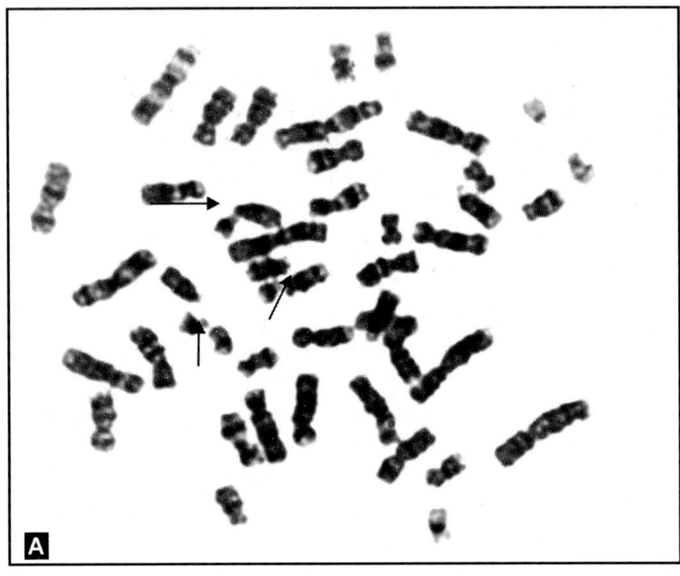
A

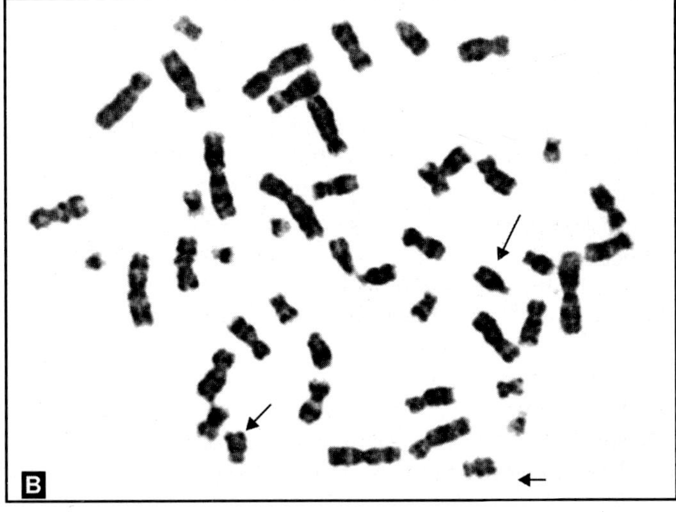
B

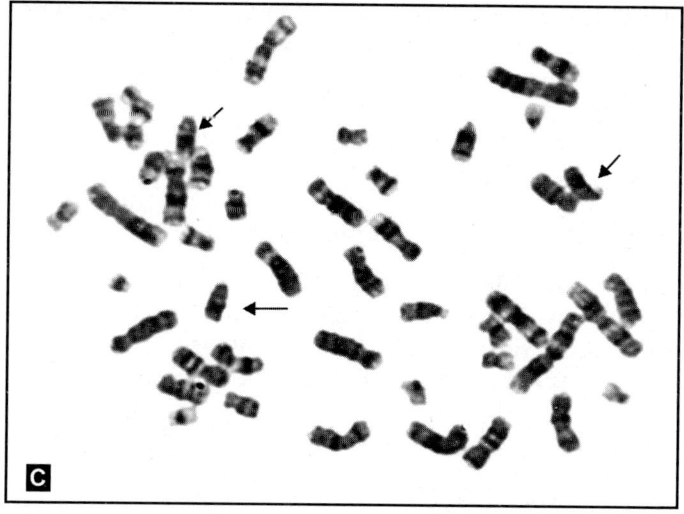

Figs 3.13A to C: Metaphase spreads showing (A) trisomy 21, (B) trisomy 18 and (C) trisomy 13

(Klinefelter syndrome), and less commonly 47, XYY. Multiples of X chromosome syndromes are known and have same phenotypic effect in males. In females 47, XXX Triple X syndrome is known. Presence of an extra sex chromosome is mostly compatible with life and has very few phenotypic effects.

Monosomy

The term monosomy is absence of a single chromosome from a normal diploid complement. Autosomal monosomies are always lethal. Sex chromosomal monosomies are compatible with life but could also result in foetal loss. The most common example is 45,X (Turner syndrome). Turner syndrome can be due to loss of either an X or Y chromosome. The cause of monosomy is non-disjunction at meiosis. If during divisions one gamete receives two copies of a homologous pair, the other gamete will have absence of a chromosome in it (nullisomy). Monosomies are also known to occur due to no anaphase lag, leading to loss of chromosomes.

Origin of Trisomies and Monosomies

Trisomies mainly occur by failure of separation of homologues chromosomes at meiosis I (anaphase) (Fig. 3.14). This is called non-disjunction. Trisomies can also occur due to non-disjunction at meiosis II. Here the sister chromatids of

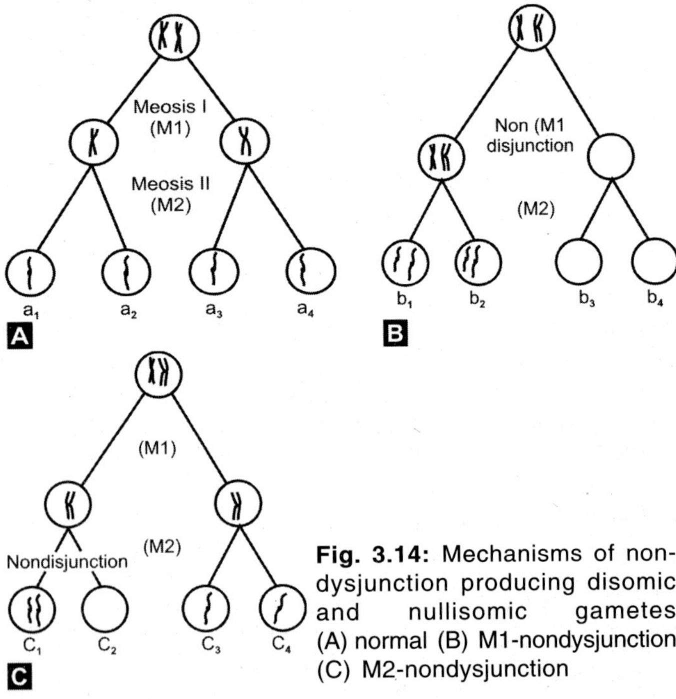

Fig. 3.14: Mechanisms of non-dysjunction producing disomic and nullisomic gametes (A) normal (B) M1-nondysjunction (C) M2-nondysjunction

a pair fail to dissociate. In both the cases, the gamete gets a pair of homologous chromosomes. At fertilization, a single chromosome from a parent results in trisomy. Most trisomies occur due to non-disjunction at maternal meiosis. Another group of trisomies resulting from non-disjunction occur in a developing zygote during early mitotic divisions. Such divisions usually lead to mosaic cell lines.

Causes of Nondisjunction

We have seen that nondisjunction leads to numerical errors of chromosomes. But what causes nondisjunction is still uncertain. Increased incidence of Down's syndrome in advanced maternal age suggests an effect of aging on the primary oocytes. Trisomy 13 and 18 can also occur with advancing maternal age. In a female the primary oocyte lies in suspended prophase stage. This means an egg of a female is as old as she is. The theory put forward for maternal age and disjunction is that there may be absence of recombination between homologous chromosomes in the ovary of the foetus. Incidence of aneuploidy is also increased when there is delay between ovulation and fertilization.

STRUCTURAL CHROMOSOMAL ABNORMALITIES

Structural rearrangements are a result of chromosome breakage and reunion at an abnormal site. Such abnormalities are usually heritable and are a cause for chromosomal aberrations in the progeny. Cells have enzymes for repair of broken strands of DNA and such repair goes on throughout the life of each cell. Some preference sites for breaks are known and are called fragile sites. Chromosome breakage is frequently accompanied by exchange of material from one chromatid to another during mitosis, when the replicated chromosomes are waiting to separate into two daughter cells. This is known as sister chromatid exchange (SCE). During meiosis, exchange of material on homologous chromosomes occurs during pachytene of the first meiotic division. This ensures mixing of the maternal and paternal gene pool and is termed crossing over. SCE and crossing over are seen in somatic and germ cells respectively. Abnormalities arise only if the chromosomes break at non-homologous sites leading to unequal exchanges.

Rearrangements can occur within a chromosome or may involve more than one chromosome. An individual with a normal chromosomal set is said to have balanced chromosomes. If some information is additional or missing, the arrangement is called an unbalanced chromosomal arrangement. Balanced rearrangements normally do not cause any phenotypic effect, as all the genetic information is present even though at a different position. The subsequent generations however, are at a risk, as such carriers are likely to produce unbalanced gametes resulting in abnormal offspring with unbalanced karyotypes.

REARRANGEMENTS INVOLVING SINGLE CHROMOSOMES

The phenotype is likely to be abnormal because of deletion, duplication, or in some cases, both. Duplication of a part of a chromosome is comparable with partial trisomy; deletion leads to partial monosomy. Any change that leads to deviation from the normal genetic complement may result in abnormal development.

Deletion

Deletion is a loss of chromosomal material causing an imbalance in the normal complement. The clinical manifestations depend on the size of the deleted portion and the function of the genes in that segment. Deletion may occur due to chromosome breakage within the chromosome. If the pieces are reconnected to the acentric material, the resultant chromosome is short (Fig. 3.15). Deletions may also be generated by abnormal segregation from a balanced translocation or inversion. This appears to be a more likely mechanism than multiple breaks in a single chromosome. A deletion may be terminal or interstitial. High-resolution banding may be used in cases of deletions that are not observable by routine metaphase studies. To be detectable by high-resolution banding, a deletion must be at least 2-3 megabases in size. FISH techniques may be

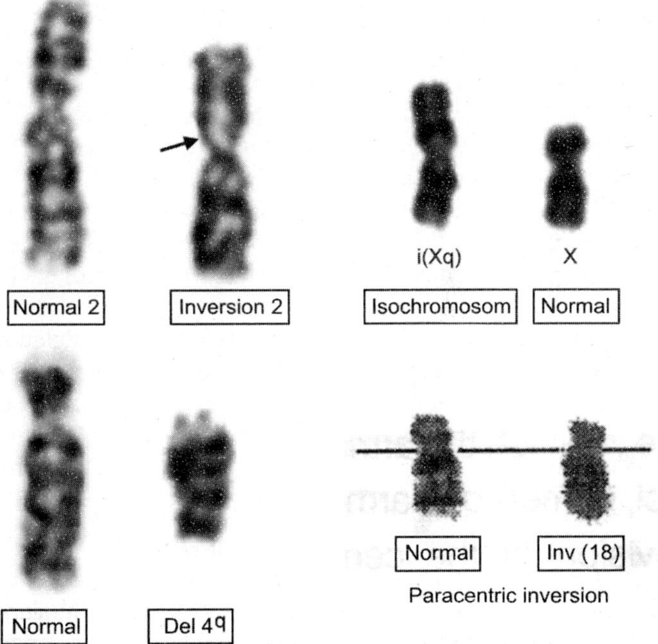

Fig. 3.15: Examples of chromosomal anomalies involving a single chromosome

used for detection of very small deletions. Specific syndromes have been ascribed to certain deletions and are described in the section on microdeletion syndromes, in the chapter on chromosomal syndromes. Deletions that appear to be identical in extent but different in parental origin may lead to differences in phenotypic expression. This is due to genomic imprinting, which marks maternal and paternal chromosomes differently. An example of this is the Prader-Willi and Angelman syndromes.

Duplication

A duplicated segment may be inserted in the same order as the original segment or may be reversed. Tandem duplications may arise by unequal crossing over during meiosis or from a rearrangement between two chromatids during mitosis. To form a reversed duplication, the segment should be inserted upside down next to the original segment. The exact mechanism of this rearrangement is not known. Duplication is usually less harmful than a deletion. However, because duplication in a gamete results in chromosomal imbalance, and because of the chromosome breaks that generate, it may disrupt genes. Duplication often leads to some sort of a phenotypic abnormality. Certain phenotypes appear to be associated with duplications of particular chromosomal regions and are functionally trisomic for the regions.

Inversion

An inversion involves two breaks in a single chromosome. The broken segment turns a complete 180° and reattaches to the points of breaks. Two types of inversions are known, paracentric or pericentric (Fig. 3.15). The centromere is not included in a paracentric inversion as both breaks occur in one arm, hence the arm ratio is unchanged. In a pericentric inversion the centromere is included in the inverted portion, causing the arm ratio to change. As no change is involved in the arm ratio in paracentric inversions, they can be detected by banded preparations. Pericentric inversions are easier to identify as the arm ratio and the banding pattern is altered (Fig. 3.16).

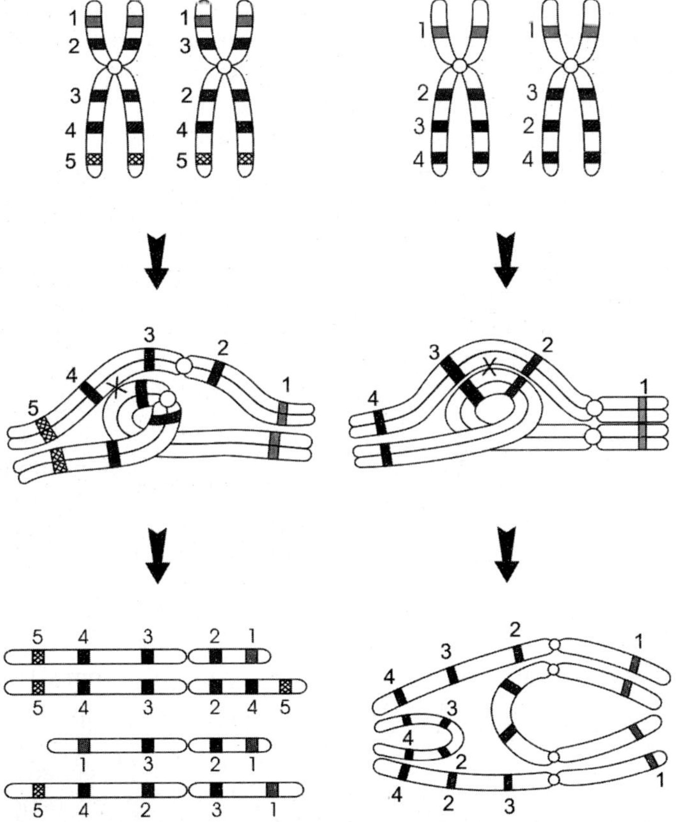

Fig. 3.16: Pericentric and paracentric inversions and mechanisms of production of recombinant chromosomes

An inversion does not usually cause any phenotypic change, as it is a type of balanced rearrangement. A carrier of either type of inversion is at a risk for producing abnormal gametes that may lead to unbalanced chromosomal complements in the offspring. The manifestation of the two types of inversions is different. A loop is formed when the chromosomes with an inversion, pair in meiosis I; if crossing over occurs within the loop, a deleted or duplicated chromosome can result (Fig.3.16). Inversions are only rarely implicated in chromosomal abnormalities in humans. Recombination which is a normal feature of meiosis I, is somewhat suppressed within inversion loops, but may occur in larger inversions. When the inversion is paracentric, acentric or dicentric chromosomes are formed on recombination and the resulting gametes with an unbalanced complement may not be compatible with the survival of the offspring. A pericentric inversion may result in unbalanced gametes with duplication or a deficiency of chromosome segments flanking the site of inversion. A particular risk is associated with pericentric inversions; the larger ones being more likely to result in viable offspring than smaller ones, because the former have smaller unbalanced segments. Pericentric inversion in chromosome 9 is the most commonly seen chromosomal inversion in humans. An increased risk of miscarriage is not commonly seen and these are considered normal variants, as there does not appear to be an increased risk of producing unbalanced gametes.

Isochromosomes

An isochromosome is one in which the arms on either side of the centromere are morphologically identical and bear the same genetic loci, namely one arm is missing while the other is reduplicated. Isochromosomes may be formed by horizontal division of the centromere instead of vertical division. Thus the two arms of the chromosome are separated instead of two chromatids. In subsequent mitosis the joint arms act as a bi-armed chromosome. Formation of isochromosomes may occur by chromatid-to-chromatid exchange, or chromatid translocations within a chromosome following breakage and loss of the distal sections of the chromatids. This may cause many isochromosomes to be dicentric. Isochromosomes appearing monocentric may have two centromeres so close to each other that they cannot be perceived as separate; special staining may be required to visualize them.

The isochromosome of the long arm of the X chromosome, denoted as i (Xq) is the most commonly seen isochromosome, observed in some individuals with Turner syndrome. Isochromosome 17q is seen in some patients with leukaemia. Solid tumours may also show isochromosomes (Fig. 3.15). Isochromosomes have also been seen in chromosome 12, 13, 18 and 21. The clinical effects manifested by isochromosomes are a result of the monosomic state of the missing loci, as well as the trisomic state of the genes on the isochromosome.

Ring Chromosomes

Ring chromosomes are a result of the joining together of the sticky ends caused by two breaks in a single chromosome (Fig. 3.17). The two terminal fragments are lost, giving rise to monosomic state of these loci. Clinical manifestations are a result of monosomy. If the centromere is within the ring, fragments lost are acentric. Disjoining of ring chromosomes at anaphase may pose a problem, especially when a twist is developed in a ring through breakage and reunion. Breakage and fusion may form larger and smaller rings. Because of mitotic instability, ring chromosomes may be seen only in a proportion of cells. Ring chromosomes have been detected for every human chromosome. Presence of a ring of any type can lead to ring syndrome, because of random duplication and deletion of genetic material in many different cell lines.

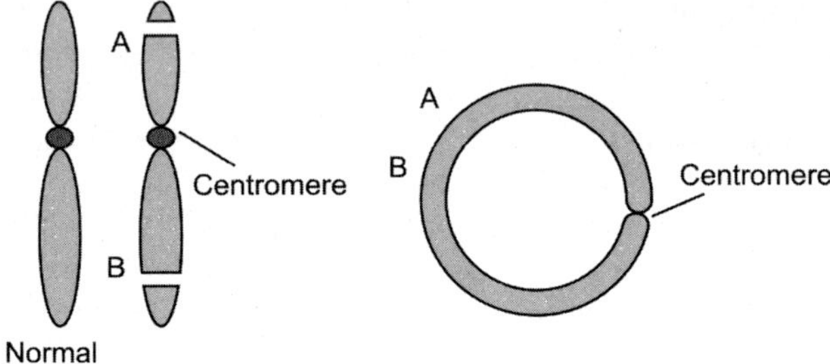

Fig. 3.17: Mechanism of formation of ring chromosomes

Dicentric Chromosomes

A dicentric chromosome possesses two centromeres, resulting from the joining of two broken fragments of chromosomes, each having a centromere. These may be formed from two different chromosomes or from two chromatids of the same chromosome. The two centromeres may act as a single large one if they are situated very near each other, or one may be inactivated in this case (sometimes called 'pseudodicentric'). If the centromeres are far apart or if both are active, they can be drawn to opposite poles of the spindle, resulting in formation of an anaphase bridge, a chromosome that makes a bridge between two daughter cells at anaphase. This may result in the dicentrics being left outside both the daughter nuclei as they form, or in breaking apart, leading to a loss or gain of chromosomal material. Dicentric chromosomes are most likely to be observed in cancer cells and represent an acquired abnormality. The most common dicentrics and pseudodicentrics are formed from the acrocentric D and G group chromosomes. Other chromosomes might be involved occasionally.

REARRANGEMENTS INVOLVING MORE THAN ONE CHROMOSOME

Translocations

Translocation involves exchange of genetic material between two or more non-homologous chromosomes. This can occur when two or more chromosomes break at the same time. Broken ends are usually sticky and the cellular enzymatic repair service usually reunites them, but occasionally a mismatch is possible. Breakage tends to occur more frequently at fragile sites at or near the centromere, at chromosome ends or at euchromatin-heterochromatin junctions.

Translocations are classified as reciprocal translocations or Robertsonian translocation.

Reciprocal Translocations

This type of rearrangement occurs when the breakage of non-homologous chromosomes results in reciprocal exchange of the broken segments. Usually only two chromosomes are involved. As the exchange is reciprocal, the total chromosome number is unchanged. In very rare situations three or more chromosomes may be involved. Reciprocal translocations are usually harmless as they are balanced rearrangements. However, they have a risk of producing unbalanced gametes and abnormal progeny. There may be meiotic complications, particularly a risk of non-disjunction.

Robertsonian Translocations

In this type of translocation two acrocentric chromosomes fuse near the centromere region with loss of the short arms. The resulting balanced karyotype has only 45 chromosomes, one of them consisting of the long arms of two chromosomes (Fig. 3.18B). Because the short arms of the acrocentric

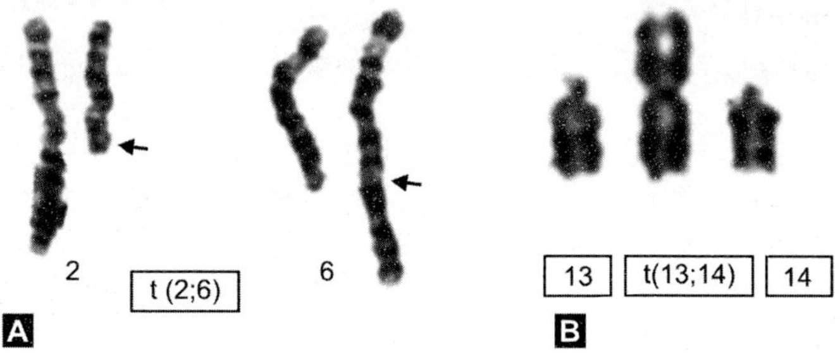

Figs 3.18A and B: Partial karyotype showing (A) Reciprocal translocation between chromosomes 2 and 6 t(2.6) and (B) Robertsonian translocation between chromosomes 13 and 14 t(13;14)

chromosomes have multiple copies of genes for ribosomal RNA, the loss of their short arms is not deleterious. Phenotypically, Robertsonian translocation carriers may be normal but there is an increased risk of production of unbalanced gametes and therefore of abnormal offspring. Of clinical importance is the one involving chromosome 21 as there is a risk of producing a child with translocation Down's syndrome. It is difficult to decide which centromere of a chromosome is involved unless C or Q banding is done. The numerical count in Robertsonian translocation is 45.

A translocation of either type can render the carrier functionally sterile, because of the complex synaptic structures formed. Complex translocations involving more than two breaks can cause serious problems in cell division. Small exchanges of the genetic material may produce viable dysmorphic infants, whereas large exchanges may lead to greater problems with spontaneous abortions. Sporadic translocation in chromosome 7;14 occurs in PHA stimulated blood samples.

Insertions

These are non-reciprocal type of translocations as a segment removed from one chromosome is inserted into a different chromosome. This insertion is either in its usual orientation or in an inverted one. Insertions are however, rare, as they require three breaks. Abnormal segregation in an insertion carrier can produce offspring with duplication or deletion of the inserted segment, as well as normal offspring and balanced carriers.

MARKER CHROMOSOMES

Marker chromosomes are occasionally seen in tissue culture, mostly in the mosaic state. They are designated as supernumerary chromosomes, as they are present in addition to the normal chromosomal complement. A marker chromosome also comprises a structural rearrangement. A marker chromosome must have a centromere. It may be derived from breakage of a chromosome with loss of the acentric fragment and non-disjunction from its homologue at meiosis. Tiny markers often consist of little more than centric heterochromatin, whereas larger ones contain some material from one or both arms, creating an imbalance for whatever genes are present. Due to problems in identification of the marker chromosomes, its clinical significance is difficult to assess, and hence poses serious problems in genetic counselling. In some cases, no phenotypic effects have been seen in individuals with small markers. Some others however produce severe clinical effects. If a marker chromosome has an identifiable centromere, it should be included as a derivative chromosome (der); if no further identification is possible, it should be denoted by the marker symbol (mar). If a marker chromosome is observed in amniotic fluid culture or chorionic villous samples, a prenatal karyotype is recommended to confirm its origin as familial or *de novo*.

BREAKS AND GAPS

Breaks can occur in chromatids or in chromosomes. In a break the chromosomal segment is completely fractured. The separate segment is either lost, or is seen as an attached fragment. In a gap, the segment appears discontinuous, but is attached by a thread like structure. Chromosomal breaks and gaps are significant, as they involve a loss of chromosomal material.

GENETIC IMPRINTING AND UNIPARENTAL DISOMY

An individual inheriting two copies of the same homologous gene from one parent due to an error at meiosis II, is an example of uniparental disomy. An individual inheriting two different homologues from any one parent and through error at meiosis I will have uniparental hetero-disomy. In both the above conditions, the conceptus would be trisomic, with loss of a chromosome resulting in a disomic State. One third of foetuses with such chromosome losses would result in uniparental disomy.

Genomic imprinting is defined as determination of the expression of a gene by its parental origin. It is generally accepted that an individual inherits one autosomal allele from each parent and that these alleles are equally expressed. Exceptions to this rule were detected for two syndromes Prader-Willi (PWS) and Angelman syndrome (AS). Both these syndromes are caused in most instances by microdeletions of the same chromosomal region on 15q11-q13. However, in PWS, the individuals inherit the deleted chromosome from their father and in AS the individuals inherit their deleted chromosome from their mother. This is thought to be due to functional inactivation (imprinting) of the nondeleted homologue (Fig. 3.19), resulting in structural monosomy, but functional nullisomy. Whereas maternal uniparental disomy resulting in PWS is common, accounting for about 20% of all cases, disomy of the paternal chromosome 15 causing as is rarer.

OTHER CHROMOSOMAL ABNORMALITIES

Mosaicism

The term mosaicism is applied to a condition where a in a body tissue, more than one cell type or line is seen. This can occur at mitosis, or any time after conception. Mosaicism can be present at two levels, in somatic cells or in gonadal cells (germ cells).

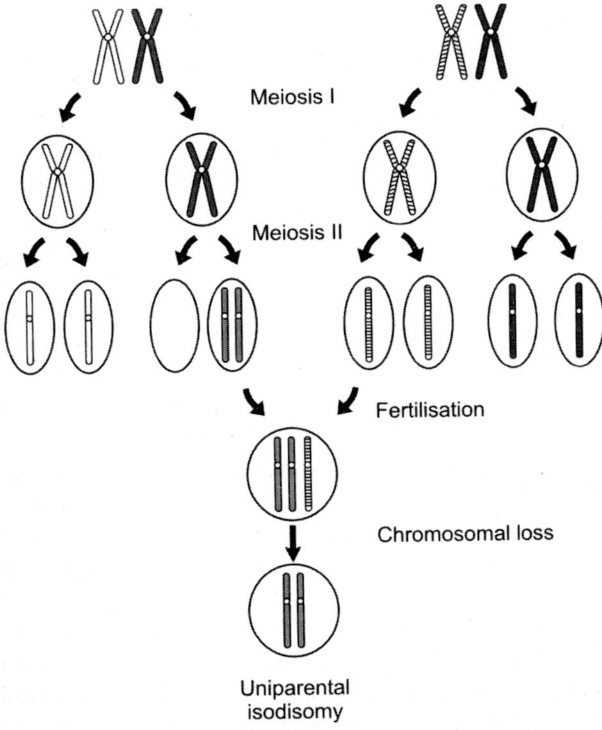

A

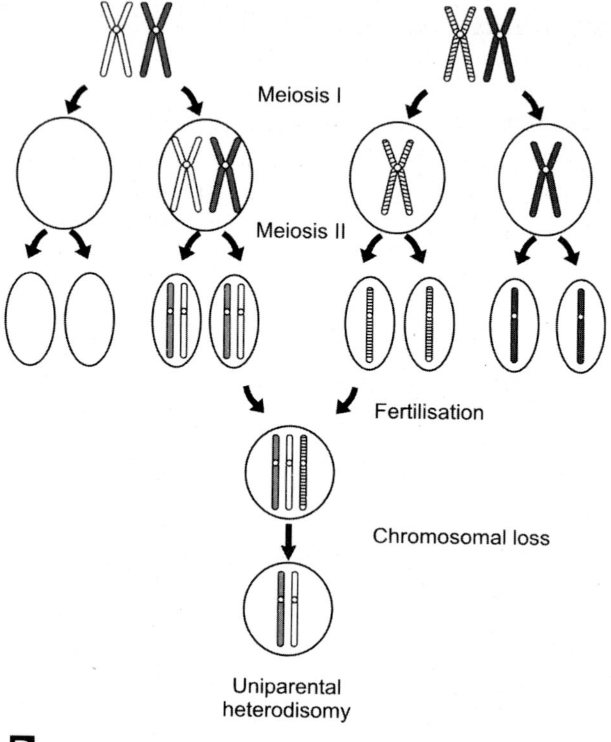

Figs 3.19A and B: Mechanism of origin of uniparental disomy (A) Uniparental isodisomy (B) Uniparental heterodisomy

Somatic Mosaicism

When the phenotype of a single gene disorder is less severe in an individual or is confined to a specific body part, somatic mosaicism should be suspected. The mutation pattern and severity will depend on the time when it arises during the developmental process. Hypomelanosis of ITO (Fig. 3.20) a disorder showing alternating patterns of pigmented and depigmented streaks corresponding to embryological developmental lines (Blaschkos lines).

Gonadal Mosaicism

There are certain families where a known genetic inheritance pattern like autosomal dominant or recessive is inherited, and more than one child is affected in spite of the parents being normal. This can be explained by gonadal mosaicism, where the mutation occurs only in the parents germ-line, and therefore the parents are not affected and are normal.

By definition, mosaicism is the presence of two or more chromosomally distinct cell lines. This may arise due to non-disjunction during early division of the zygote, or due to anaphase lag. In anaphase lag, there is a delay in chromosome movement on the spindle, and it does not reach the daughter cell before the nuclear membrane closes. In such a type of mosaicism, this is transmitted as an abnormal cell line, but the other cells of the embryo are normal.

If during chromosomal counting a mosaic cell line is observed, additional cells (a total of up to 100) should be counted, to ascertain the percentage of mosaicism. The level of mosaicism depends on when the misdivision occurs. If it is at the first cell division after fertilization, most of the body tissues will be affected. If the misdivision occurs after the formation of three germ layers ectoderm, mesoderm and endoderm, the abnormal cell line may be present in only one cell type.

Mosaicism can also be acquired. This is noted in cytogenetic analysis of malignant tissues or because of the impact of viruses and chemicals. It is recommended that 20 cells be counted and if they have an equal modal number, it is sufficient to give a diagnosis. If at any time, clinical diagnosis suggests the presence of a syndrome, additional cells are to be counted. In case of cancer patients or for investigating fragile site or

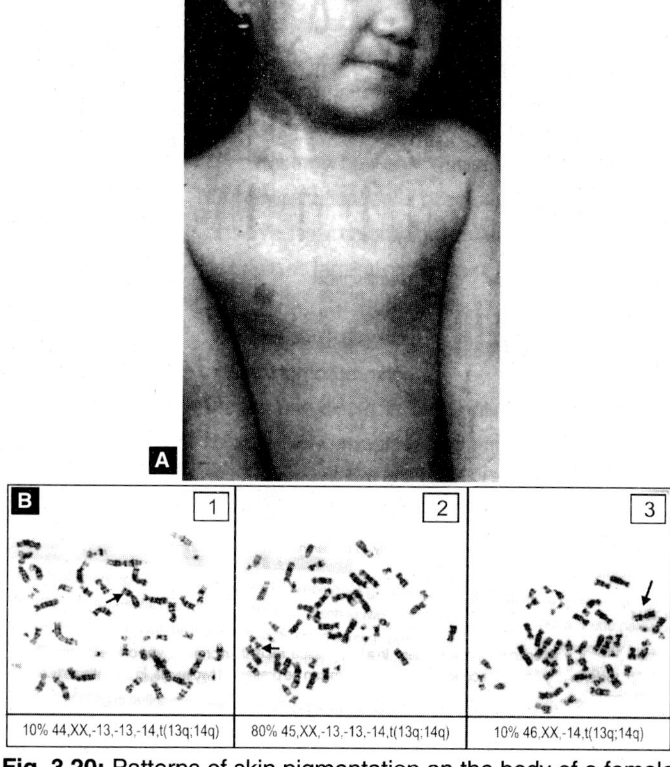

Fig. 3.20: Patterns of skin pigmentation on the body of a female child having mosaic cell line Metaphase spreads below.The skin conditions is called hypomelanosis of ITO *(Figure 3.20A for color version see Plate 2)*

chromosomal instability syndromes it is necessary to analyse more cells. If a single cell with a different modal number is found in the usual counting of 20 cells, an additional counting of up to 30 cells is indicated. If no further cells are noted mosaicism can be assumed to be an artefact.

In case of prenatal diagnostic samples, mosaicism for chromosome number 2 and 16 is observed as a common artefact. With bone marrow samples even if a single aberrant cell is observed, it needs to be reported, as it can be significant. The term pseudomosaicism is used for sporadic artifactual changes. It is important to differentiate between the two.

Chimera

Another condition of a mosaic cell line is known as chimera. A chimera has cells of different genetic constitutions. Here, two cell lines originate from two separate zygotes by fertilization of a polar body and the ovum. These two subsequently fuse. Chimeras can also arise by fertilization of two ova, which then fuse for example an XX / XY cell line.

Hydatidiform Moles

Paternally derived genes are responsible and essential for trophoblast development and maternally derived for early embryonic development. In hydatidiform moles, the pathology lies in the placental tissue. The placental morphology is completely distorted. Hydatidiform mole can be classified as a partial or a complete mole. In a partial mole, the foetus is always present but it rarely survives to term. In partial moles the conceptus is always triploid. Using DNA polymorphism studies it has been shown that the father contributes 46 chromosomes. This diploid paternal chromosome is either due to fertilization by two sperm or dispermy or duplication of haploid sperm chromosomes by endoreduplication.

Complete Hydatidiform Mole

Complete moles have 46 chromosomes exclusively of paternal origin. The condition is caused by fertilization of an empty ovum by two sperms or endoreduplication of a single sperm as in a partial mole. Complete moles are of importance in obstetric management as they are liable to undergo malignant change into invasive choriocarcinoma. Successful management of choriocarcinoma is possible by chemotherapy, but in untreated patients the outcome is fatal.

KARYOTYPE REPORTING

There is a refined system for reporting a karyotype (Table 3.3). The first point is to give total number of chromosomes including sex chromosomes, followed by a comma (,), the sex chromosomes are given next. If there is an abnormality of autosomes, that is specified next. Thus, a normal female karyotype is reported as 46,XX normal female and that of a normal male as 46,XY normal male.

If there is sex chromosomal aberration, it is written first. In addition, if autosomal abnormalities are noted they are written next in numerical order e.g. 47,X, t (X; 13) (q27; q12)

In uncomplicated cases a karyotype is written as follows:

- First the total number of chromosomes is written, then the sex chromosomes and next the addition of any chromosome if present.
- 45,X - (loss of one 'X' chromosome as in Turner's Syndrome)
- 47,XX, +21 (for Down's Syndrome)

In a mosaic cell-line, both the cell lines are separated by a slash.

- 45,X/46,XY. In case of mosaic cell line the major cell line is described first and the number of cell counted is given in the following square brackets 45,X [27]/46,XY [23].

In addition, symbols are used in rearrangements. The symbol is placed ahead of the chromosome involved and the involved chromosome is written in the parenthesis. 46,XX, r(20), means a female karyotype with a ring form of chromosome 20.

Table 3.3: Common nomenclature symbols and abbreviation

Symbol or Abbreviation	*Description*
p	short arm of chromosome
q	long arm of chromosome
s	satellite
t	translocation
ter	terminal end of chromosome
slant line	
/	separates cell lines in describing mosaicism
plus	
+	gain of material
add	additional material of unknown origin
cen	centromere
del	deletion
der	derivative chromosome, result of a translocation
parentheses	
( )	enclose structurally altered chromosome
question mark	
?	origin unknown
fra	fragile site
inv	inversion
mar	marker chromosome
mat	maternal origin
pat	paternal origin
semicolon	
;	separates region of structural alteration
colon, single	
:	break
colon, double	
::	break and rejoin
minus	
–	loss of material
arrow	
→	from - to
rob	Robertsonian translocation

For Banded Chromosomes

Regions and bands are numbered from the centromere. The symbol p is designated to the short arm and q to the long arm of the chromosome. The centromere is designated as 10. The part adjacent it on the short arm is p10 and on the long arm, q10. The regions adjacent to the centromere are labelled 1 on both the arms, the distal regions as 2 and so on. The band designation is written as follows:

1. Chromosome number
2. Arm symbol
3. Region number
4. Band number within the region.

There is no spacing or punctuation. For example, 1p31 indicates chromosome 1, short arm region 3, band 1, if the band has a subdivision, a decimal point is placed after the band description e.g. 1p3 is subdivided further in to three sub-bands 1p31.1, 1p31.2 and 1p31.3.

CHAPTER 4

MOLECULAR BASIS OF INHERITANCE

INTRODUCTION

The information regarding the expression of the genome is revealed by the analysis of chromosomes, and the DNA contained within them, using techniques at the molecular level. Chromosomes are the inherited elements through which the genetic material is transmitted. Within the chromosomes, the information-carrying component is DNA. Therefore the study of inheritance involves the study of the DNA sequence in genes. In order to understand genetic basis of a disease, and to use this information for diagnosis, possible treatment and the prevention, it is essential to know the structure and function of genes.

STRUCTURE OF A CHROMOSOME

The compact DNA forming a chromosome is composed of acidic chromosomal proteins called histones, and other heterogeneous proteins, non-histones. This DNA and protein complex is called chromatin. Histones are of five major types, and are termed as H1, H2A, H2B, H3 and H4, and they help in proper packaging of the chromatin. Two copies of these four histones form an octamer around which DNA winds. Each histone is associated with 140 base pairs, making two turns. Each DNA core complex is spaced by 20-60 base pairs. Thus the appearance of chromatin is like a beaded string. The complex of DNA and histones is called a nucleosome. Out of the five histones mentioned above, amino acid sequence of H1 varies more between species, while the other four show a conservation of amino acid sequences. The helical structure of the nucleosome is compacted into secondary chromatin structure, called solenoid. Under the electron microscope the chromatin structure appears three times thicker than the nucleosome fibre. Each turn of solenoid contains six nucleosomes. The solenoids are packed into loops, which are attached to non-histone proteins. The light and dark bands seen in prophase and metaphase chromosomes reflect the folding of clusters of loops, and also define functioning regions of the genome.

STRUCTURE OF DNA

Deoxyribonucleic acid (DNA) or nucleic acid is the hereditary material, which is transmitted faithfully from parents to offspring during reproduction. First identified by F. Miescher in 1869, nucleic acids were first called "nuclein" because they were isolated from cell nuclei. In 1953, James Watson and Francis Crick on their X-ray diffraction studies, proposed a double helix model of DNA described below. For their work Watson and Crick, received a Noble Prize for Medicine and Physiology in 1962.

DNA is tightly bound coil, and lies in the condensed form within the nucleus of a cell in the form of rod shaped bodies called chromosomes (Fig. 4.1). DNA is composed of repeating subunits called nucleotides. Each nucleotide is composed of a phosphate group, a five-carbon sugar (pentose), and a cyclic nitrogen-containing compound called a base. In DNA, the sugar is 2-deoxyribose. The DNA molecule consists of two complementary strands twisted in the form of a double helix. These complementary strands are chains composed of two types of nucleotide bases, pyrimidines and purines. The pyrimidine bases are thymine (T) and cytosine (C), and the purine bases are adenine (A) and guanine (G). The DNA model resembles a twisted ladder. The sides of the ladder form a backbone, and the links of DNA consist of deoxyribose residues linked by phosphate. The rungs of the ladder are made up of the bases purines and pyrimidines. Two strands of DNA are joined with each other by hydrogen bonds, which are present between the purine and pyrimidine bases. In a DNA molecule, adenine pairs with thymine (AT) and guanine with cytosine (GC). The ends of the DNA strands are designated as 5' and 3'. The 5' end is written to the left and indicates the sequence near the beginning of the gene, and 3' is written to the right indicating the sequence near the end of the gene (Fig. 4.2).

THE GENETIC CODE

The genetic information is stored in the DNA molecule in a sequence of three bases, and this is referred to as the triplet code (Fig. 4.3). The coding unit, codon consists of three nucleotide bases each signifying an amino acid. For example, the codon UUC is the code for pheohis flexibility in third position in referred to as the wobble. The DNA code is said to be universal code and is same for all organisms, except is yeast mitochondria and mycoplasma. The complete 'genetic code" was established by Nirenberg, Khorana and co-workers for which they were awarded Nobel prize in 1968 for physiology and medicine. The genetic message in the genetic code needs to be transmitted. The stages involved in this are replication, transcription and translation (Fig. 4.4).

Replication

In order to transmit genetic information from one generation to the next, the DNA molecule replicates. It is the process by which each strand of the parental DNA duplex is copied precisely by base pairing with complementary nucleotides. If

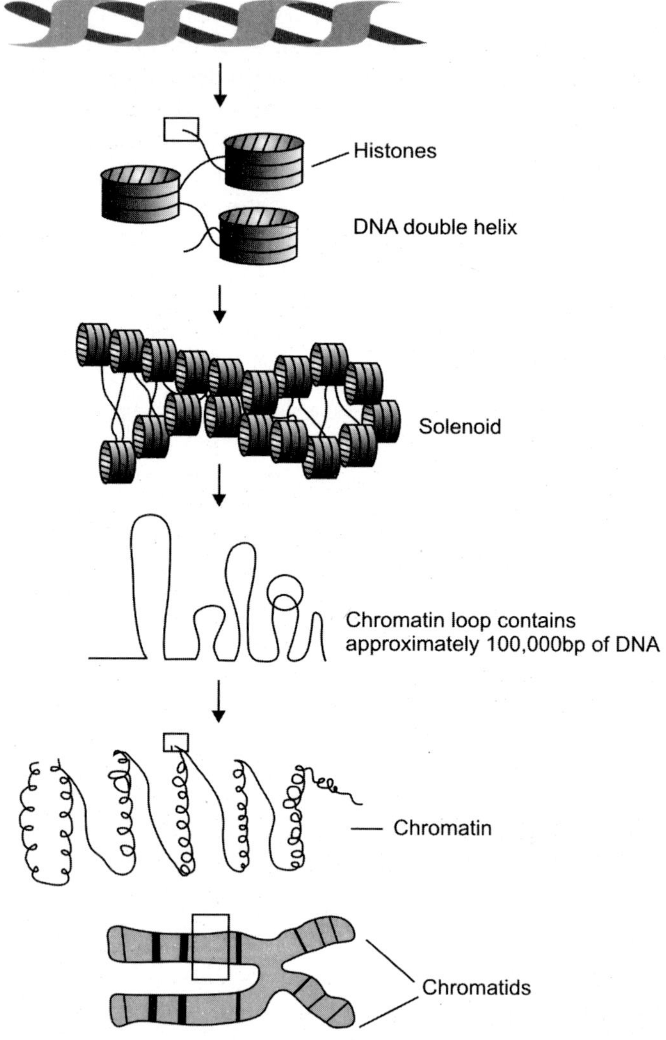

Fig. 4.1: Structure of chromosome

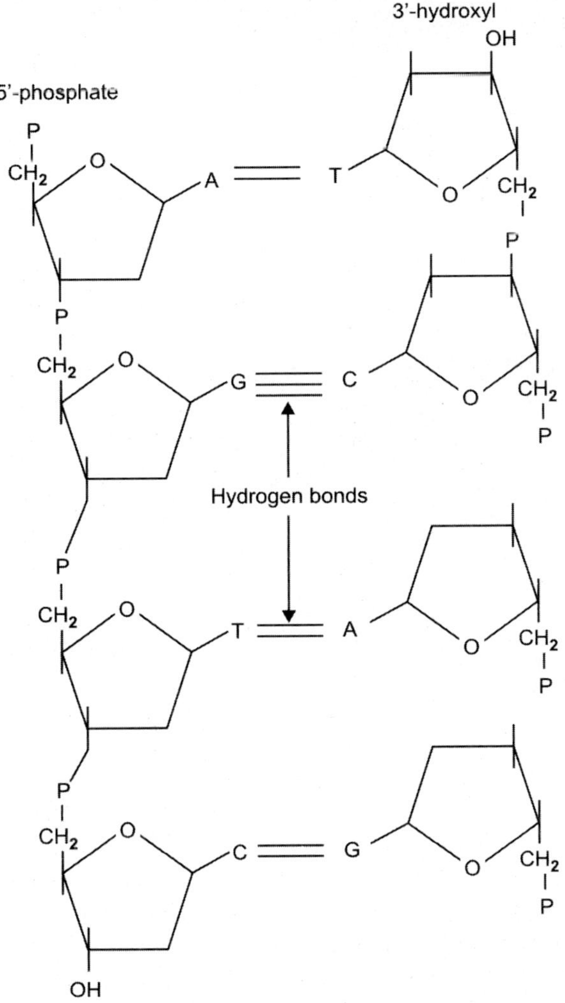

Fig. 4.2: DNA molecule showing the sugar phosphate backbone and nucleotide pairing of A,G, C and T

First position (5' end)	*Second position* U	C	A	G	*Third position (3' end)*
U	Phe (F)	Ser (S)	Tyr (Y)	Cys (C)	U
	Phe (F)	Ser (S)	Tyr (Y)	Cys (C)	C
	Leu (L)	Ser (S)	Term	Term	A
	Leu (L)	Ser (S)	Term	Trp (W)	G
C	Leu (L)	Pro (P)	His (H)	Arg (R)	U
	Leu (L)	Pro (P)	His (H)	Arg (R)	C
	Leu (L)	Pro (P)	Gln	Arg (R)	A
	Leu (L)	Pro (P)	His (H)	Arg (R)	G
A	Ile (I)	Thr (T)	Asn (N)	Ser (S)	U
	Ile (I)	Thr (T)	Asn (N)	Ser (S)	C
	Ile (I)	Thr (T)	Lys (K)	Arg (R)	A
	Met (M)	Thr (T)	Lys (K)	Arg (R)	G
G	Val (V)	Ala (A)	Asp (D)	Gly (G)	U
	Val (V)	Ala (A)	Asp (D)	Gly (G)	C
	Val (V)	Ala (A)	Glu (E)	Gly (G)	A
	Val (V)	Ala (A)	Glu (E)	Gly (G)	G

Fig. 4.3: Genetic code

the replication is errorless, the product is two duplexes identical in nucleotide sequence to the parental duplex. The genetic code is maintained during cell division. The new cell contains newly synthesised strands of DNA. This means, when a cell divides, genetic information encoded on the DNA is conserved and transmitted without change to daughter cells. The process is termed as semi-conservative replication. Two enzymes are required for this, DNA polymerase, and ligase. In a DNA molecule the replication starts at multiple points, which appears

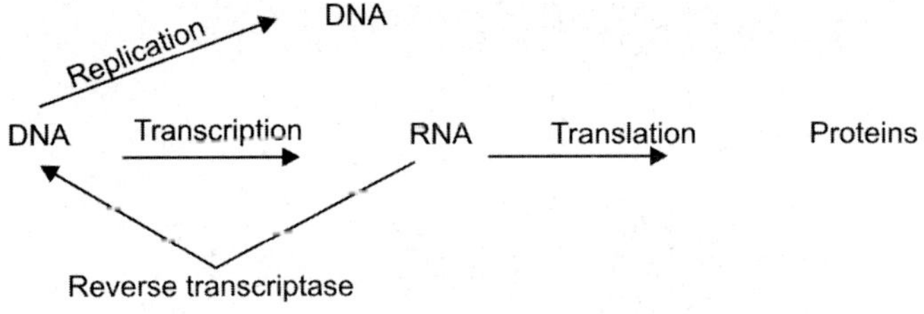

Fig. 4.4: Steps in the transfer of genetic information

as a forked structure called the replication fork (Fig. 4.5). This occurs in both directions. Replication origins are usually 30-300 kb apart, and each replication unit is 20-80 bp. Replication takes place during "S' phase of the cycle until the total DNA is copied. Any damage that occurs in a DNA strand gets repaired and reconstituted the same way.

Transcription

This is a process by which information contained in a DNA molecule is copied by base pairing, to form the complementary sequence of ribonucleotides. This is called messenger RNA (mRNA). The mRNA gets transported from nucleus to cytoplasm. Only 10% of DNA is transcribed into mRNA. The chemical difference between RNA and DNA is that sugar in RNA is ribose in place of deoxyribose in DNA, and the pyrimidine base is uracil (U) in RNA place of thymine (T). In retroviruses, the genetic material is in the form of RNA. This RNA is transcribed into DNA by the action of an enzyme called reverse transcriptase. This enzyme is of great practical value, as with the help of this DNA probes can be produced from RNA that corresponds to a coding sequence of a human gene.

During transcription, the two strands of DNA separate in

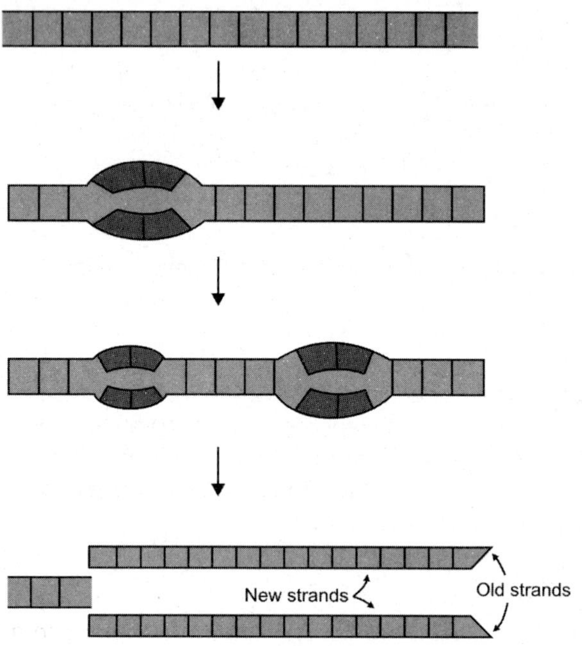

Fig. 4.5: Replication fork

the area to be transcribed. One strand (the sense strand) functions as the template, and mRNA is formed under the influence of RNA polymerase. Transcription proceeds in a 5' to 3' direction. After some processing and modification, the mRNA molecule diffuses to the cytoplasm and the DNA strands reassociate.

Translation

Translation is a complex process that occurs on the ribosomes in the cytoplasm. In this step, information transcribed from DNA into messenger RNA (mRNA) directs the order of polymerisation of specific amino acids for the synthesis of proteins. Each mRNA molecule becomes attached to one or more ribosomes. As the ribosome moves along the RNA from the 5' to the 3' end, each codon is recognized by a matching transfer RNA (tRNA), which contributes its amino acid to the end of a new growing protein chain. Amino acids are successively added to the polypeptide chain till the stop codon is reached.

THE STRUCTURE OF A GENE

Introns and Exons

The sequences of most vertebrate genes are split into coding sequences called exons, which are separated by noncoding intervening sequences called introns. It was in 1977 that the intron-exon structure of genes was discovered. Introns are transcribed into the primary RNA transcript, but are spliced out of the mRNA before translation. A group of DNA sequences known as consensus sequences precisely control this process. Most eukaryotic genes are mainly composed of introns. The exact function of introns is not known but it is suggested that they increase the length of genes, so that reshuffling of genes between the homologous chromosomes during meiosis becomes easier. It is also suggested that introns may help to modify the time required for DNA replication. Exons are segments of the gene that remain after splicing of the primary RNA transcript (5' untranslated sequences, coding sequences and 3' untranslated sequences) (Fig. 4.6).

Promoters and Enhancers

Promoters and enhancers are responsible for regulation of transcription. A promoter sequence is a combination of short sequence elements to which RNA polymerase binds in order to initiate transcription of a gene. Common promoter sequences are GC, TATA, CCAAT (these are called boxes). Transcription of genes starts in different places, thus producing different proteins. The same gene sequence is therefore known to code for a variety of proteins in different tissues. Any mutation in the promoter sequence will therefore reduce the transcription level.

Another group of regulatory sequences are called enhancers. Enhancers are *cis* acting DNA sequences that can direct a significant increase in transcription, independent of their respective position and orientation within a given gene. Enhancers could be located thousands of base pairs away from promoters, but can interact with promoter sequences by a mechanism of DNA that allows multiple loop formation, which can permit interaction of many regulatory elements.

EXTRAGENIC REPEATED DNA SEQUENCES

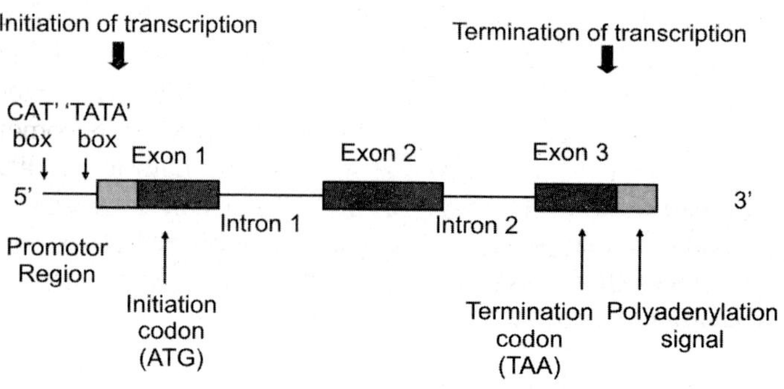

Fig. 4.6: Structure of a gene

The human nuclear genome contains a large amount of highly repeated DNA sequence families, which are largely transcriptionally inactive. A wide variety of different repeats are known. Noncoding repetitive DNA shows two major types of organization: tandemly repeated and interspersed.

NONCODING REPETITIVE DNA

Tandemly Repeated Noncoding DNA

Such families are defined by blocks or arrays of tandemly repeated DNA sequences. Depending on the average size of the repeat units, highly repetitive noncoding DNA belonging to this class can be grouped into satellite (blocks from 100 kb to several Mb in length), minisatellite (blocks within the 0.1-20 kb) range and microsatellite DNA (blocks often less than 150 bp in range) (Fig. 4.7).

The major chromosomal location of satellite DNA is the centromeric chromatin of chromosomes and includes alphoid DNA and the Sau3A family. The major chromosomal location of the minisatellite DNA is at the telomeres and includes the hypervariable family and the telomeric family of minisatellite sequences.

Microsatellite sequences are dispersed throughout the human genome.

Repetitive Interspersed DNA

Two major classes of interspersed repetitive DNA families have been discerned on the basis of repeat unit length, SINES (Short interspersed repeated sequences) and LINES (Long interspersed repeated sequences).

Short Interspersed Repeated Sequences (SINES)

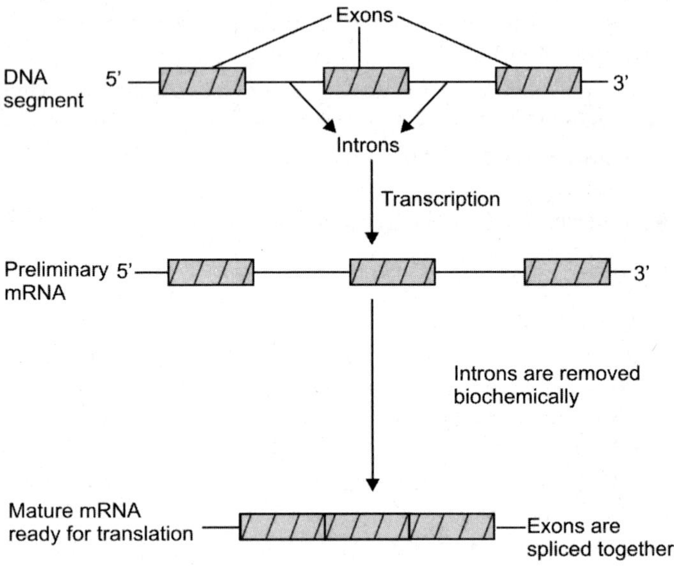

Fig. 4.7: Removal of introns and splicing of exons during formation of a mature mRNA

The most conspicuous human SINE is the *Alu* repeat family (so called because of the early attempts at characterizing the sequence using the restriction endonuclease *Alu* I). The size of the repeat unit is ~0.3 kb, and there are about 1,000 000 copies present.

Long Interspersed Repeated Sequences (LINES)

Human LINES are exemplified by the *LINE-1* or *L-1* element. The size of the full length repeat unit is 6.1 kb, but the average size is ~0.8 kb. They are present at 200,000-500,000 copies per haploid genome.

MUTATIONS

The term mutation refers to a sudden, heritable change in the genetic material of an organism or an individual. Such a newly formed phenotype is called a mutant. Mutants may result from faulty replication, movement, or repair of DNA and occur with a frequency of about one in every 10^6 cell divisions. Mutational changes in genetic material include changes in chromosomal number (aneuploidy, euploidy), structure, or in individual genes. Mutations can occur in the coding or non-coding regions of DNA molecule, and are of significance when they occur in the coding region. Mutations in the germ line may lead to inherited genetic diseases. If the mutation is dominant it will be passed on to half the germ cells, affecting half the progeny. If the mutation is recessive, it must be in the homozygous form to be expressed. When a child inherits identical mutations from both the parents he or she will become homozygous for that mutation. Mutations often affect somatic cells and so are passed on to successive generations cells within an organism. For example, most cancers are due to horizontal transmission of induced mutations, initially restricted to only that differentiated colony of cells. Mutations can occur spontaneously or may be induced by physical or chemical mutagens or by ionising radiations.

IMPORTANCE OF MUTATIONS

Mutation is the source of all genetic variation, and thus is the ultimate potential source for evolution. Alterations in alleles are mainly responsible for adaptation of individuals to the surrounding and for evolution in nature. On the other hand, mutations may be lethal to an individual, or may be responsible for disease.

Types of Mutations

Mutations can be divided into single base substitutions, which can be classified into silent, missense, and nonsense mutations. Other types of mutations include deletions, insertions, frameshift mutations, (which can be produced by deletions, insertions or splicing errors) and dynamic mutations, which include the triplet repeat mutations.

Single base Substitutions

Substitutions are the most common types of mutations, and as the name suggests it is the replacement of a single nucleotide by another. If a substituted nucleotide is replaced by the same type of nucleotide namely C for T or vice-versa, or A for G and vice-versa, it is called a transition. (a pyrimidine by pyrimidine or a purine by purine substitution). When a pyrimidine is substituted by a purine it is known as transversion. C to U transitions are more common and result in CpG dinucleotides. CpG dinucleotides get methylated in genomic DNA, with cytosine converting to thymine, and are called 'hot spots'.

Silent Mutation

A mutation that does not alter the polypeptide product of the gene is termed as a synonymous or silent mutation. There is no alteration in the properties when a single base pair occurring in the third position of a codon results in another triplet coding for the same amino acid.

Missense Mutation

In a missense mutation, there is a single nucleotide substitution, which results in the coding for a different amino acid, resulting in the synthesis of an altered protein. The chemically dissimilar amino acid alters the protein structure. This is also known as non-conservative substitution, leading to a reduction or loss of biological function. Missense mutations lead to qualitative and not quantitative changes in protein function. So, even though the biological activity is maintained, there is a difference in the behaviour of the protein, an example of this being that of abnormal haemoglobins. The term conservative substitution is applied to a condition where chemically similar, but different amino acids are produced with no functional effect.

Nonsense Mutation

It occurs when a base pair substitution leads to the generation of a premature stop codon resulting in truncated proteins, and usually a dramatic reduction in gene function.

Deletions

A deletion involves the loss of one or more nucleotides. If the deletion occurs in a coding sequence and involves a single or multiple nucleotides, but not multiples of three, the reading frame is disrupted.

Insertions

An insertion can be an addition of one or more nucleotides in a particular gene. The situation is similar to a deletion whether it involves one or multiple nucleotides but not multiples of three, thus disrupting the reading frame.

Frameshift Mutation

Any mutation involving the insertion or deletion of one or a few nucleotides which are in the coding region, can change the triplet code. The reading frame being shifted, this constitutes a frameshift mutation.

Dynamic Mutations

Mutations can be passed unaltered to the next generation thus called stable mutations, or they may further alter during the process of transmission when they are called dynamic or unstable mutations. Triplet repeat expansions are included in the class of dynamic mutations.

In 1991, the genes for fragile X syndrome and spinobulbar muscular atrophy were found to contain unstable expanded trinucleotide repeats. This mechanism has now been implicated in several other diseases. The discovery of triplet repeat expansions finally allowed a molecular explanation for the inheritance pattern of anticipation. Anticipation is a phenomenon in which the age of onset of a disorder is reduced, and/or the severity of the phenotype is increased in successive generations. Anticipation has been observed in myotonic dystrophy, fragile X syndrome, Huntington disease, and autosomal dominant spinocerebellar ataxia, all of which are known to be caused by a similar mechanism.

Triplet repeats can be found in transcribed RNA destined to be untranslated (either 5' or 3' such as in fragile X syndrome or myotonic dystrophy respectively), spliced out intronic sequence (such as Freidreich ataxia) or coding exonic sequence (such as the dominant ataxias). In general non-coding repeats are able to undergo massive expansions from a normal number of 6-40 repeats to an abnormal range of many hundreds or thousands of repeats. This leads to either transcriptional suppression as in the case of fragile X syndrome or abnormal RNA processing limiting the amount of cytoplasmic message as in the case of myotonic dystrophy. In contrast, the coding expansions undergo much more modest expansions from a normal range of approximately 10-35 repeats to an abnormal range of approximately 40-90 repeats. Since these are CAG repeats coding for polyglutamine tracts, constraints of the individual protein structures significantly modify this range. CGG expansions occur in the 5'untranslated region in fragile X syndrome. Freidreich ataxia contains an intronic GAA repeat, and myotonic dystrophy contains a CTG expansion in the 3' untranslated region. The expansion of CAG repeats within a coding segment of an exon is seen in Huntington's disease, dentatorubral pallidoluysian atrophy (DRPLA), spinobulbar muscular atrophy (SBMA) and the spinocerebellar ataxias (SCAs). This results in proteins with elongated glutamine (Q) tracts.

FUNCTIONAL EFFECTS OF MUTATIONS

Mutations of a gene might cause a phenotypic change in either of two ways:

1. The product may have reduced or no function, called a loss of function mutation. The alleles generated will be termed as null alleles (an allele that produces no effect) or hypomorphic alleles (an allele that produces a reduced amount or activity of a product)
2. The product may do something positively abnormal, called a gain of function mutation. The alleles generated will be termed as hypermorphic alleles (an allele that produces an increased amount or activity of the product) or neomorphic alleles (an allele with a novel activity or product).

Loss of Function Mutations

Loss of function mutations most often produces recessive phenotypes. For most gene products especially enzymes, the precise quantity is not crucial and we can get by on reduced levels of the product, up to half the normal amount. For some gene products however, 50% of the normal level is not sufficient for normal function. This is termed as **haploinsufficiency** and produces an abnormal phenotype, which is inherited in an autosomal dominant manner. Sometimes a non-functional mutant polypeptide interferes with the function of the normal allele in a heterozygous person. This is called the **dominant negative effect**.

Gain of Function Mutations

Gain of function mutations usually cause dominant phenotypes, because the presence of the normal allele does not prevent the mutant allele from behaving abnormally.

MUTAGENS

Mutations can arise spontaneously or due to environmental agents, which can alter the DNA or a chromosome. Such environmental agents are known as mutagens, and can be chemical, or ionising radiations (natural or artificial).

CHEMICAL MUTAGENS

There are 4 main groups of chemicals, which cause DNA mutations. Base analogues which mimic standard bases but pair improperly (5-bromouracil), alkylating agents which add alkyl groups to bases and so hamper correct pairing (nitrogen mustard), intercalating agents which intercalate with DNA and distort its structure (acroline dyes), and other agents which act directly on DNA (deamination by hydroxylamine).

Mustard gas, formaldehyde, and benzene are mutagenic in animals. Environmental chemicals that one can be exposed to, through use of pesticides in agriculture, industrial and pharmaceutical chemicals used commonly can be harmful. The Bhopal poison gas leakage in 1984 in India, is an example of a chemical mutagen, methyl isocynate which was responsible for chromosomal aberrations seen in affected survivors, and their offspring.

IONISING RADIATION

Ionising radiation consists of short wave length X-rays, gamma rays and high-energy particles (alpha, beta and neutrons). X-rays, gamma rays and neutrons have high penetrating capacity but beta particles penetrate a few millimetres while the alpha particle penetrates only a fraction of millimetres, thus both penetrate only soft tissues. Heat, light and invisible radiation which man constantly receives from ground, air or from food and drink are also present. In the process of penetration, they produce ions by colliding with atoms of the material through which they penetrate and release electrons. The released electrons collide with other atoms releasing further electrons. The change in electron number, transforms a stable atom or molecule into a reactive ionic state. Thus along the tract of each high-energy ray, a train of reactive ions is formed, which can initiate a variety of chemical reactions affecting biological processes. Such an irradiation is called ionising radiation.

The effect of radiation always depends on the dose of radiation and the measure used to calculate the radiation absorbed dose is called as rad. 1 rad measure denotes 100 ergs of energy actually absorbed by per gram of tissue exposed. Radiation for diagnostic purpose is a mixture of radiation measured as rem (roentgen equivalent for man). One rem is equivalent to 1 rad of plain X-ray. The amount of radiation received by an individual is measured in millisieverts (mSv), which is the commonly accepted unit. (100 Rem = 1Sv). Rem is the biological equivalent of Rad or Gray and is the accepted unit, and the term used in cases of medical exposure. [100 Rad=1Gray]. The critical dose in an adult is 500 Rads and more. However, for treatment of malignant illnesses, the dose far exceeds this, and may be as high as 5000-10000 Rads.

While studying mutations, exposure measurements in gonads are important as these effects are transmitted to progeny. These are of great significance in people who are exposed to X-rays as an occupation. Average human generation time is taken as 30 years approximately and gonadal dose of radiation is expressed as amount of rads in that period.

NATURAL SOURCES OF RADIATIONS

These include cosmic radiations from the earths atmosphere, from the sun and the galaxy around it, the crust of the earth and rocks, the most important being Radon, which is emitted by rocks and can be trapped in buildings, and finally from our food and drink. The spontaneous rate of chromosomal breakage may be markedly increased due to exposure to ionising radiation or mutagenic chemicals. UV light causes formation of a pyrimidine dimmer in which pairs of adjacent pyrimidine bases become linked by carbon-carbon bonding. Dimerization produces a bulge in the affected DNA region, and cross links form interfering with DNA synthesis and RNA transcription. However there are naturally occurring DNA repair mechanisms and these mechanisms involve enzymes such as DNA glycosylases and nucleases.

ARTIFICIAL SOURCES OF RADIATIONS

Doses from artificial sources of radiation are for most of the population much smaller than those from natural radiation. The artificial sources are the ones used for diagnostic and therapeutic purpose and those generated due to nuclear explosion.

Maximum Permissible Dose

The female oocyte is especially radiosensitive around the time of fertilization. An accidental diagnostic X-ray during the early stages of pregnancy results in the total added risk of 1 in 1000 to the fetes for congenital malformation, mental retardation or cancer. Neither termination of pregnancy or amniocentesis is indicated. Termination may be indicated if the fetes is less than 8 wks and the mother is exposed to 0.25 Gy or 25 rads. Exposure to 2-4 Gy results in female sterility. Exposure of either sex to therapeutic doses of radiation results initially in structural chromosomal abnormalities (rings, dicentrics, translocations) in 25-35% of lymphocytes. These tend to resolve by two years although translocations may persist.

The IAEA has recently updated its Basic Safety Standards together with the WHO, FAO and other such organisations. The occupational exposure permitted for a worker is 20 mSv per year. For the general public, the dose is 1 mSv per year, or in special circumstances up to 5 mSv in a single year provided the average over 5 years does not exceed 5mSv in 5 years. In the UK exposure limit is 15 mSv in a year. 1 mSv is approximately equal to 50 times the dose received in a single chest X-ray.

CHAPTER 5

RECOMBINANT DNA TECHNOLOGY AND ITS APPLICATIONS

INTRODUCTION

Recombinant DNA technology involves techniques of uniting two heterologous DNA molecules using *in vitro* ligation. The desired fragment of specific DNA sequence within a complex DNA population is selectively amplified using either cell based DNA cloning or polymerase mediated cloning using the polymerase chain reaction (PCR). Cell based DNA cloning involves attaching foreign DNA fragments (target DNA) to DNA sequences capable of independent ligation called vectors or replicons. This is done using an enzyme called DNA ligase, and the process is called ligation. Cutting the target DNA and the vector, with specific restriction endonucleases facilitate this step (Fig. 5.1A). Following ligation, the next step is called transformation, where the recombinant DNA molecules are transferred into host cells in which they can undergo DNA replication independent of host cell chromosomes. Recombinant screening and identification of cells containing recombinant DNA (vector molecules with inserts) is accomplished by insertional activation of a marker gene. The vector molecule is designed to have a multiple cloning site called the polylinker within the marker gene.

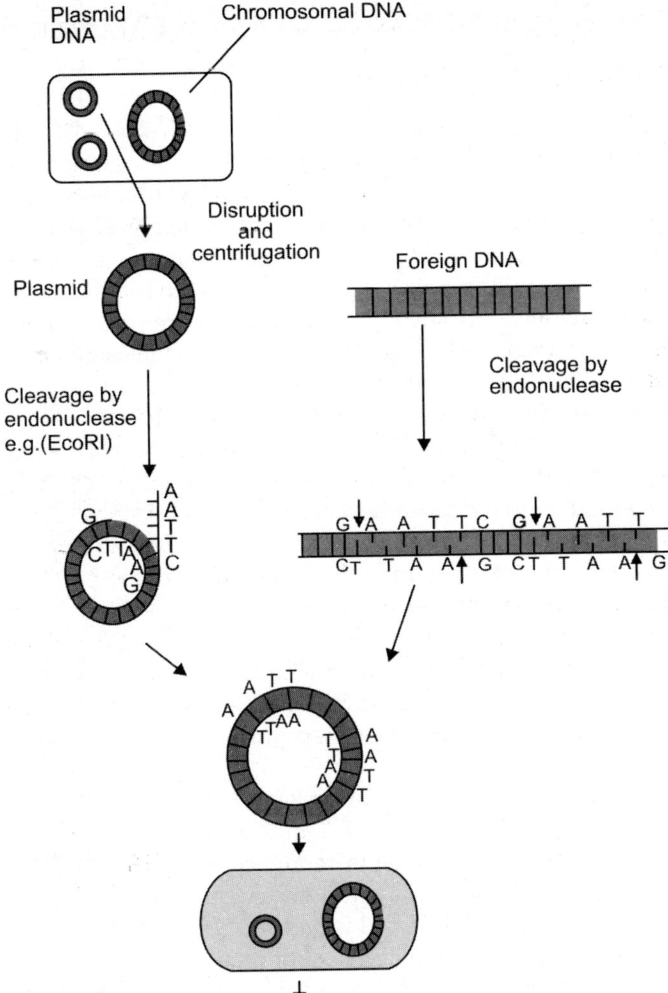

Fig. 5.1A: Steps in recombinant DNA technology generation of a recombinant plasmid by ECORI

TOOLS OF RECOMBINANT DNA ANALYSIS

Restriction Endonucleases

Restriction endonucleases are enzymes, which cleave DNA at specific recognition sequences, usually 4-8 base pairs long. A DNA sequence that is recognized by a restriction enzyme is called a restriction site. Restriction endonucleases enable the target DNA to be cut up into pieces and facilitate ligation into similarly cut vector molecules. The recognition sequences for a vast majority of restriction endonucleases are palindromes. A palindrome is a DNA sequence that reads the same when read in the 5' to 3' direction on each strand. Restriction fragments generated after cleavage with restriction endonucleases can be blunt ended or possess 5' or 3' overhangs called sticky ends. Restriction endonucleases that happen to recognise the same target sequence are called isoschizomers. A restriction enzyme is named according to the organism from which it was isolated. The first letter of the name is from the genus of the bacteria, the next two letters are from the name of the species, an additional subscript letter indicates the type of strain and the final number is the order in which the enzyme was discovered in the particular organism. Some examples of restriction endonucleases, their source, and recognition sequence are given below.

*Alu*I is derived from *Arthrobacter luteus* and the recognition sequence is AGCT; *Taq*I is derived from *Thermus aquaticus* and the recognition sequence is TCGA; *Hind*III is derived from *Hemophilus influenzae* Rd and the recognition sequence is AAGCTT; *Eco*RI is derived from *Eschericia Coli* R factor and the recognition sequence is GAATTC; *Bam*HI is derived from *Bacillus amyloliqueficans* H and the recognition sequence is GGATTC; *Sma*I is derived from *Serratia marcescens* and the recognition sequence is CCCGGG; and *Not*I is derived from *Nocardia otitidis caviarium* and the recognition sequence is GCGGCCGC.

VECTOR SYSTEMS

A vector is a molecule of DNA to which the fragment of DNA to be cloned is attached. The vector should be capable of autonomous replication, it must contain specific nucleotide sequences recognized by restriction endonucleases, and it must carry a gene that confers the ability to select for the vector such as an antibiotic resistance gene. Cloning vectors that can accept large DNA inserts have been used in general physical mapping of genomes and have permitted the characterisation and expression of large genes or gene complexes. Figure 5.1B some of the commonly used vectors are described below.

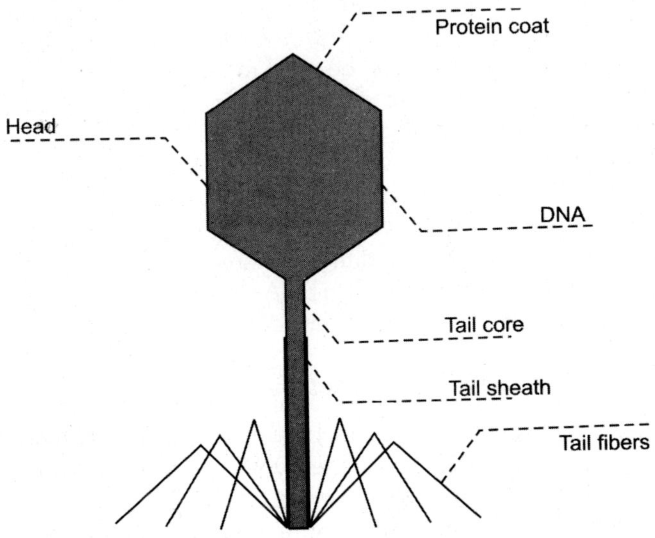

Fig. 5.1B: Components of bacteriophage vector

Plasmids

Bacteria contain single large circular chromosomes. In addition, most species also contain small circular extra chromosomal double stranded DNA molecules called plasmids, which individually contain very few genes. Their existence is intracellular and they are vertically distributed to daughter cells following host division, or they can be transferred horizontally to neighbouring cells during bacterial conjugation. Plasmid DNA undergoes replication that may or may not be synchronised to chromosomal division. Plasmids may carry genes that convey antibiotic resistance to the host bacterium and may facilitate the transfer of genetic information from one host to the other. If a DNA fragment is inserted into the middle of such an antibiotic resistance gene, then cells carrying the recombinant plasmid will be sensitive to this antibiotic. Thus the pattern of antibiotic resistance can be used to select for and identify bacterial cells carrying recombinant plasmids. Another method is using β-*galacatosidase* gene complementation. Plasmids can be readily isolated from bacterial cells, their circular DNA cleaved at specific sites by restriction endonucleases, and foreign DNA inserted into them. The hybrid plasmid can be reintroduced into a bacterium and large numbers of copies of plasmid containing the foreign DNA can be produced. Foreign DNA molecules 0-10 kb in size can be cloned using such vectors.

Bacteriophage λ/Phage Vectors

Phages, also known as bacteriophage λ are viruses, which infect bacteria, and are 45 kb in size. DNA is cloned in and the chimeric DNA is collected after the phage proceeds through its lytic cycle and produces mature infective phage particles. In order to design suitable cloning vectors based on λ, foreign DNA needs to be attached to the λ replicon *in vitro*, and the resultant recombinant DNA be able to be transformed into

E. coli cells at a high efficiency. DNA is packaged in a protein coat resulting in high infection efficiency. Modification of the λ results in two types of vectors. One is the replacement λ vector, which lacks the central segment of the λ genome, which can be replaced by a foreign DNA fragment. These vectors can be used to clone DNA fragments up to 23 kb in length, and such vectors are used to make DNA libraries. The other type is the insertion λ vector, where the λ genome is modified to permit insertional cloning into the cI gene. These vectors are used to make cDNA libraries and can be used to clone fragments up to 10 kb in length.

Cosmid Vectors

Cosmid vectors contain cos sequences inserted into a small plasmid vector. Cos sites are required for packaging λ DNA into the phage particle. Foreign DNA molecules 30-44 kb in size can be cloned using such vectors.

BAC Vectors

Bacterial artificial chromosomes (BACs) contain a low copy number replicon and only very low yields of recombinant DNA can be recovered from host cells. An example is the *E. coli* fertility plasmid, the F factor. The plasmid contains two genes parA and parB, which makes the copy number of the F factor at 1-2 per *E. coli* cell. Vectors based on the F factor system are able to accept large foreign DNA fragments greater than 300 kb. The resulting recombinants can be transferred with efficiency into bacterial cells using electroporation, resulting in BACs.

Bacteriophage P1 vectors and PACs

Bacteriophages have relatively large genomes, which allow development of vectors that can accommodate large foreign

DNA fragments. An example is the bacteriophage P1 that packages its genome in a protein coat. P1 cloning vectors are designed in which components of P1 are included in a circular plasmid and can accept up to 100 kb of foreign DNA. The features of the P1 and F factor systems have been combined to produce P1 derived artificial chromosome (PAC) cloning systems. Foreign DNA molecules up to 150 kb in size can be cloned using PACs.

YACs

Cloning of very large fragments involves the construction of yeast artificial chromosomes (YACs) due to the finding that the great bulk of DNA in the chromosome is not required for normal chromosome function. The DNA segment necessary for functional activity *in vivo* in yeast is limited to a few hundred base pairs of DNA. As a result a novel cloning system was generated based on the use of ARS (autonomous replicating sequence) elements, which are elements required for autonomous replication of chromosomal DNA. To make a YAC, two telomeres, one centromere and one ARS element along with an up to 2 Mb suitably sized foreign DNA fragment is used. The overall transformation efficiency for YACs is very low and so is the yield of cloned DNA (up to one copy per cell). Foreign DNA molecules 0.2 to 2 Mb in size can be cloned into YACs.

GENOMIC AND cDNA LIBRARIES

DNA libraries are comprehensive collections of DNA clones (cloned restriction fragments) from complex starting DNA populations. There are two types of libraries, genomic DNA libraries and cDNA libraries (Fig. 5.2).

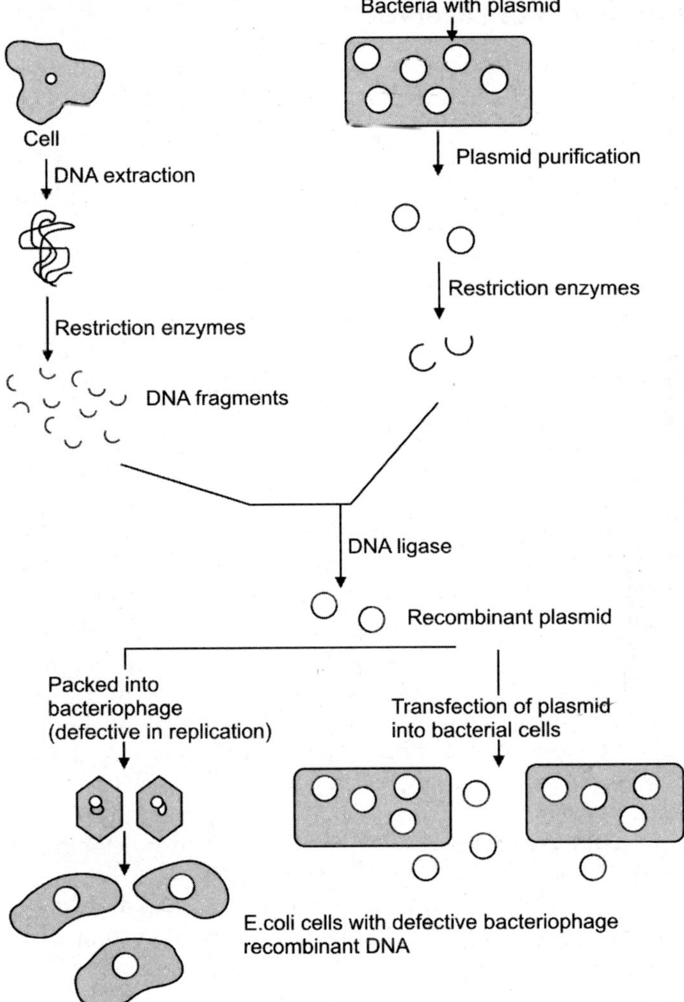

Fig. 5.2: Genomic and cDNA libraries

Genomic DNA Libraries

Genomic libraries are collections of fragments of double stranded DNA obtained by digestion of total DNA of an organism with a restriction endonuclease, and subsequent ligation into an appropriate vector. The recombinant DNA molecules are replicated within host bacteria. The amplified DNA fragments represent the entire genome of the organism and are called a genomic library. The complexity or number of independent DNA clones of a genomic DNA library can be defined in term of genome equivalents (GE). A genome equivalent of one, which is a so-called one fold library is obtained when the number of independent clones is equal to genome size/average insert size.

cDNA Libraries

The enzyme reverse transcriptase (RNA dependant DNA polymerase) can be used to make a DNA that is complementary in base sequence to the mRNA called cDNA (complementary cDNA) If a gene of interest is expressed at a very high level in a particular tissue, the mRNA corresponding to that gene is also likely present at high concentrations in the cell. The starting material for making cDNA libraries is total RNA from a specific tissue or specific developmental stage of embryogenesis. The mRNA is used as a template to make a cDNA library using reverse transcriptase and the cDNA can be amplified by cloning or PCR. These mixtures of heterogeneous cDNAs can be cloned to make a cDNA library. To assist cloning, oligonucleotide linkers which contain suitable restriction sites are ligated to each end of the cDNA.

NUCLEIC ACID HYBRIDISATION

Nucleic acid hybridisation is a method for identifying closely related nucleic acid molecules within two populations. One is the target of a complex, heterogeneous population of nucleic acid molecules, such as total genomic DNA or RNA. The other, called a probe, is a homogenous population of cloned DNA or chemically synthesized oligonucleotides. The rationale of hybridisation is to use the probe to identify related fragments from the complex target molecules and anneal to them. There are two types of hybridisation assays, standard and reverse assays. Standard nucleic acid hybridisation assays consist of the labelled probe in solution, and the unlabelled target bound to a solid support. Reverse nucleic acid hybridisation assays consist of the labelled target (complex DNA in solution) and unlabelled probes such as oligonucleotides or DNA clones bound to solid support. Examples of standard nucleic acid hybridisation assays include Southern blotting, Northern blotting, and dot blots using allele specific oligonucleotides (ASOs). Examples of reverse nucleic acid hybridisation assays include reverse dot blots, DNA microarrays, and oligonucleotide microarrays. Some examples of these assays are described below.

Dot Blot Hybridisation Assay

Dot blot assay is a screening method in which an aqueous solution of target DNA like total human genomic DNA is spotted onto a nitrocellulose or nylon membrane and allowed to dry. The target sequence is heat or alkali denatured and is exposed to a solution containing single stranded labelled probe. The probe target heteroduplex is allowed to form and the membrane is washed to remove excess non-specific probe, dried and exposed to autoradiographic film. This method employs specific oligonucleotides probes (ASOs) to discriminate between alleles differing at a single nucleotide position. ASO dot blot hybridisation is used to identify common mutations in sickle cell anaemia, and other commonly seen mutations.

Southern Blot Hybridisation Assay

Target DNA is digested with restriction endonucleases, size fractionated by agarose gel electrophoresis, denatured and transferred to a nitrocellulose or nylon membrane for hybridisation. The immobilized single stranded target DNA sequences are allowed to associate with labelled single stranded probe DNA. The radiolabel led probe binds only to complementary sequences in target DNA and can be detected by exposure to autoradiographic film (Fig. 5.3).

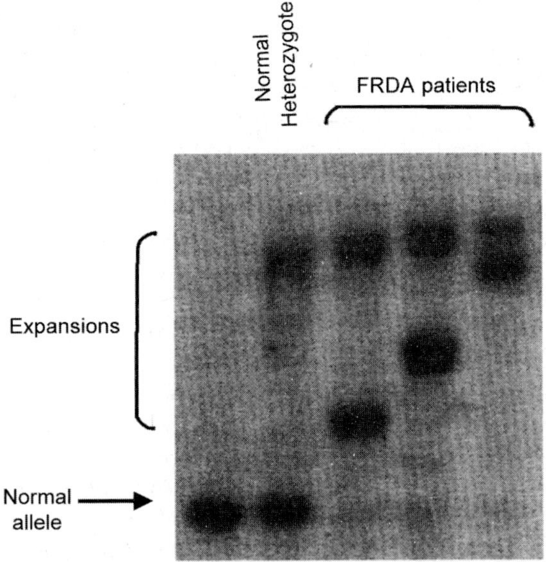

Fig. 5.3: Shows a diagrammatic representation and an example of a Southern blot assay

Northern Blot Hybridisation Assay

Northern blotting is a variant of Southern blotting in which the target nucleic acid is RNA instead of DNA. This method is used to obtain information on the expression patterns of specific genes. RNA isolated from a variety of tissues can be run in different lanes and size fractionated. This can be transferred to a membrane and hybridisation carried out with a suitable labelled nucleic acid probe. The data obtained can provide information on the range of tissues in which the gene is expressed and the abundance of transcripts. Different sizes of transcripts are produced due to alternative splicing and can be detected on a Northern blot. Figure 5.4 shows an example of the use of labelled factor IX cDNA probe, and levels of

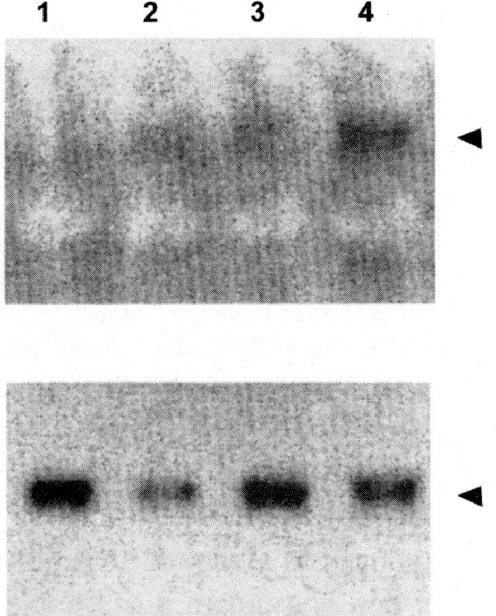

Fig. 5.4: An example of the use of labelled factor IX cDNA probe, and levels of expression detected

expression detected in lanes in the upper panel. The lower panel shows hybridisation of the same blot with a universally expressed GAPDH probe showing equal expression in all lanes, which also confirms equal loading of RNA in all lanes.

In situ Hybridisation

In situ hybridisation involves hybridisation of a nucleic acid probe to the denatured DNA of a chromosome preparation, and example of which is fluorescent *in situ* hybridisation (FISH) described elsewhere. Nucleic acid probes (double stranded cDNAs or single stranded RNA probes called riboprobes, labelled isotopically or non-isotopically) can also be hybridised to RNAs of tissue sections fixed onto slides called tissue *in situ* hybridisation or whole organs or embryos called whole mount *in situ* hybridisation.

Microarray Hybridisation Assay

DNA micro array technologies (DNA chips) employ a reverse nucleic acid hybridisation approach. The probes consist of unlabelled DNA fixed to a solid support (oligonucleotide or DNA arrays) and the target is labelled in solution. Micro arrays of DNA clones are generated by micro spotting, and micro arrays of oligonucleotides are generated by combining photolithography and *in situ* synthesis of oligonucleotides. The applications of micro array technology include large scale screening of gene expression at the RNA level and screening of DNA variation, including assaying for known mutations in genes and identification of single nucleotide polymorphisms (SNPs).

Western Blotting

This method is used to detect protein expression using cell extracts fractionated according to size using a form of polyacrylamide gel electrophoresis using SDS-PAGE and transfer (blotting) to a membrane. The proteins are detected using antibodies specific to regions of the protein such as specific domains or C or N terminal domains. Antibodies to human gene products are obtained by injecting suitable animals with immunogens such as synthetic peptides or fusion proteins, or by using genetic engineering methods such as phage display technology.

Polymerase Chain Reaction

The polymerase chain reaction (PCR) is a rapid *in vitro* method for amplifying defined target sequences present within a source of DNA. The method is designed to permit selective amplification of a specific target DNA sequence within a heterogeneous collection of DNA sequences like total genomic DNA or a complex cDNA population (Fig. 5.5).

Basic Features of PCR

PCR uses a DNA polymerase to repetitively amplify targeted portions of DNA. Each cycle of amplification doubles the amount of DNA in the sample leading to an exponential increase in DNA with repeated cycles of amplification. In order to perform a PCR it is necessary to know the nucleotide sequence of short sequences flanking the region of interest to be amplified. The nucleotide sequences of the flanking regions are used to design and construct two single stranded oligonucleotides, usually 20-30 nucleotides long that are complementary to the respective flanking sequences. These synthetic oligonucleotides are called primers.

There are three steps in a PCR reaction, denaturation, annealing and extension. For denaturation, the DNA to be amplified is heated to separate the double stranded target DNA into single strands. This involves heating the PCR mixture

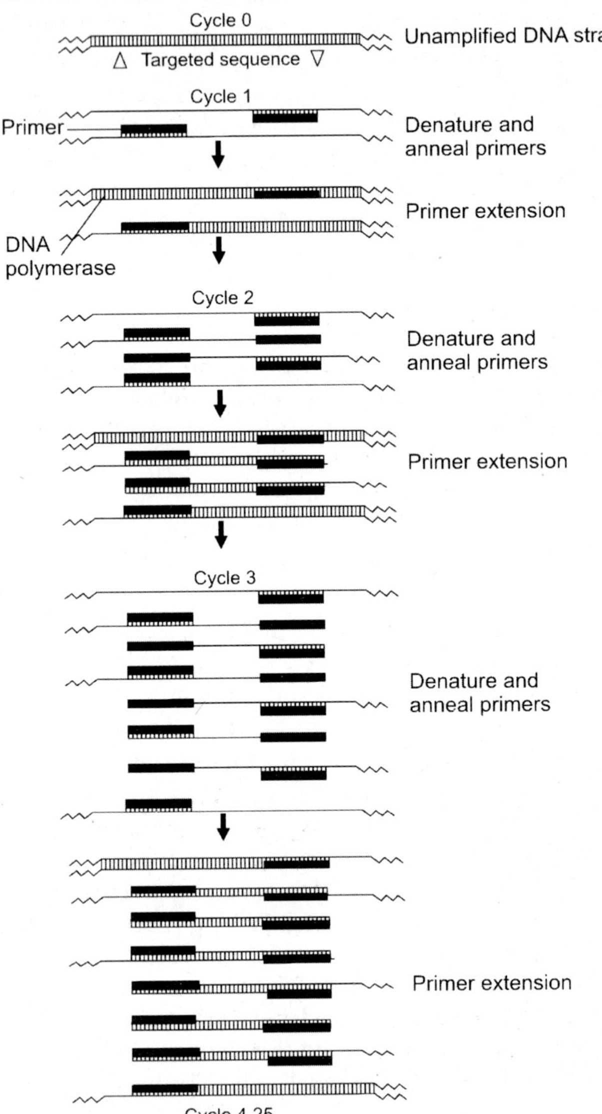

Fig. 5.5: Polymerase chain reaction (PCR)

to 93°C for human genomic DNA template. Annealing of primers to single stranded DNA occurs when the temperature is lowered to the temperature that is approximately five degrees below the melting point (Tm) of the primers used in the reaction. For the extension reaction, DNA polymerase and an excess of deoxyribonucleoside triphosphates (dATP, dGTP, dCTP, dTTP) are added to the mixture to initiate the synthesis of two new chains complementary to the original DNA. This is done at 70°C. DNA polymerase adds nucleotides to the 3' hydroxyl end of the primer, and strand growth extends across the target DNA making complementary copies of the target. At the completion of one cycle of replication, the reaction mixture is heated again to denature the DNA strands, both the original target strand and the newly generated strands. Each strand binds a complementary primer and the cycle of chain extension is repeated. Typically 20-30 cycles are run during DNA amplification. Each newly synthesised polynucleotide can act as a template for successive cycles, which leads to an exponential increase in the amount of target DNA with each cycle. After about 25 cycles of DNA synthesis the products of the PCR will include in addition to the starting DNA about 105 copies of specific target sequence. This amount is easily visualised as a discrete band of specific size when subjected to agarose gel electrophoresis.

The major advantages of PCR are its rapidity, sensitivity, and robustness. The major disadvantages of PCR are the general requirement for prior target sequence information, the size of the DNA fragments generated and the limited amount of PCR product that is obtained. Another disadvantage is the infidelity of *Taq* polymerase, which has no associated 3' to 5' exonuclease activity to confer a proofreading function, which means the error rate due to misincorporation during DNA replication is high. This can be overcome by using other polymerases such as *Pfu* polymerase.

Applications of PCR

1. PCR enables rapid amplification of numerous DNA templates for screening of uncharacterised mutations. The identification of exon-intron boundaries and sequencing at the end of introns of a gene of interest offers the possibility of genomic mutation screening by amplification of individual exons by PCR and screening by various mutation screening methods such as single stranded conformational polymorphism analysis (SSCP), heteroduplex analysis, or chemical cleavage mismatch analysis. PCR can also be used to provide amplification of cDNA sequences for mutation screening. To do this mRNA is isolated and converted to cDNA using reverse transcriptase, and the cDNA is used as a template for a PCR reaction. This is called reverse transcriptase PCR or RT-PCR.
2. PCR can be used for rapid typing of polymorphic genetic markers such as RFLPs (restriction fragment length polymorphisms) and STRPs (short tandem repeat polymorphisms).

   RFLPs result in alleles possessing or lacking a specific restriction site. Such polymorphisms can be detected using Southern blotting. RFLPs are genetic variants that examined by cleaving DNA into fragments (restriction fragments) with a restriction enzyme. The length of the restriction fragment is altered if the genetic variant alters the DNA to create or abolish a restriction site. Mutation of one or more nucleotides at a restriction site can render the site unrecognisable by the enzyme or create a new restriction site. Cleavage with the enzyme will result in fragments of lengths differing from normal that can be detected by DNA hybridisation. PCR can be used to type RFLPs by designing primers that flank polymorphic restriction sites, amplifying from genomic DNA, and cutting the PCR product with appropriate restriction enzymes and separating the fragments by agarose gel electrophoresis.

STRPs are also called microsatellite markers and consist of short sequences that are tandemly repeated several times. An example of these is dinucleotide repeats such as CA repeats, trinucleotide and tetranucleotide repeats. Primers are designed from sequences known to flank a specific STRP locus, permitting amplification of alleles whose sizes differ by integral repeat units. The PCR products can be size fractionated by polyacrylamide gel electrophoresis. An example of the use of a CA repeat marker in an autosomal dominant pedigree is shown in Figure 5.6.

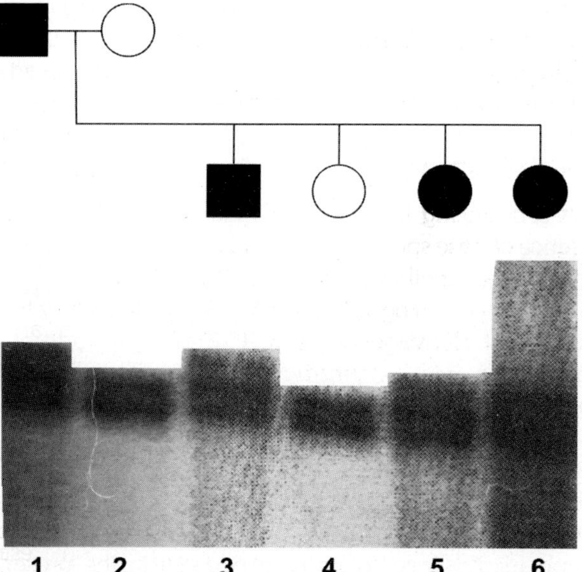

Fig. 5.6: An autoradiograph of a polymorphic tetranucleotide repeat co-segregating in a family with a dominant disorder

3. Use of PCR in genomic DNA cloning and cDNA cloning. Cloning of new members of a DNA family or cloning of cDNAs from amino acid sequence can be carried out by using DOP-PCR. DOP-PCR (degenerate oligonucleotide PCR) is a form of PCR using partially degenerate oligonucleotides to permit searching of a new or uncharacterised DNA sequence that belongs to a family of related sequences either within or between species.
4. PCR can be used for gene expression studies using RT-PCR. Spatial patterns of expression are provided efficiently by tissue *in situ* hybridisation. Quantitation of expression of a particular gene can also be provided by a Northern blot, which requires large amounts of starting material in the form of RNA. RT-PCR provides a rough quantitation of expression of a particular gene using very small amounts of starting material. RT-PCR can also be useful for identifying and studying different isoforms of an RNA transcript produced due to alternative splicing.

DNA Sequencing

DNA sequencing involves enzymatic DNA synthesis in the presence of base specific dideoxynucleotide chain terminators. Prior to these methods, chemical DNA sequencing methods were employed using base specific chemical modification and subsequent cleavage of DNA. Current methods of DNA sequencing use enzymatic methods. The DNA to be sequenced is provided in a single stranded form, from which DNA polymerase synthesises new complementary DNA strands. The subsequent DNA sequencing reactions involve DNA synthesis using one or more labelled nucleotides and a sequencing primer. In addition to the normal nucleotide precursors, DNA synthesis is carried out in the presence of base specific dideoxynucleotides (ddNTPs). The principle of dideoxy sequencing is that the sequencing primer binds specifically to a region 3' of the desired DNA sequence and primes synthesis of a complementary DNA strand in the indicated direction. Four base specific reactions are carried out in parallel each with all four dNTPs and one ddNTP. Competition for incorporation into the growing DNA chain between a ddNTP and its normal dNTP analogue results in a population of fragments of different lengths. The fragments have a common 5' end defined by the sequencing primer and variable 3' ends depending on where the dideoxynucleotide has been inserted.

Traditional dideoxy sequencing methods employed radioisotope labelling (35S labelled oligonucleotides) using a dNTP mix that contains a proportion of radiolabel led nucleotides, which are incorporated within the growing DNA chains. Size fractionation of products of the four reactions is carried out in separate wells of a polyacrylamide gel. The gel is dried and subjected to autoradiography allowing the complementary strand to be read from top to bottom. Figure 5.7 shows an example of a sequence within the gene for neurofibromatosis type-1.

Cycle Sequencing

Cycle sequencing is also called linear amplification sequencing. It is a PCR sequencing approach, which uses a thermostable DNA polymerase and a temperature cycling format of denaturation, annealing and DNA synthesis. However, cycle sequencing employs only one primer and includes a ddNTP chain terminator in the reaction. Therefore the product accumulates linearly instead of exponentially as seen in a conventional PCR reaction. Double stranded plasmids, cosmids, and PCR products can be sequenced using this method.

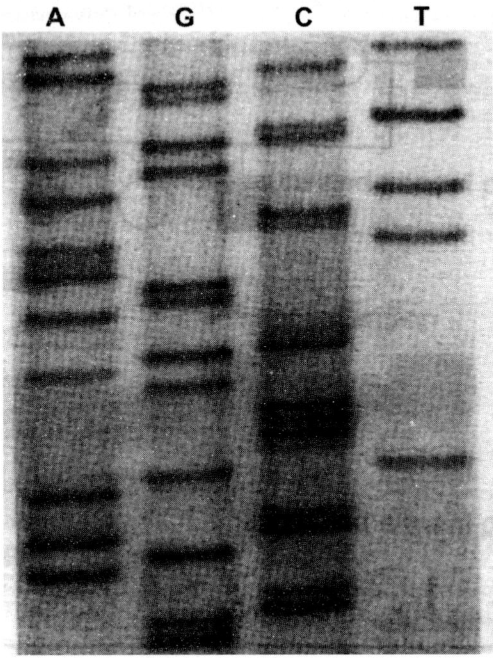

Fig. 5.7: A portion of the sequencing gel showing the nucleotide sequence of a single stranded DNA template from the neurofibromatosis type-1 gene

Automated DNA Sequencing Using Fluorescent Labelling Systems

These procedures use primers or dideoxynucleotides, which have attached chemical groups called flurophores, which are capable of fluorescing. Different flurophores are used for the four base specific reactions, and therefore all four reactions are loaded in a single lane. During electrophoresis a monitor detects and

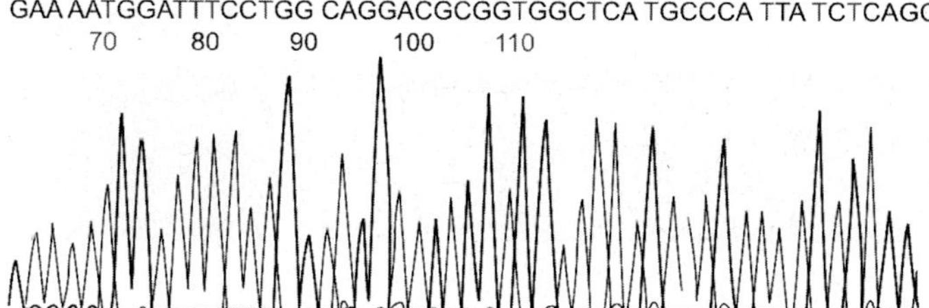

Fig. 5.8: Automated DNA sequencing using fluorescent primers showing output of sequence data from an automated DNA sequencer and dye and basic specific probes

records a fluorescent signal as the DNA passes through a fixed point in the gel. As individual fragments migrate past this position, the laser causes the dyes to fluoresce. Maximum fluorescence occurs at different wavelengths for the four dyes and the information is recorded electronically. An example of automated DNA sequence using fluorescent primers is shown in Figure 5.8.

CHAPTER 6

DEVELOPMENTAL GENETICS

INTRODUCTION

Progress in *in vitro* fertilization has helped many couples achieve parenthood. The process of embryonic development is very complex and depends on the genetic and environmental factors at the time of fertilization, which occurs when the egg and sperm meet at the optimal time of a woman's menstrual cycle. Fertilization takes place in the Fallopian tubes, and the fertilised egg contains the full complement of maternal and paternal genes. With the process of cell division, this fertilized egg forms a small cluster of cells, which are undifferentiated. With appropriate environmental interaction and with an inherent genetic constitution, a cell differentiates, and by the end of 12 weeks from the first day of the last menstrual period (LMP), the foetus is formed. After formation, maturation of the various physiological processes takes place and growth is established. The study of human development from fertilization to the various foetal stages is the field of embryology. The field of developmental genetics involves study of the genetic mechanisms behind this development.

MAIN EVENTS IN THE DEVELOPMENT OF A HUMAN FETUS

There are three main stages in prenatal life, pre-embryonic, embryonic and foetal (Fig. 6.1).

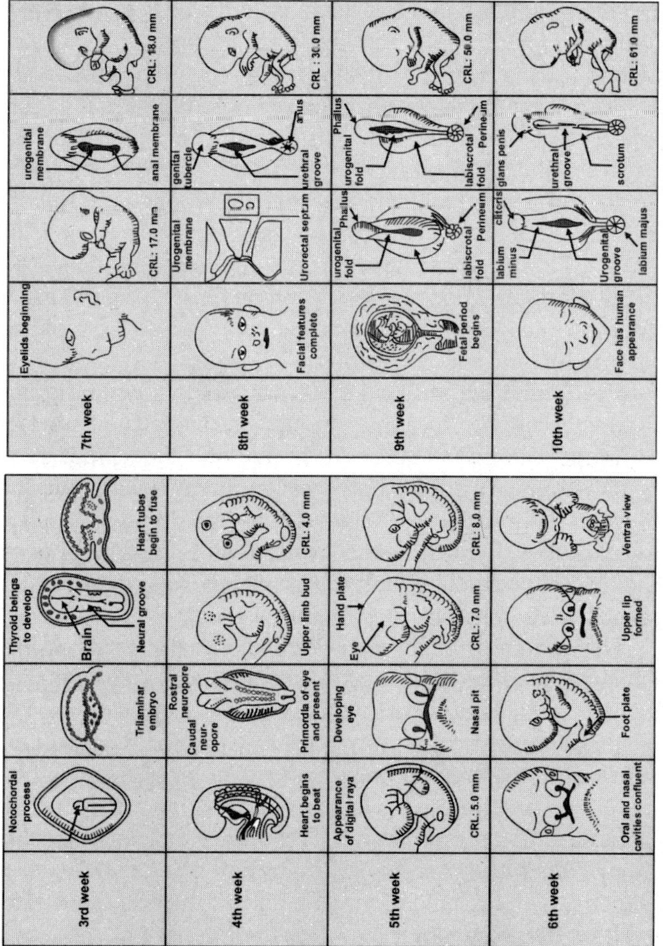

Fig. 6.1: Important landmarks in fetal development

Fertilisation occurs when the male and female gametes fuse in the Fallopian tube. The number of spermatozoa reaching a single egg is over 100 million. They are deposited in the female genital tract and reach the site of fertilization. Of these only a single spermatozoon is successful in penetrating the corona radiata and zona pellucida of the oocyte. The sperm pierces the oocyte, and it is only then that the second meiotic division takes place. This completes the process of meiosis. The newly formed cell now consists of two nuclei, which are called pronuclei. Each pronucleus contains a haploid set of chromosomes (23). The pronuclei then fuse and a diploid set of chromosome (46) is restored.

The fertilized egg also known as a zygote goes through a series of mitotic divisions. The two-cell stage is reached by 30 hours, four-cell stage by 40 hours, and the 12-cell stage by 163 hours. This last stage is called the morula. Up to this stage, an embryo is in the fallopian tube and during this period any pathology in the tube may result in an ectopic pregnancy. The field of preimplantation diagnosis involves a study of the genetic material from these pre-embryos.

This pre-embryonic stage of development is successfully achieved *in vitro*. A process of cell division and cavitation forming a blastocyst further develops in an embryo. The blastocyst consists of an inner cell mass called embryoblast, which forms the embryo proper, and an outer cell mass, which forms the trophoblast. The trophoblast gives rise to the placenta and its membranes. The inner cell mass further divides into bilaminar and trilaminar discs. This occurs between the beginning of the second and the end of the third week of development.

The bilaminar embryo is oriented dorsoventrally with the yolk sac below and amniotic cavity above. Epiblast cells migrate through the primitive streak, and gastrulation begins. The notochord formation demarcates the midline. Embryonic regions differentiate and anterior structures like the forebrain and heart, dorsal structures like the neural crest and neural tube, ventral structures like the foregut, lungs and thyroid and posterior structures like the hindgut and allantois are formed. The body form is completely established by 4 to 8 weeks of gestation. The primitive streak appears at the caudal end of the embryo. The three germinal layers ectoderm, endoderm and mesoderm are now formed. The ectoderm develops into skin, teeth, sweat glands and neural tissue. The mesoderm is divided into three parts, paraxial mesoderm forming the skeleton, muscles and dermis, the intermediate mesoderm forms urogenital tissues and lateral mesoderm forms the heart, limbs, and lateral body wall. The endoderm forms the gastrointestinal system, the pharynx, trachea and lungs at the anterior end and the cloaca and urogenital system at the posterior end. Once the body plan and the germ layers are formed, by 4-8 weeks organ systems are formed by cell growth, differentiation and cell migration. The neural tube is formed next and the neural crest cells migrate to form parts of the nervous system - the sympathetic nervous system, sensory ganglia, and pigment cells. The bone and cartilage part of the branchial arches and face are also formed at the same time. Any error at each stage of this minute developmental process can lead to a developmental defect. For example, disorders of nerve cells of neural crest lead to neurofibromatosis type 1.

MOLECULAR ASPECTS OF HUMAN EMBRYONIC DEVELOPMENT

Three developmental biologists and geneticists, who shared the 1995 Nobel prize for physiology/medicine, Lewis, Volhard, and Wieschaus, described how specialized cells are derived from a fertilized egg in a multicellular organism. Their discovery was the finding of pattern-forming genes that control the overall organization of the body. These genes also control development of body segments and the special features of a fruitfly like its legs and wings.

It is well known that most genes produce proteins called transcription factors. Transcription factors control RNA transcription from the DNA template by virtue of a binding process to specific regulatory DNA sequences. These sequences form complexes, which initiate transcription by RNA polymerase.

Developmental Genes

Genes can get switched on and off by transcription factors which in turn, activate or repress gene expression. It is assumed that transcription factors control many different genes in coordinated sequences, which in turn control basic embryologic processes of apoptosis or programmed cell death. It is also presumed, that these processes are mediated by growth factor cell receptors and chemicals, collectively known as morphogens. We are now aware that morphogenesis is the result of intricately regulated pathways of gene expression. For a normal developmental sequence to take place, appropriate genes should be should be expressed at the correct time and in the correct sequence to produce proteins.

A study of human malformation syndromes has shown that various gene families are responsible for isolated malformations or multiple anomaly syndromes.

Segmentation Genes

Segmentation genes have been studied in insect bodies. Insects have many body segments which are repeated and which differentiate into various structures according to their body position. Three main groups of segmentation determining genes are known and are subdivided according to their mutant phenotypes. They are classified as *gap* mutants

that delete groups of adjacent segments, *pair rule* mutants that delete alternate segments, and *segment polarity* mutants, which cause portions of each segment to be deleted and duplicated on the wrong side.

Segment polarity genes are responsible for two morphogenes, hedgehog and *wingless* and are maintained in evolution. Three mammalian hedgehog homologues are known. They are *sonic hedgehog*, *desert hedgehog*, and *indian hedgehog*. Holoprosencephaly, a developmental defect of the ventral neural tube is a lethal condition. In this condition the forebrain is not divided into cerebral hemispheres. Patients with holoprosencephaly have been shown to have loss of function mutations in the *sonic hedgehog* gene.

Homeobox (HOX) Genes

Mutations in the class of genes known as the homeotic genes are responsible for major structural anomalies determining segment identity in *Drosophila* or fruitfly. Development of a leg instead of antenna can occur with such a mutation. Homeobox genes are responsible for spatial pattern development and control. In humans four homeobox gene clusters have been identified, Table 6.1 each inherited in an autosomal dominant fashion. About 30 *HOX* genes are known. Homeobox specifies a homeodomain of ~60 amino acids (Fig. 6.2).

Table 6.1: Chromosomal location of homeobox gene clusters in humans

Gene cluster	*Chromosomal location*	*Genes involved*
HOX 1(HOXA)	7p	11
HOX 2(HOXB)	17q	9
HOX 3(HOXC)	12q	9
HOX 4(HOXD)	2q	9

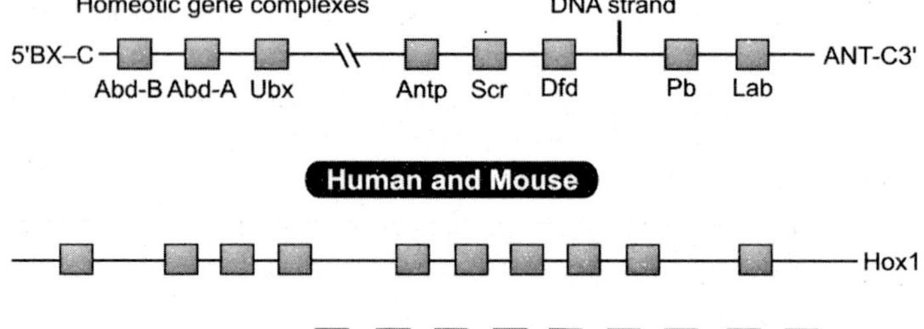

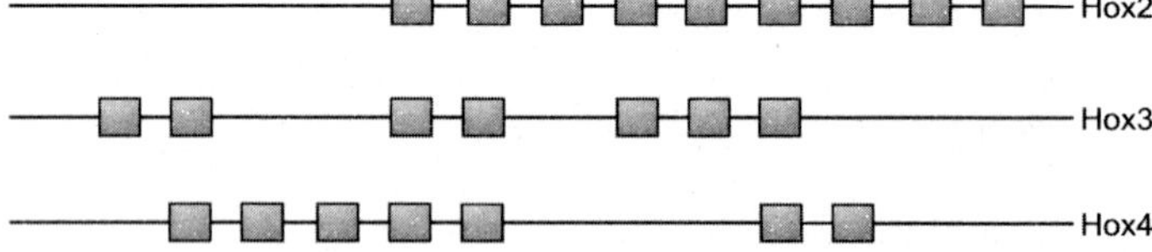

Fig. 6.2: Homeobox genes in Drosophila, mouse and human

Syndactyly and polydactyly occur due to a mutation in the *HOXD13* genes (Fig. 6.3). Synpolydactyly is a rare developmental anomaly in which an additional digit originates between the webbed third and fourth digits. The severity increases in homozygotes, with short metacarpals and metatarsals that appear almost like carpal and tarsal bones.

Paired Box (PAX) Genes

Paired box genes were first identified in *Drosophila*. Paired box encodes a paired domain of ~130 amino acids. *PAX* genes often have in addition a type of homeodomain known as paired-type homeodomain. These genes encode DNA binding proteins, which are transcription control factors and are of great significance in developmental processes. Nine *PAX* genes have been identified so far in mice and humans.

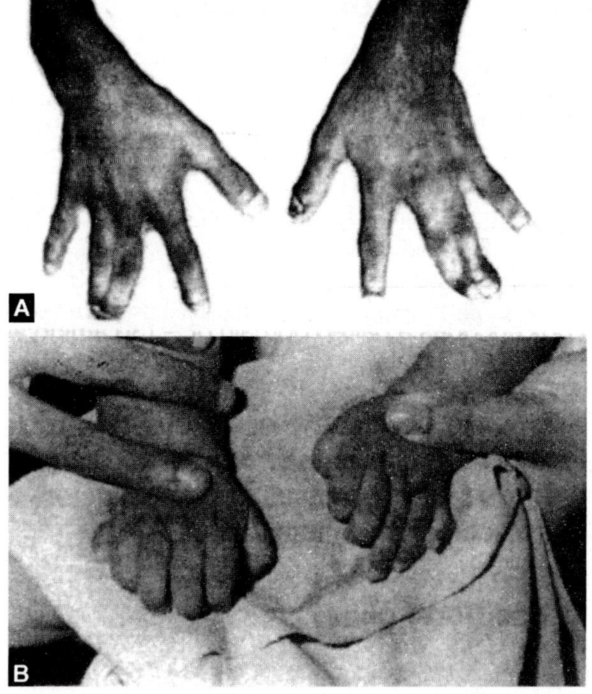

Figs 6.3A and B: (A) Syndactyly (B) Polydactyly

The development of nervous system and vertebral column is dependent on these genes. In humans loss of function mutations of *PAX3* lead to Waardenburg's syndrome type 1 and *PAX6* mutations cause aniridia. Waardenburg syndrome is inherited as an autosomal dominant condition. The clinical features of the syndrome are sensorineural hearing loss, areas of depigmentation and heterochromia of the iris. Aniridia results from gene deletion involving PAX6 locus on chromosome 11p13.

SRY Genes, (HMG BOX) SOX Genes

SRY genes are Y linked genes that play a major role in male sex determination.

The *SOX* genes have an *SRY* like HMG box which encodes a domain of ~ 70 amino acids. The *SOX* genes are transcription regulators. Genes *SOX1*, *SOX2*, and *SOX3* are expressed during embryogenesis at specific times. About 15 *SOX* genes have been identified so far.

In humans, loss of function mutations in *SOX19* located on chromosome 17 cause campomelic dysplasia. Campomelic dysplasia is a rare disorder characterized by bowing of long bones, sex reversal in XY males and a poor life span. *In situ* hybridisation in mouse showed the gene to be expressed in the developing embryo in primordial skeletal tissues and on genital ridges.

T-box (TBS) Genes

These genes play an important role in the development and formation of mesoderm and notochord differentiation in mice. The *TBX* genes encode a transcription factor, which contains activator and depressor genes. Loss of function or mutation leads to mice with short tails and small sacral vertebrae.

The *TBX* genes are dispersed in the human genome. Approximately 15 genes are known, and the sequence domain is the *T-box* which encodes a domain of ~ 170 amino acids. The cluster of genes located on chromosome 12 contains the *TBX3* and *TBX5* genes. Loss of function mutations in *TBX5* cause Holt Oram Syndrome, characterized by congenital heart disease (atrial septal defect) and upper limb reduction, which can present as mild hypoplasia of the thumbs due to absence of forearms.

Zinc Finger Genes

The term zinc finger genes refers to genes with a finger like loop formed by a series of four amino acids forming a complex with zinc. Genes containing zinc finger motifs act as transcription factors.

A zinc finger motif containing gene is *GL13* on chromosome 7, and is the cause of two known developmental disorders. Large deletions or translocations, which involve GL13, lead to Greigcephalopolysyndactyly. The clinical features include a large head, and hand and foot abnormalities like polydactyly and syndactyly. Frameshift mutations in *GL13* lead to Pallister-Hall syndrome. The clinical features of this syndrome are polydactyly, hypothalamic hamartomata and imperforate anus.

Another gene with zinc finger motifs, *WT1* is located on chromosome 11. It is responsible for some cases of Wilm's tumor and Denys-Drash syndrome. In Denys-Drash syndrome the patient has ambiguous genitalia and nephritis leading to renal failure.

SIGNAL TRANSDUCTION GENES

These genes are involved in the processes responsible for extra-cellular growth factors regulating cell growth and differentiation. The pathway is complex and genetically determined, with intermediary steps being involved. Mutations in these genes cause developmental abnormalities and may also be responsible for malignant processes.

The RET Proto-oncogene

This gene is located on chromosome 10q11.2 and encodes a cell surface tyrosine-kinase. Gain of function mutations lead to thyroid cancer, while loss of function mutations has been identified in 50% of familial cases of Hirschsprung's disease.

In this disease ganglionic cells fail to migrate to the submucosal and myenteric plexuses of the large bowel. Symptoms appear after birth, when the child suffers from intestinal obstruction, and abdominal distention. Multiple endocrine neoplasia (MEN2) characterized by familial clustering of phaeochromocytoma, medullary thyroid carcinoma and parathyroid adenoma and is caused by mutations in the *ret* oncogene.

Fibroblast Growth Factor Receptors (FGFRs)

This factor plays a principal role in embryogenesis, cell division, migration and differentiation. Nine fibroblast growth factor genes have so far been identified.

Mutations in these genes are seen in two disorders, craniosynostosis syndromes and achondroplasia. An example of a craniosynostosis syndrome is Apert's syndrome, (Figs 6.4A and B) characterized by premature fusion of cranial sutures and hand or foot abnormalities. Apert's syndrome is caused by mutation in *FGFR2*, in peptides linking the second and third immunoglobulin loops. Mutations in the third

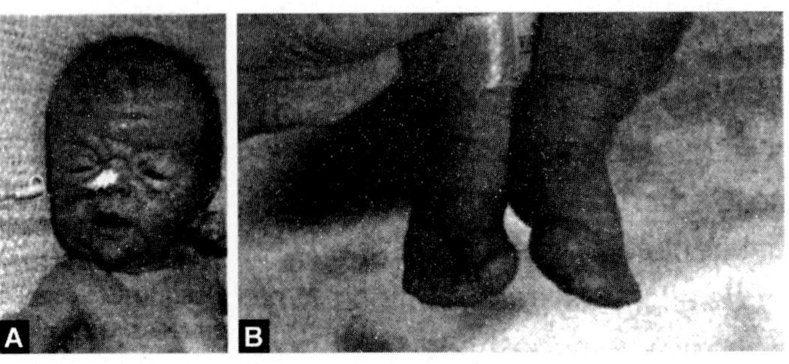

Figs 6.4A and B: (A) Apert's syndrome (B) Abnormalities in the feet in the same patient

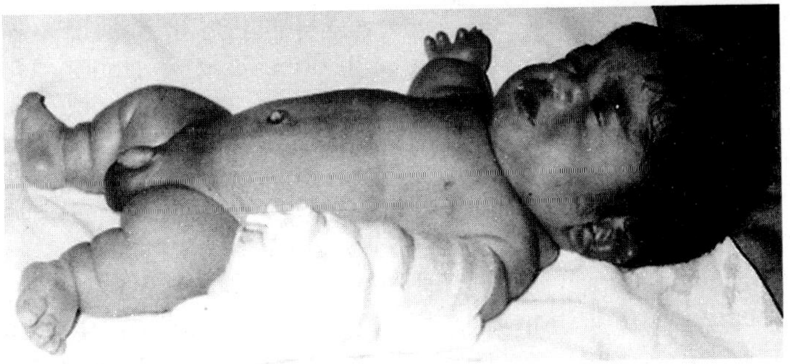

Fig. 6.5: Thanatophoric dysplasia
(For color version see Plate 3)

immunoglobulin loop cause Crouzon's syndrome where the limbs are normal, or Pfeiffer's syndrome where only the thumbs and great toes are abnormal.

A commonly known skeletal dysplasia is achondroplasia, leading to short stature. The limbs have rhizomelic (proximal) shortening, and the head is enlarged with frontal bossing. The patient has normal intelligence and a normal life span. The mutated gene involved is *FGFR3*. Another mutation in the proximal tyrosine kinase residues of the *FGFR3* gene results in skeletal dysplasia of a similar phenotype, except for a normal size and shape of the head. Thanatophoric dysplasia (Fig. 6.5) is a lethal skeletal dysplasia caused by mutations in the second and third immunoglobulin domains of *FGFR3*.

SEXUAL DIFFERENTIATION AND X-INACTIVATION

The sex of an individual is determined by the sex chromosomes X and Y. The Y chromosome is responsible for maleness, irrespective of number of X chromosomes. In the absence of the Y chromosome the foetus by default develops into a female.

However, sex determination and differentiation are two different processes and do not occur until 6 weeks of gestation. Up to this stage the gonads possess both the cortex and the medulla but are undifferentiated. The Wolfian and Mullerian ducts are present at this stage and the actual differentiation starts only when the testes determining gene starts an initiation process, which differentiates the so far undifferentiated gonads into testes. The gene responsible for this was discovered in 1990 and is located on the short arm of the Y chromosome adjacent to the pseudoautosomal region. This gene is now labelled as the *SRY* gene. This *SRY* (sex regulator gene) gene encodes the code for masculinity (Fig. 6.6).

The role of the SRY gene in sex differentiation is appreciated by studying individuals with sex chromosomal abnormalities such as the presence of the *SRY* gene in phenotypic males with a 46 XY karyotype, and the deletion of the *SRY* gene in XY females. During the process of meiosis 1 all the chromosomes pair with homologous chromosomes that have corresponding gene locations. Sex chromosomes are unequal in size, and have small homologous regions, which can pair at meiosis. However, the *SRY* gene is in close proximity to the pseudoautosomal region and hence there is a chance that it can get caught in a process of recombination, which is what happens in XX males. The frequency of sex reversal is 1 in 20,000 births. Molecular studies and FISH analysis show the presence of the Y chromosome sequence on the distal end of the short arm of one of the X chromosomes. This region is 140 kilobase pairs long, which is almost .2 percent of the Y chromosome.

X Chromosome Inactivation

X-linked disorders are expressed in males through carrier females. However, it has been observed that occasionally

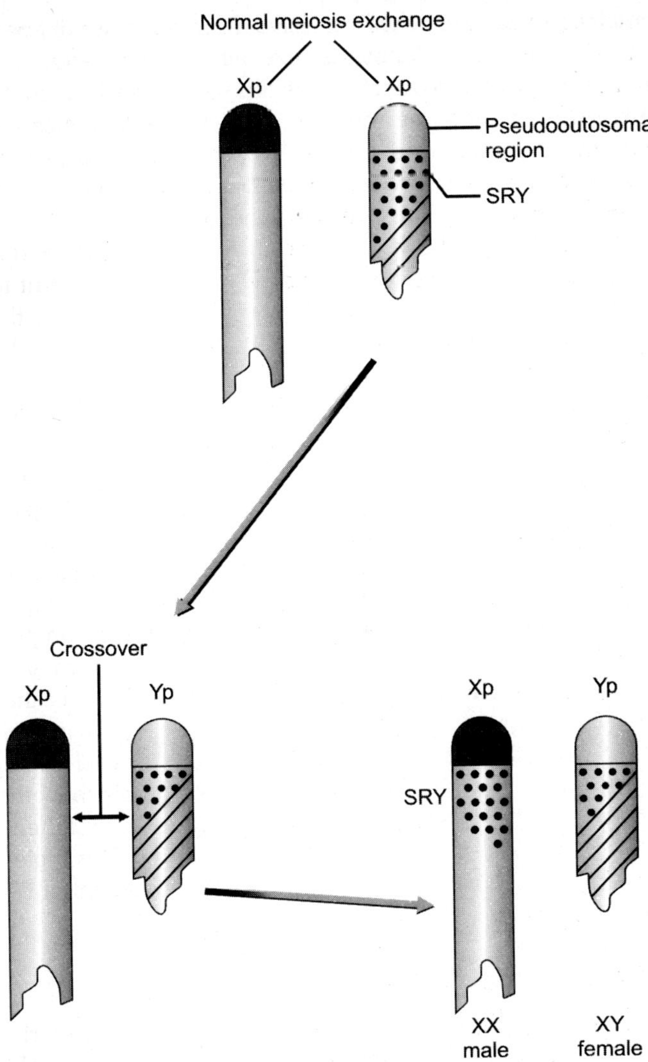

Fig. 6.6: Generation of XX males and XY females due to recombination events involving the SRY gene

females can have X linked recessive disorders in a mild or a full form (for example female carriers with Duchenne muscular dystrophy). This can occur if there is a structural abnormality of the X chromosome involving that region, or there is involvement of a normal gene in the process of inactivation. The latter is called skewed X inactivation. In females with 46Xr(X) karyotype, typical Turner syndrome features appear as the ring lacks the X sequence, which is normally not inactivated, and appears to be responsible for normal phenotype.

CHAPTER 7

PATTERNS OF INHERITANCE

INTRODUCTION

Human beings show a great degree of variation in their genetic patterns, which show classical patterns of inheritance. As these disorders follow the laws of Mendel, they are often referred to as Mendelian inheritance, though some exceptions are noted. Genes are responsible for a particular pattern, and alternative forms of genetic patterns at a specific locus are referred to as alleles. Some genes have only one pattern and this pattern is called the wild type, while some gene loci exhibit different forms called polymorphisms. Genetic patterns and disorders are transmitted from one generation to the other. The study of patterns of inheritance is important for the diagnosis, prognosis, and estimation of the recurrence risk in other family members. In order to study genetic diseases, certain terminologies and methods in history taking are used, which are described below.

The genetic constitution of a person is called a genotype, which may be considered collectively, or may be specific for a single locus. The phenotype is a term is used for expression of a genotype at a morphological, molecular or biochemical level. The term single gene disorder is used, when there is disorder arising from a mutation at a single locus on one or both members of a chromosome pair. A person having a pair of identical alleles is called a homozygote, and if the alleles are different, the person is called a heterozygote. Another term, compound heterozygote is used when two different mutant alleles are present at the same locus.

A family history is recorded by drawing a family tree. This is called pedigree charting. Various symbols are used in this process, and are described in Figure 7.1. The importance of taking a family history needs to be stressed in genetics, as this by itself can be useful as a screening test, or help in providing a diagnosis on the basis of pattern of inheritance or familial occurrence. An example is a disorder called osteogenesis imperfecta. In this condition, the child has a tendency to get fractures even with a history of minor injury, and the first fracture may be passed off as an accidental fracture. A detailed family history of a similar episode in another child with blue sclerae, would direct a geneticist towards the possibility of a genetic disorder. If such history is absent, it could be due to a new mutation. Confirmation of the diagnosis is not only important for the index case for management, but also for estimating a recurrence risk, and for planning future prenatal diagnostic tests.

PEDIGREE CHARTING AND SYMBOLS

Family history taking in genetics starts from an index case. The index case is the person through whom the family came to be investigated. This index case is called a proband, or propositus. A female propositus is called the propositi. The proband is indicated by an arrow in the pedigree chart. This means the whole family is studied through this case. The details of other family members, brothers, sisters, parents and relatives on both sides are noted.

MENDELIAN INHERITANCE

There are over 8,000 genetic traits, which are known to follow the Mendelian pattern of inheritance, though some common

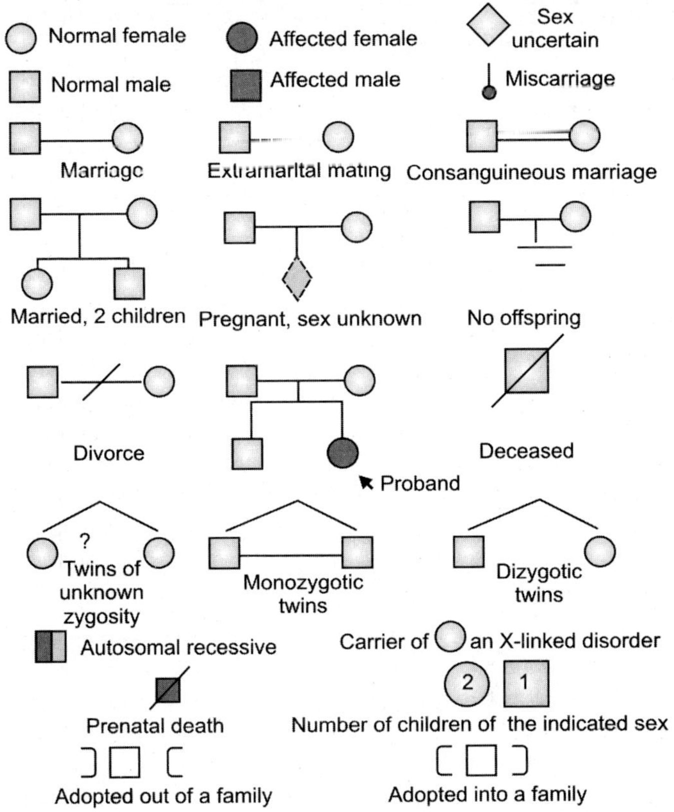

Normal female
Affected female
Sex uncertain
Normal male
Affected male
Miscarriage
Marriage
Extramarital mating
Consanguineous marriage
Married, 2 children
Pregnant, sex unknown
No offspring
Divorce
Proband
Deceased
?
Twins of unknown zygosity
Monozygotic twins
Dizygotic twins
Autosomal recessive
Carrier of an X-linked disorder
Prenatal death
2
1
Number of children of the indicated sex
Adopted out of a family
Adopted into a family

A

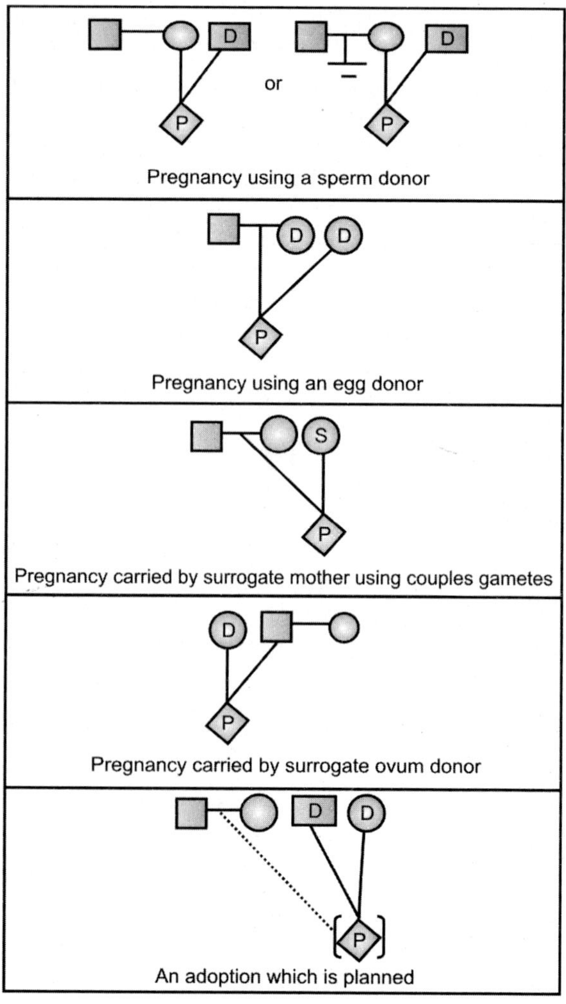

Figs 7.1A and B: (A) Pedigree drawing and terminology used in history taking. (B) Pedigree symbolisation of assisted reproductive technology

familial traits or disorders do not follow this pattern. If a gene responsible for a disorder or a trait is located on an autosome, it is said to follow autosomal inheritance and if located on a sex chromosomes is said to follow a sex-linked inheritance.

These single gene inheritance patterns are further classified into autosomal dominant, autosomal recessive and X-linked (recessive and dominant). All such traits or disorders are enlisted in a catalogue entitled Mendelian inheritance in Man. This catalogue is now available on line.

Autosomal Dominant Inheritance

If a trait manifests itself in a heterozygous state, and only one copy of the mutant gene is needed for manifestation of disease. This means the affected person carries a single copy of the affected gene, and the other copy is normal. The disorder is transmitted vertically, and seen in every generation. In some cases, a dominant trait or a disorder may not have a family history, it is called a new mutation. The propositus may be the first person to manifest the trait. Some of the dominant conditions occur at a relatively high frequency, presumably because they have little effect on reproductive fitness and are passed on to next generation. There are however a few rare disorders, which can be incapacitating thus are not passed on by an affected individual (Table 7.1). The gametes from

Table 7.1: Characteristic criteria of autosomal dominant inheritance

- Shows vertical pattern of transmission in a pedigree, appears in every generation.
- Inheritance is from 1% (heterozygote) only.
- Risk of transmission is 50%.
- There is no sex preference, male and female offsprings are equally affected.

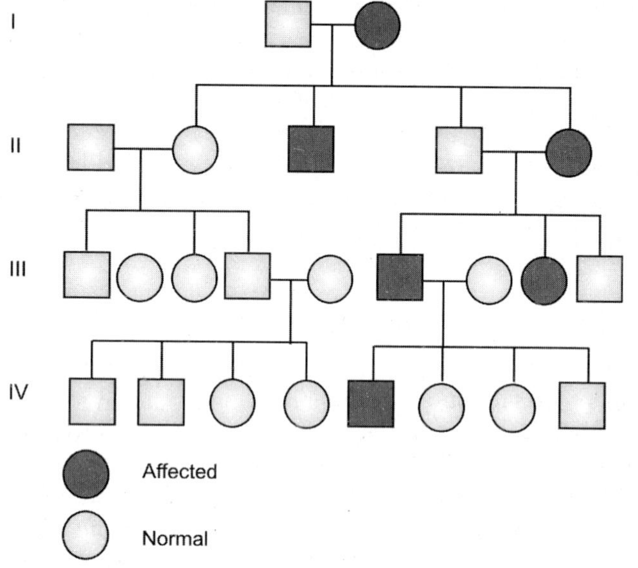

Fig. 7.2: Autosomal dominant inheritance

an individual with a dominant trait will contain one abnormal and one normal gene and therefore his chances of transmitting the affected gene to his progeny are 50%. It can affect both the male or female offspring equally, there is no sex preference (Fig. 7.2).

Pleiotropy

Autosomal dominant traits can involve one organ, or different systems and different organs. This is called pleiotropy.

Reduced Penetrance

The mutant phenotype may or may not be expressed fully and identically in all disorders. When classical features of a syndrome are minimal, this may be due to reduced penetrance. If classical features are totally absent, it is called non-penetrance, a condition where the abnormal gene may be present but not expressed. The calculation of penetrance is done by studying the number of individuals expressing the disease divided by the total number of individuals inheriting the alleles. A common example of an autosomal dominant condition is Polydactyly. This is expressed in 65% of those inheriting the allele. Some autosomal dominant traits like Huntington's disease need other influencing conditions factors like age. Huntington's disease is a severe degenerative neurological disease caused by a triplet repeat expansion of the CAG trinucleotide repeat in the coding region of the Huntington's gene on chromosome 4. The neurological condition is expressed in middle to late adult life, even though the individual is born with the mutation.

Variation in Severity, Dependent on Sex

The severity of a dominant condition may depend on the sex of an affected parent. For example, in individuals with myotonic dystrophy of early onset, it is usually inherited from an affected mother, while in Huntington's disease those with early severe disease are likely to have an affected father.

Variable Expressivity

In many dominant disorders, there can be a wide variation between the clinical features of persons suffering from same trait or a disease. This is called variable expressivity.

New Mutations

Many autosomal dominant disorders can appear in an individual where parent is not affected. This is due to a new mutation arising in the offspring.

Co-dominance

This terminology is used for traits, which are expressed in the heterozygous state. For example, in a person with AB blood group it is possible to demonstrate that their red blood cells have both A and B blood group antigens. This is an example of co-dominance.

AUTOSOMAL RECESSIVE CONDITIONS

Every gene from one parent is matched with a gene with the same function on the matching chromosome of the other parent. The actual function controlled or directed by matching genes is a reflection of their combined action. If one of the matching genes inherited from one parent is defective, then the other normal gene provides half the needed function, usually enough to keep the functioning normally (called the carrier or heterozygous state). So a recessive gene may have no effect, if it is paired with a normal gene from the other parent, though the genetic function expected of this pair of genes (one defective, one normal) will probably be half of what is normally found. Autosomal recessive disorders are transmitted horizontally which means that in a particular family there may not be any affected member in the previous generation but the siblings of the proband may be affected (Fig. 7.3). Like autosomal dominant disorders both the sexes are affected equally. Thalassaemia is an autosomal recessive inherited genetic disorder, common in the Mediterranean region as well as in India (Table 7.2). A simple screening test for carrier detection, and prenatal screening can help reduce the incidence of such births. The risk of recurrence in recessive disorders is 1 in 25 for each pregnancy.

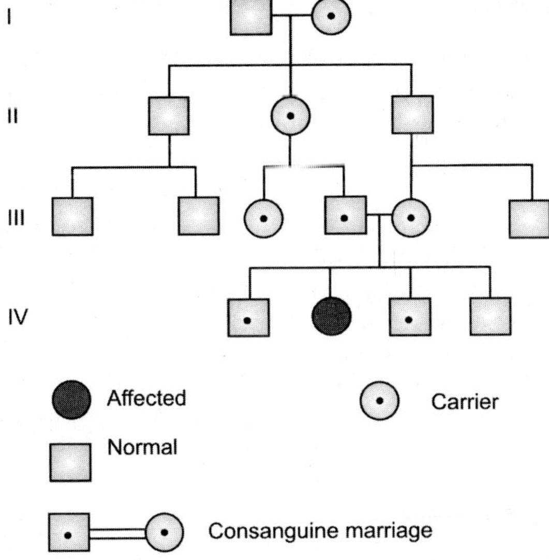

Fig. 7.3: Pedigree showing autosomal recessive inheritance

Table 7.2: Characteristic criteria of autosomal recessive inheritance

- The disorder has horizontal pattern of transmission.Siblings are affected.
- Both the parents are obligatory carriers but are unaffected.
- The offspring of the carrier parents has 1 in 4 chance of getting affected.
- Half of the sibling of carriers will be carriers and remaining will not carry the trait.
- Consanguinity, inbreeding and ethnicity increases the frequency of trait

Consanguinity

Many autosomal recessive traits occur due to consanguinity. Any individual though apparently normal, has 4-8 abnormal genes in his or her body. In random marriages it is a matter of chance that two individuals carrying the same abnormal gene will marry, thus reducing any chances of a recessively inherited genetic disorder in their progeny. Families with consanguine marriages are more likely to share the same abnormal gene resulting in an increase in the incidence of recessive genetic disorders. In the case of consanguine marriages, the more rare the recessive trait or disorder, the greater the chance of transmitting it to the progeny. In oculo-cutaneous albinism, 1 in 20 parents of the affected children are first cousins.

Pseudo-dominance

If an individual affected with an autosomal recessive disorder marries another carrier individual of the same disorder their progeny will have 50% risk of being affected. Such a pedigree is said to exhibit pseudo-dominance.

Genetic Heterogeneity

Many genetic disorders are inherited in a variety of ways due to genetic heterogeneity. Genetic heterogeneity may result from the existence of a series of different mutations at a single locus (allelic heterogeneity) or from mutations at different genetic loci (non allelic or locus heterogeneity). For example, phenotypes such as Charcot-Marie tooth disease, retinitis pigmentosa, and congenital sensory neural deafness all have autosomal dominant, autososmal recessive and X-linked forms. For example, in sensory neural hearing impairment, a couple with deaf mutism can have normal children, as their deaf mutism could be due to genetic heterogeneity. The normal offspring may be double heterozygotes for mutations in two different genes. If two homozygotes with deaf mutism marry all their children would be affected, as the offspring would have two copies of the affected genes. A number of genes can cause autosomal recessive sensory neural deafness, and to date several loci have been shown to be involved. A genetic disorder with a phenotype due to different genetic loci is known as a genocopy. If the same phenotype is due to an environmental cause, it is known as a phenocopy.

Compound Heterozygotes

Heterogeneity can occur at an allelic level. For example, in beta thalassaemia a large number of mutations have been identified. Individuals having 2 different mutations at the same locus are known as compound heterozygotes. The heterozygosity can be common to a particular community.

Sex-linked Inheritance

Sex-linked inheritance is a type of inheritance occurring as a result of mutant genes located on the X or Y chromosomes. The disorders, which occur due to mutant genes located on one of the X chromosomes, are referred to as sex-linked disorders. The Y chromosome does not have any such genes, but has certain traits that are passed from father to son. This is called holandric inheritance.

X-linked Recessive Inheritance

A female can pass either her normal X or the X carrying the abnormal gene to her sons. Thus half the sons will be normal and the other half affected. The female offspring of such carrier females will have one normal X from the father to balance the defective gene. They will therefore be carriers like their mothers. There is also a 50% chance of daughters getting a normal gene and being totally normal (Table 7.3). An example of an X linked recessive disorder is Haemophilia A. The carrier mother has an abnormal gene on one of her X chromosomes. This gene on her X chromosome is expressed only in males. The female child who receives the mutant gene from the mother also receives a matching normal gene from the father and will be a carrier. The inheritance pattern in X linked disorders in males can be summarized as disorders being transmitted from the affected person to his carrier daughters and then to his grandsons (Fig. 7.4).

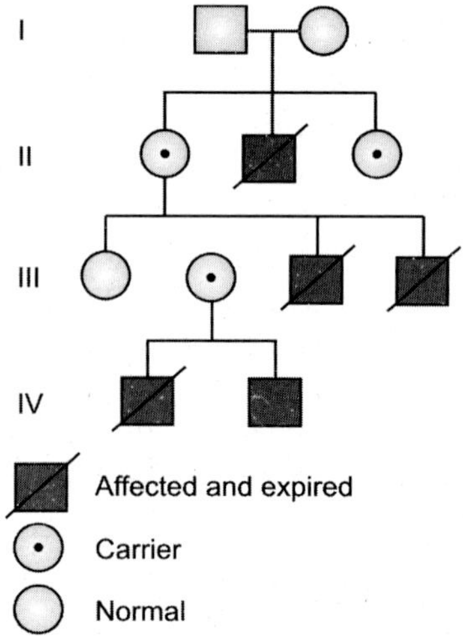

Fig. 7.4: Pedigree showing X-linked recessive inheritance

Table 7.3: Characteristic criteria of sex linked inheritance

- Females have two X chromosomes so they can be homozygous or heterozygous for the genes located on them.Males have one X chromosome thus will be hemizygous for X linked genes.
- One X chromosome of the females is inactivated in female embryos (Lyon Hypothesis) thus a heterozygous female is an actual mosaic for abnormal allele.
- Male to male transmission is not possible as father transmits only Y chromosome to his son.
- Unaffected males will not transmit the diseased gene.
- All the daughters of the affected male will carry the gene and will be affected if the gene is dominant.
- A carrier mother will transmit the mutated gene to 50% of the offspring of either sex.
- For Y linked inheritance only male to male transmission is possible.

Some X linked genetic recessive disorders such as Duchenne muscular dystrophy (DMD) are not transmitted through affected males, as the affected male does not survive up to reproductive age. 2/3 of DMD cases are new mutations. In most cases, symptoms in the affected males start in early childhood by the age of three and as the muscular weakness progresses the child is confined to the wheel chair. Death is commonly due to affection of the respiratory muscles.

Variable Expression in Heterozygous Females

There are several X-linked recessive disorders in which heterozygous females show a mosaic phenotype (mixed features of normal and mutant alleles) e.g. X-linked ocular albinism. In this condition affected males totally lack pigment in their iris and ocular fundi. Mothers of such children show a mosaic pattern of pigmentation. Such a pattern is explained by the process of X-inactivation in females and is based on the Lyon Hypothesis. In the pigmented areas the normal gene is on the active X chromosome and in the depigmented area mutant allele is on the inactive X chromosome.

Homozygosity for X-linked Recessive Disorders

Red green colour blindness is a condition, which affects about 8% of males while in females its incidence in 1 in 150. This shows that females do get affected with X-linked recessive trait. Homozygosity in a female is due to an affected father and carrier mother or a new mutation occurring in the father's X chromosome and carrier mother.

Symptomatic Carrier Female (Skewed X-inactivation)

This can occur due to the possibility of inactivation of the normal X chromosome in most cells of a female and expression of X chromosome with a mutant allele. A carrier female can then show symptoms of the disease. This has been reported in female carriers of haemophilia and Duchenne muscular dystrophy (DMD).

X-chromosomal Abnormalities and X-linked Inheritance

A female can manifest an X-linked disorder in a carrier state if she has only one X chromosome, as in Turner syndrome. Haemophilia and DMD in Turner females has been reported in the literature.

X-autosome Translocation

If a break point in an X-autosome translocation occurs at a position where the gene in question is located on the X-chromosome, females can be affected with an X-linked recessive disorder. This happens because the X-chromosome involved in the translocated chromosome maintains the functional disomy of the autosomal genes. Mapping of the gene for Duchenne Muscular Dystrophy was aided by this observation in females with X-autosome translocations (Fig. 7.5).

X-linked Dominant Inheritance Disorders

This is an uncommon pattern. However there are X-linked dominant traits, which manifest in the heterozygous female as well as in the male having a mutant allele on his X chromosome. This condition appears as an autosomal dominant trait since both male and female offspring are affected. An important point to note here is in all X-linked dominant conditions the affected male will transmit the disorder to female offspring only and never to a male (Fig. 7.5). Some X-linked disorders are lethal in utero in males and severely or completely impair reproduction in females. An example of an X-linked dominant disorder is incontinentia pigmenti.

Y-linked Inheritance

Y linked or holandric inheritance suggests that, only males are affected. The Y chromosome is exclusively transmitted from

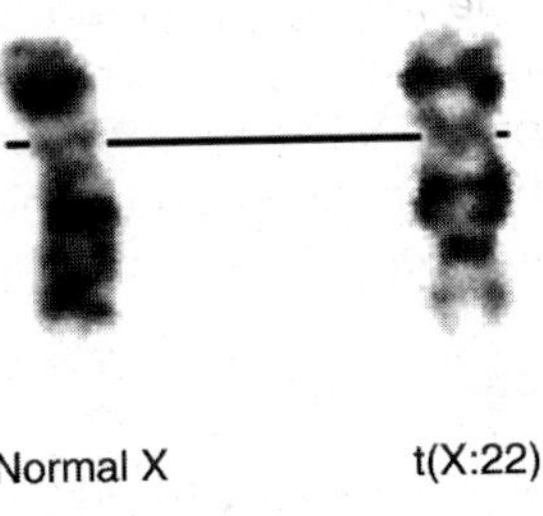

Fig. 7.5: X-autosomal translocation

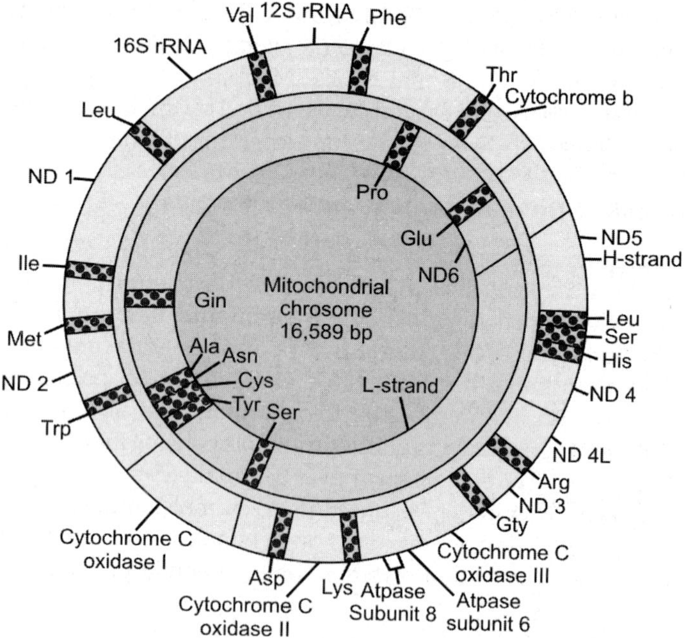

Fig. 7.6: The human mitochodrial genome with various gene positions

father to son, and the daughters are not affected (Fig. 7.6). The commonest known traits are hairy pinna and baldness. Ongoing research on the Y chromosome clearly indicates that H-Y histocompatibility antigen and genes responsible for spermatogenesis are located on the Y chromosome.

Partial Sex Linkage

This refers to the linkage of genes located on the homologous portion of the X chromosome with that of Y chromosome. At meiosis these homologous regions on the X and Y pair at the pseudo-autosomal region. Due to this, during crossing over, genes located on X chromosome can transfer to the Y chromosome.

Some confusing patterns of 'X' or 'Y' linked inheritance have utilised this possible explanation for diseases like colour blindness and rare skin disorders, though more work and family studies are necessary in these areas.

Influence of Sex on Inheritance Patterns

Sex-influenced patterns of autosomal dominant inheritance are observed in conditions like gout and pre-senile baldness, males being affected the most. This may occur through the effect of male hormones. In females, gout is rarely seen before menopause.

MITOCHONDRIAL INHERITANCE

Mitochondria are small organelles located in the cytoplasm of all eukaryotic cells, and are mainly responsible for the generation of ATP in the body, which is the main source of energy for all metabolic activities. As per the metabolic and energetic requirements of the organ, the number of mitochondria in the respective cells varies. This means organs showing high metabolic activity such as brain, liver, germ cells, skeletal muscles, have the largest number of mitochondria. These organs are mainly affected by dysfunctioning of mitochondria. Mitochondria possess their own genome, mitochondrial DNA (mtDNA) that is responsible for ATP synthesis and different RNA forms such as mitochondrial ribosomal RNA (rRNA) and transfer RNA (tRNA). The size of the mitochondrial genome is 16-17 kb and it is circular and double stranded.

Mitochondria contain several (2 to 10) copies of circular chromosomes (mtDNA) that contain genes. The cytoplasmic localization and high copy numbers of mtDNA result in a characteristic non-Mendelian inheritance pattern termed "maternal" or mitochondrial inheritance. Because the sperm contains hardly any cytoplasm the mitochondria in a zygote originate almost exclusively from the cytoplasm of the ovum. Therefore mitochondrial inheritance of a trait is exclusively maternal, inherited by all offspring, with males and females being equally affected. However mutations are only present in a proportion of cellular mitochondrial chromosomes (heteroplasmy) and cellular function is affected only if a significant proportion is mutated (threshold expression).

Dysfunction of mitochondria leads to degenerative diseases. Clinical manifestations due to mitochondriopathies depend not only on mutation of genes, but also upon energy requirement of organs. Mitochondrial diseases are mainly classified into two categories: 1) deficiencies that arise due to disturbance in respiratory chain function leading to mitochondrial myopathies, 2) deficiencies of enzymes for metabolic functions and substrate transport across the mitochondrial membrane. Several diseases have been identified that result due to mitochondrial mutations. Diseases such as myoclonic epilepsy and ragged red fibres (MERRF), mitochondrial encephalomyelopathy with lactic acidosis and stroke like episodes (MELAS), amino-glycoside-induced deafness (AID) are due to mitochondrial tRNA mutations. Leber's hereditary optic neuropathy (LHON), neurogenic muscle weakness, ataxia and retinitis pigmentosa (NARP) are as a result of mutations in the coding sequence. Point mutations in the *ATPase 6 gene* leads to Leigh syndrome, which is maternally inherited. Pearson disease, Wolfram syndrome, Kearns-Sayre syndrome and ocular myopathies are due to deletions.

CHAPTER 8

POPULATION GENETICS

INTRODUCTION

Population genetics is that branch of medical genetics, which deals with distribution of inheritance of genes and inherited traits in the population. It also studies the factors that maintain or change the frequency of genes. These factors are mutational events, natural selection and genetic drift. The studies are based on mathematical calculations, environmental factors, and population migration. Population genetic studies are important for the calculation of autosomal recessive gene carrier frequencies, for an understanding of linkage disequilibrium, and for its implications for human evolution.

THE HARDY-WEINBERG PRINCIPLE

In the absence of forces that change gene ratios in populations, when random mating is permitted, the frequencies of each allele (as found in the second generation) will tend to remain constant throughout the generations. This led to the concept of Hardy-Weinberg equilibrium, which shows that the frequency of alleles for any character will remain unchanged in a population through any number of generations, unless this frequency is altered by some outside influence, such as non random mating, selection, small populations, migration leading to gene flow or mutations.

Ova	Sperms	
	H(p)	H(q)
H(p)	HH(p^2)	Hh(pq)
H(q)	Hh(pq)	HH(p^2)

Fig. 8.1: Punnett's square showing genotype frequencies for the alleles H and h in the first generation

Punnett Squares and Probability

A Punnett square is a grid named after its inventor RC Punnett in 1905. This can be used to predict the results of genetic crosses. The alleles that could be present in the female gamete are placed on the left of the grid and the alleles that could be present in the male appear on top of the grid (these could be reversed). The alleles from both are combined in the relevant squares of the grid. This shows all the different possibilities for pairing, hence the different possible genotypes of the offspring. It also gives the probability for each pairing. In the Figure 8.1, we have a gene locus with two alleles H and h, which have the frequency of p and q. p + q = 100% or 1.

The Hardy-Weinberg Law and its Extensions

Given the existence of a population, there are implications of Mendelian genetics for the distributions of genotypes in the population. The Hardy-Weinberg law shows that in a population in which individuals mate at random with respect to their genotype, and in the absence of selection, the frequencies of genotypes MM, MN and NN in the population are p2, 2pq and q2 respectively, where p and q are the frequencies of the genes M and N respectively. Counting the genes in the population gives the following result:

p = (frequency of MM) + ½ (frequency of MN)

q = 1–p = (frequency of NN) + ½ (frequency of MN)

This distribution is achieved in one generation and remains the same for all future generations. The result of the Hardy Weinberg law is that random mating is equivalent to the random union of gametes, namely those of the M and N genes.

The Hardy Weinberg law has another very important implication, namely, genetic variability once it is established in a population tends to remain, and is not dissipated. This is effectively a result of Mendelian segregation. Maintenance of variability in a population is an essential requirement for Darwin's theory of evolution by natural selection. Evolution is simply defined as a change in genetic frequencies as a result of selection and genetic variation.

DISTURBANCE OF GENE FREQUENCIES IN A POPULATION

These can occur in the following ways:

1. Non-random mating
2. Selection
3. Small population
4. Migration leading to gene flow

Non-random Mating

Random mating is the selection of a mate irrespective of the spousal genotype. In practice, mating is probably never entirely random, as inherited factors such as height, weight, race and intelligence tend to play a role. This is called **assortive mating**. Consanguinity or mating between genetic relatives is also an example of non-random mating. The offspring of consanguineous mating are at an increased risk of homozygosity for recessive alleles carried by common ancestors.

Selection

Selection can alter gene frequencies and can reduce (negative selection) or increase (positive selection) a particular genotype. Selection acts by modifying an individual's biological fitness, f. Selection may act on the recessive heterozygote, and this is seen in sickle cell disease. The area where sickle cell disease is most prevalent corresponds geographically with the distribution of plasmodium falciparum malaria. In the sickle cell disease heterozygote, red cells parasitized by plasmodium falciparum undergo sickling and are destroyed. The sickle cell heterozygote thus overcomes malarial infection and is at a reproductive advantage. Heterozygotes for β thalassaemia and G6PD deficiency also have a selective advantage over homozygous normals by virtue of malarial resistance.

Small Communities

With only a small number of individuals in a breeding population, the actual frequencies of alleles varies widely from one generation to the next. This is known as **random genetic drift**. By chance an allele may fail to be passed on to the next generation and may disappear. This is known as **extinction**.

Gene Flow (Migration)

Due to migration or intermarriage, a new allele can get introduced into a population and there will be a change in the relevant allele frequencies. This type of slow diffusion is known as gene flow. The blood group B is given as an example, and it is seen throughout the world. It is thought to have its origin in Asia, and has spread slowly towards the west through invasion.

APPLICATIONS OF THE HARDY-WEINBERG EQUILIBRIUM

Application of Hardy-Weinberg principle is important in genetic counseling where estimation of recurrence is to be calculated in various patterns of inheritance. An example of estimation of carrier frequencies is discussed below:

For an autosomal recessive trait, if p is the frequency of the normal allele and q is the frequency of the mutant allele, then the frequency of the recessive homozygote is equal to the square of the mutant allele frequency (q2). An example that can be used is that of cystic fibrosis.

Recessive homozygote frequency $q^2 = 1/1600$

$q = \sqrt{1/1600} = 1/40$

$p = 1 - q = 39/40$

The heterozygote frequency (carrier frequency) is $2pq = \sim 1$ in 20

THE BALANCE BETWEEN MUTATIONS AND SELECTION

The ultimate source of all genetic variation is mutation, namely an alteration in the DNA sequence. The vast majority of deleterious mutations in expressed genes are likely to disrupt the function of a gene, and therefore lead to a selective disadvantage. The disadvantage will lead to the disappearance of the mutant gene from the population. However, new mutations arise continuously each generation. Therefore a balance is achieved between mutations giving rise to new deleterious variants of a gene, and selection removing them from the population.

ESTIMATION OF MUTATION RATES

The mutation rate (m) is the frequency of a change in the genetic material. It is expressed as the number of mutations at a locus per million gametes produced.

For rare autosomal dominant traits, the mutation rate may be calculated as:

$m = n/2N$, where n = number of affected children with normal parents, and N = total number of births.

If an autosomal dominant condition does not prevent reproduction, then some new cases will inherit the trait from an affected parent. Here the birth frequency is given by:

$2m/(1–f)$, where f is the biological fitness.

If affected individuals cannot reproduce, $f = 0$, and the birth frequency is twice the mutation rate.

For an autosomal recessive trait, the birth frequency is $m/(1–f)$. If the affected homozygote never reproduces ($f = 0$), the birth frequency equals the mutation rate.

For an X-linked recessive trait, the birth frequency in the population is $3m/(1–f)$. Thus for individuals with a biological fitness of zero, the birth frequency equals 3 times the mutation rate.

GENETIC POLYMORPHISMS

The extent of genetic variability in human populations is very high and it is reflected in the unique characteristics of all individuals. This variability includes differential disease susceptibility for both common and rare diseases. It was recognized by Fisher and Haldane in the 1930s that linkage analysis using common polymorphisms is a very powerful tool for the analysis of genetic diseases.

A genetic polymorphism in a population is when two or more discontinuous traits appear at a frequency where the rarest cannot be explained by the mutations. A locus is considered as polymorphic when at least two alleles at the same locus with a frequency greater than 1%. If the frequency is less than 1% it is considered as rare variant. In the normal population about 30 gene loci are considered to be polymorphic. Each individual is 10 to 20% heterozygous for structural gene loci.

Polymorphisms at the DNA level can be used to trace diseases within families. This establishes the position of a mutated gene along a chromosome and is the basis for positional cloning. Polymorphisms that can be detected using PCR include polymorphisms at positions of CA repeats. More variation is identified at the level of single nucleotides called SNP or single nucleotide polymorphisms. The study of polymorphisms provides a basis for understanding genetic variability in the human population as it relates to disease.

CHAPTER 9

POLYGENIC AND MULTIFACTORIAL INHERITANCE

INTRODUCTION

There are many disorders, which have familial clustering, but do not follow a Mendelian pattern of inheritance. Many common congenital malformations and some diseases of adulthood fall into this group. Family studies show more than one family member or near relative affected with a disorder but their percentage is much lower than single gene disorders. The underlying cause is not known but it is believed that many genes are responsible, which can get triggered by environmental factors. These gene loci each act in an additive fashion, and no one gene is responsible.

An inheritance is called **polygenic,** when many genes present at different loci, with each gene having some additive effect, control a trait. In a **multifactorial disorder**, both genetic and environmental factors contribute, where genetic contribution is from both the parents. Thus genes and environmental factors as multifactorial traits can vary in different individuals.

QUANTITATIVE AND QUALITATIVE TRAITS

Quantitative traits are measurable, and some examples are serum cholesterol, height and weight. This means there exists an unlimited value between the upper and lower limits of a value, which has definite range. In qualitative traits, the phenotypes are either present or absent. An example of this is achondroplasia. The inheritance pattern in quantitative phenotypes (normal variation) is inherited as a multifactorial trait.

Normal Variation

The majority of phenotypic differences among normal persons are due to multifactorial traits, for example height, intelligence, and skin colour. In normal quantitative traits a child's phenotype is normally the average of his parents' value, which is often referred to as a midpoint value.

Linkage Studies

Linkage studies are of great value in identifying contributory genes by molecular methods. They are useful in identifying underlying causes in multifactorial diseases.

Characteristics of Multifactorial Disorders

a. Diseases appear familial, but there is no monogenic pattern.
b. Frequency is higher in one sex than in the other. Examples include pyloric stenosis, which is more common in males, while systemic lupus erythematosis (SLE) is more common in females.
c. Recurrence risk is same for all the relatives. It is dropped when relationship is more remote.
d. Recurrence risk in multifactorial inheritance is lower in a population where incidence is lower.

The normal incidence of multifactorial disorders is 1 in 1000. The recurrence risk in siblings or children of affected is 2-4%. Multifactorial diseases of adult origin have a 1% population risk. The risk to siblings and children is 5 - 10%. Multifactorial diseases are more common in the progeny of consanguineous marriages as their genetic pool contains similar abnormal genes.

FACTORS INFLUENCING RECURRENCE RISK

Familial Clustering

The recurrence risk is increased if more than one near relative is affected, as well as if more than one child is affected. This is different from monogenic inheritance, where recurrence risk is totally dependant on parental genotypes, and is independent of previously affected children.

Recurrence risk is higher if a proband is more severely affected. The recurrence risk is also higher in relatives of an affected person, if the sex involved is less frequently associated with the disease. For example, if an affected child with pyloric stenosis is male, the recurrence risk to his brother is 3-8% and 9.2% if the affected child is female. These examples are different from monogenic and chromosomal disorders, where severity of the disorder in the proband does not affect the recurrence risk.

The Diagnosis is Always Made by Exclusion

Isolated cleft lip and cleft palate individually or in combination exhibits multifactorial inheritance, may be part of a chromosomal syndrome, or may occur due to teratogenic factors. Spina bifida is another condition, which is mostly inherited as a multifactorial disorder but could be associated with a chromosomal disorder.

As multifactorial diseases are caused by a combination of genes and environment, environmental factors have a great effect when genetic predisposition factors prevail. Prevention of this is possible. An example of this is use of periconceptional folic acid in the prevention of neural tube defects.

Studies in twins are often used to distinguish between multifactorial traits, Mendelian traits or nongenetic factors.

SOME COMMON MULTIFACTORIAL DISORDERS

These could be categorized into two groups on the basis of the age of onset, in adulthood or those that present at birth (Table 9.1). The group of disorders characteristically present at birth or early childhood are: anencephaly and neural tube defects, pyloric stenosis, cleft lip and cleft palate and congenital heart defects. These have been discussed below.

The second group of disorders includes the common chronic conditions that are responsible for morbidity and mortality in adult life. Hypertension, cancer, schizophrenia, coronary artery disease, obesity, and diabetes mellitus. These are discussed on the chapter on genetics of common diseases.

Table 9.1: Common multifactorial disorders

Diseases present at birth
- Neural tube defects
- Pyloric stenosis
- Congenital heart defects
- Cleft lip and Cleft palate

Adult onset diseases
- Diabetes mellitus
- Hypertension
- Coronary artery disease
- Epilepsy
- Alzheimer disease
- Obesity
- Asthma

DISEASES PRESENTING AT BIRTH

Neural Tube Defects

This is the most common congenital malformation seen in clinical practice, comprising mainly of anencephaly and spina bifida and is a leading cause of mortality and morbidity in children, and leads to stillbirth, early infantile death and handicap in surviving children. When it is not part of a syndrome, there is an increased recurrence risk in subsequent pregnancies. Incidence of neural tube defects has a higher distribution pattern in certain geographical areas. For example Sikhs in Britain, Columbia and Canada have twice the overall population rate.

Anencephaly is characterized by the absence of the vault of the skull, the meninges, the forebrain and the overlying skin (Fig. 9.1A).

In Spina bifida there is failure of fusion of the arches of the vertebrae typically in the lumbar region, with severity varying from spina bifida occulta where the defect is only in the bony arch, to spina bifida presenting with meningocele and meningomyelocele (Fig. 9.1B). Other defects like clubfoot may be associated with NTD.

Pyloric Stenosis

This condition results due to hyperplasia and hypertrophy of the smooth muscles of the pyloric end of the stomach causing narrowing of the antrum of the stomach leading to recurrent obstruction. The male to female ratio per thousand is 1: 5. Increased incidence of pyloric stenosis in males suggests they have a lower liability threshold as compared to the females. Since this condition is surgically correctable, prior consultation with a paediatric surgeon in case of high-risk families during

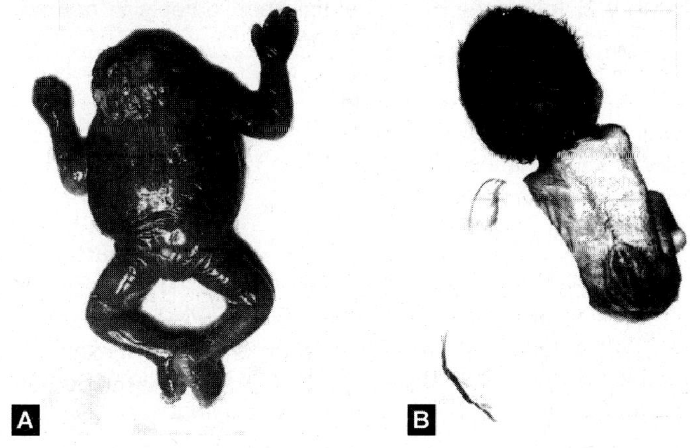

Figs 9.1A and B: Neural Tube defects (A) Anencephaly: note the absence of skull vault. (B) Spina bifida: meningomyelocele

or before pregnancy helps in timely intervention and prevention of complications. Awareness of the existence of the condition and prompt treatment is necessary to avoid lethal complications in the child like aspiration pneumonia.

Congenital Heart Defects

Congenital heart defects have a frequency of 8 per 1000 live births. These form a heterogeneous group of disorders caused by a single gene defects or maternal diseases like rubella infection or diabetes in pregnancy. The incidence of some commonly seen congenital heart diseases are described in Table 9.2.

Table 9.2: Incidence of congenital heart defects in normal population

Defect	*Population*
Ventricular septal defect (VSD)	1/575
Patent ductus arteriosus (PDA)	1/1200
Atrial septal defect (ASD)	1/1500
Aortic stenosis (AS)	1/2250

The incidence and relative risk among relatives of the affected sibling decreases with degree of relationship. With high-resolution ultrasound, prenatal diagnosis of major defects is possible by foetal Echocardiography at 18-20 weeks gestation, or slightly earlier at 14-16 weeks with vaginal sonography.

Cleft Lip and Cleft Palate (CL, CP)

One of the most common of congenital malformations, cleft lip and cleft palate result from failure of fusion of the frontal process with the maxillary process at the 35th day of gestation (Fig. 9.2). 60-80%-affected individuals are males. The causative

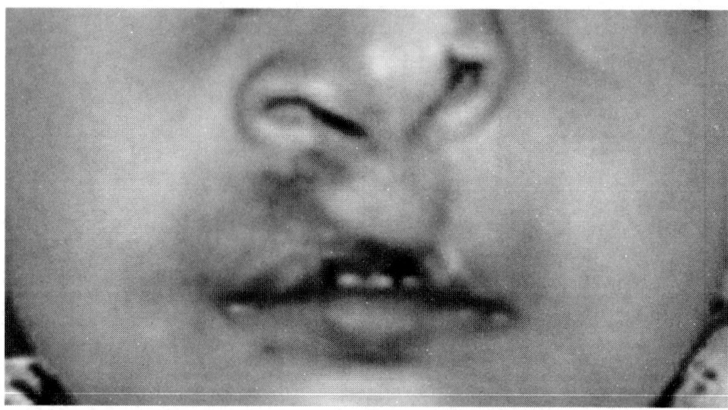

Fig. 9.2: Cleft lip with cleft palate
(For color version see Plate 3)

factor comprises of a heterogeneous group that includes single gene defects, chromosomal disorders (trisomy 13) and teratogenic exposure (rubella embryopathy, thalidomide, and anticonvulsants). The recurrence risk increases with increasing severity. From unilateral to trilateral and from isolated CL to both CL and CP. Analysis of population at large with CL (P) reveals that in certain populations there might be a major gene for liability to CL (P) in addition to multiple minor genes.

Chapter 10

BIOCHEMICAL GENETICS

INTRODUCTION

The way in which a mutation causes disease is largely related to deviations in the biochemical pathway. The path of molecular and biochemical events leading from a mutant gene to a disease gives us information not only about normal functioning but also about its deviation. Understanding these events can therefore help plan therapy for genetic diseases. Study of proteins and their metabolism constitutes the discipline of biochemical genetics.

The term "inborn error of metabolism" was established in 1902 by Sir Archibald Garrod when he observed that the urine of certain individuals turned black when exposed to air. Later it was observed that this was a genetic condition resulting from deficiency of a specific enzyme, causing a block in the normal metabolic pathway – in this case the protein being tyrosine. In another commonly known condition albinism, the deficiency of the enzyme tyrosinase in the hair, skin and eye prevents the synthesis of melanin leading to typical melanin deficient skin and irises. One has to understand that mutations producing biochemical defects do not always cause disease; they are biochemical traits detected in screening tests or when there is an offspring with a biochemical disease. In any population there is a normal variation in DNA sequences, which does not alter the quality of function of the polypeptide, irrespective of nucleotide changes being present in the coding region.

Genetic disease occurs when such alterations of vital genes reduce the quantity and function of the gene products (mRNA and protein). Single gene diseases occur due to alterations in DNA sequences controlling gene expression or encoding the structure of the protein.

In order to understand the pathogenesis of genetic disease, the primary biochemical abnormality must be understood. Till date 4,500 single gene disorders are known (autosomal and sex linked) and the specific protein deficiency has been identified in 500 such disorders. Inborn errors of metabolism are commonly caused by mutant genes, which generally result in abnormal proteins, most often enzymes. The inherited defects may be expressed as a total loss of enzyme activity or a partial deficiency of catalytic activity. Without treatment, the inherited defects often result in mental retardation or other developmental abnormalities due to harmful accumulation of metabolites. Some genetically determined enzyme deficiencies are discussed below (Fig. 10.1).

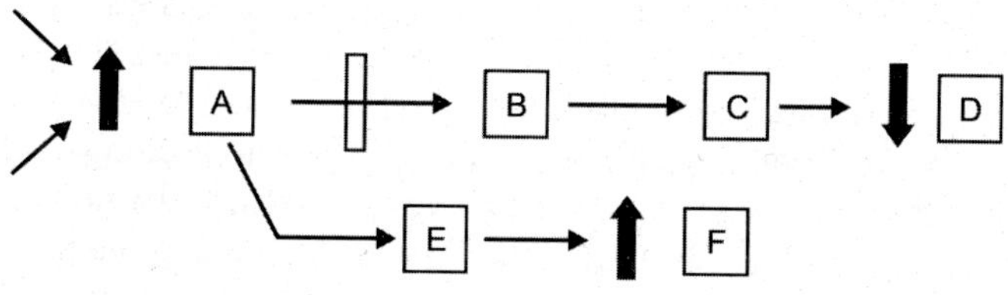

Fig. 10.1: Mechanism of genetic defect in metabloic pathway. Substrate A is converted to series of intermediate to final product D. Arrows indicate the inzymes catalyzing the reactions. A can converted to F by altering pathway. Genetic defect in the enzyme coverting A-B results in pathological consequences like 1. Accumulation of A, 2. Overflow of F, 3. Reduced formation of D, 4. Combination of these

DISORDERS OF AMINO ACID METABOLISM

Phenylketonuria (PKU)

PKU is caused by a deficiency of phenylalanine hydroxylase, and is the most common clinically encountered inborn error of amino acid metabolism, with a prevalence of 1:11,000. Hyperphenylalaninemia may also be caused by a deficiency in the enzymes that synthesize or reduce the coenzyme tetrahydrobiopterin. Phenylalanine is present in elevated concentrations in tissues, plasma and urine. Phenyllactate, phenylacetate and phenylpyruvate are also raised. Clinically patients have mental retardation, failure to walk or talk, seizures, hyperactivity, tremor, microcephaly, and failure to grow. Virtually all untreated patients show an IQ below 50. Patients also show a deficiency of pigmentation (fair hair, light skin, and blue eyes). The high levels of phenylalanine present in PKU competitively inhibit the hydroxylation of tyrosine by tyrosinase, which is the first step in the formation of the pigment melanin. Classic PKU is caused by mutations in the gene that codes for phenylalanine hydroxylase (PAH) and is inherited in an autosomal recessive manner.

Regarding the treatment of PKU, blood phenylalanine is maintained by feeding synthetic amino acid preparations low in phenylalanine. The earlier the treatment is started, the more completely neurologic damage can be prevented. Treatment should not be delayed beyond the first month of life. Patients with PKU cannot synthesize tyrosine, and it should be supplemented in the diet.

Maternal PKU: When women with PKU who are not on a low phenylalanine diet become pregnant, the offspring are affected with maternal PKU syndrome. High blood levels in the mother cause microcephaly, mental retardation and congenital heart disease. Thus dietary control of phenylalanine must begin prior to conception.

Oculocutaneous Albinism (OCA)

This autosomal recessive disorder occurs due to deficiency of the enzyme tyrosinase, which is responsible for the formation of melanin pigment from tyrosine. OCA patients have lack of pigment in the skin, hair, iris and fundus of the eye (Fig. 10.2). The lack of pigment in the eye results in poor vision and nystagmus. OCA is a heterogeneous condition varying from tyrosine negative to tyrosinase positive form (measurable as tyrosinase positive and negative activity). DNA studies have shown that both these conditions occur due to mutations in the tyrosinase gene on the long arm of chromosome 11. Another condition called albinism type 2, OCA-2, has a mutation in the P gene located on chromosome 15.

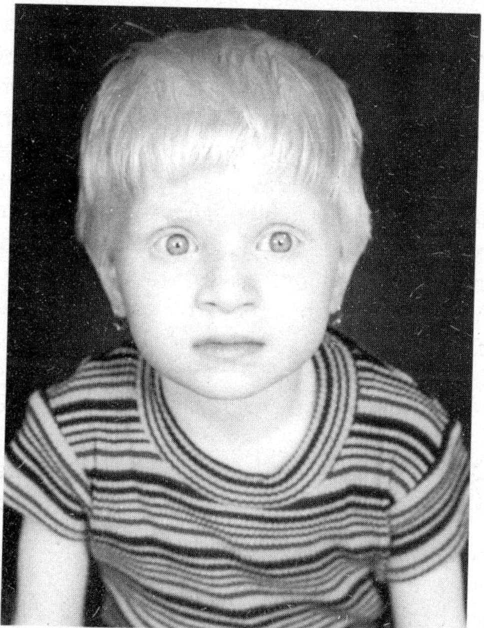

Fig. 10.2: Oculocutaneous albinism *(For color version see Plate 4)*

Alkaptonuria

Alkaptonuria was the first autosomal recessive inborn error of metabolism described by Garrod. It is caused by a deficiency in homogentisate oxidase. Homogentisic acid accumulates and is excreted in the urine. On exposure to air, it imparts a dark colour to the urine. The pigment also gets deposited in the wax of the ear, cartilage and joints. The condition is known as ochronosis and leads to arthritis in later life. Alkaptonuria is a benign condition and has a prevalence of 1 in 250,000.

Homocystinuria

This is inherited as an autosomal recessive disorder. The classical variety characterized by mental retardation, dislocation of the lens, convulsions, thromboembolic phenomena and osteoporosis. Arachnodactyly, kyphoscoliosis, and pectus excavatum may also be present.

The enzyme deficiency in homocystinuria is a lack of the enzyme cystathionine-B-synthetase. Accumulation of homocysteine occurs in the urine and methionine and its metabolites are elevated in blood. A positive nitroprusside test needs to be confirmed with plasma homocysteine levels. Treatment of homocystinuria is diet therapy, which involves low methionine, with supplements of cystine. Homocystinuria may be caused by decreased affinity of cystathione synthetase for its coenzyme pyridoxal phosphate (B6). This form may respond to megadoses of pyridoxine.

DISORDERS OF BRANCHED CHAIN AMINO ACID METABOLISM

The essential branched acids are leucine, isoleucine and valine. They share a common metabolic pathway in part and deficiency of this leads to maple syrup urine disease.

Maple Syrup Urine Disease

This is an autosomal recessive disorder and presents in the first week of life. Vomiting starts in the neonatal period and the neonates are alternately either hyper or hypotonic. If untreated, death is likely to occur in first few weeks. Neurologic problems are common and the prevalence of this disease is 1 in 200,000. The diagnosis is made initially by the typical smell of maple syrup in the urine. The deficiency of branched chain ketoacid dehydrogenase produces increased excretion in the urine of the branched chain amino acids valine, leucine and isoleucine. The confirmation is done by presence of these amino acids in urine and blood, and aminoacidograms by TLC and HPLC. The treatment is limiting dietary intake of these branched chain amino acids to the extent of the need of these essential amino acids for growth.

UREA CYCLE DISORDERS

Urea cycle disorders are inherited as autosomal recessive disorders except for ornithine transcarbamylase deficiency, which is inherited as a X-linked disorder. The overall prevalence is 1 in 30,000 live births. The metabolic process of the urea cycle is a five step pathway, taking place primarily in the cells of the liver where waste nitrogen is removed from the amino groups of amino acids in normal protein turn over. In this reaction, two molecules of ammonia and one molecule of bicarbonate are converted into urea. The five enzyme deficiencies include carbamyl synthetase deficiency, ornithine carbamyl transferase deficiency, citrullinemia due to argininosuccinic acid synthetase deficiency, argininosuccinic aciduria due to argininosuccinic acid lyase deficiency and hyperargininaemia due to arginase deficiency. Deficiencies of enzymes in the cycle result in hyperammonemia due to intolerance of protein, and resulting mental retardation. High levels of ammonia are harmful to the central nervous system resulting in coma and death if untreated.

DISORDERS OF CARBOHYDRATE METABOLISM

These include disorders of monosaccharide metabolism including galactosaemia, and hereditary fructose intolerance, and glycogen storage disorders.

DISORDERS OF MONOSACCHARIDE METABOLISM

Galactosemia

This is an autosomal recessive disorder, with a prevalence of 1:40,000 live births and occurs due to deficiency of the enzyme galactose-1-phosphate uridyl transferase, which is necessary for galactose metabolism. Untreated galactosemia presents with lethargy, feeding intolerance, vomiting hyperbilirubinemia, and liver dysfunction with coagulopathy. If not treated, 25% will develop sepsis in first 1-2 weeks. Mental retardation, cataracts and cirrhosis of the liver are the complications. Screening is by measurement of galactose and galactose-1-phosphate, and confirmation is by measurement of the enzyme in erythrocytes. Early diagnosis can help in preventing complications, which also include speech abnormalities, behaviour problems, visual perceptual learning abnormalities and ovarian failure in affected females. The affected infants are treated with milk substitutes free of galactose and lactose, the common sugars found in milk (lactose is further broken down into galactose). Three other inborn errors of galactose metabolism are known, including variant forms of transferase deficiency, which occur with 10-35% of normal transferase activity, galactokinase deficiency, and uridinediphosphate-galactose-4-epimerase deficiency.

Hereditary Fructose Intolerance

This condition is inherited as an autosomal recessive manner occurring due to a deficiency of the enzyme fructose-1 phosphate aldolase. The normal source of fructose in the diet is honey, sucrose containing baby foods for example milk powder or cereals, fruits and certain vegetables. Fructose is also present in cane sugar with the disaccharide sucrose. Fructose intolerance can present at different ages. The symptoms are milder than those of galactosemia. It may present with hypoglycaemic coma, convulsions and death. The diagnosis can be confirmed by urine examination for fructose, by enzyme assays of the intestinal mucosa or by a liver biopsy sample. Restriction of fructose in the diet has a good long-term prognosis.

GLYCOGEN STORAGE DISEASES

These are a group of diseases that result from a defect in an enzyme required for either glycogen synthesis or degradation. They result in either formation of glycogen that has an abnormal structure or the accumulation of excessive amounts of normal glycogen in specific tissues. Due to block in the metabolic pathway the normal source of glucose is unavailable and this leads to hypoglycemia, liver function impairment and neurological abnormalities. There are six major types of glycogen storage disorders and there is one specific enzyme defect involving any one of the steps in the metabolic pathways of glycogen storage disorder. The glycogen storage diseases primarily affecting the liver are described first followed by those primarily affecting muscle.

Glycogen Storage Disease Affecting the Liver

von Gierke's Disease (GSD I)

von Gierke's disease is one of the first described disorder of glycogen metabolism is due to a deficiency of the enzyme glucose-6-phosphatase. This deficiency results in normal glycogen structure, but increased storage of glycogen. Affected infants have hepatomegaly, tachycardia due to severe fasting hypoglycemia, fatty liver, hyperlacticacidemia, and hyperuricemia. Treatment is offering frequent feeds and avoiding fasting.

Cori Disease (GSD III)

Deficiency of the debrancher enzyme amylo-1-6 glucosidase results in accumulation of glycogen in the liver and other tissues. Affected infants present with hepatomegaly and muscle weakness. The treatment is the same as that for GSDI.

Anderson Disease (GSD IV)

Deficiency of glycogen brancher enzyme leads to Anderson disease. In this disorder there are long chains of glycogen, as very few branches are formed. Affected infants have abnormal liver function and hypotonia in first year of life, progressing rapidly to failure. There is no effective treatment except liver transplant.

Hepatic Phosphorylase Deficiency (GSD VI)

This multimeric enzyme complex is coded with subunits for both autosomal and X-linked genes. Deficiency of hepatic phosphorylase obstructs degradation of glycogen. Affected children present in the first 2 years with hepatomegaly, hypotonia and failure to thrive. Improvement in growth can occur with carbohydrate supplement.

Glycogen Storage Disease Affecting the Muscle

Pompe's Disease (GSD II)

Infants with Pompe's disease present in the first few months of life as floppy infants, with delayed motor milestones due to weakness of muscles. The heart is enlarged due to cardiac failure in the first or second year of life. Cardiac and skeletal muscles accumulate glycogen due to deficiency of lysosomal enzyme $\propto$ - 1, 4 glucosidase needed to break down glycogen. Excessive glycogen concentrations are found in abnormal vacuoles in the cytosol. The diagnosis is confirmed by enzyme assay on white blood cells or cultured fibroblasts.

McArdle's Disease (GSD V)

These patients present in teenage years with complaints of muscle cramps on exercise. The symptoms appear due to deficiency of muscle phosphorylase, an enzyme necessary for degradation of muscle glycogen, the liver enzyme is normal. There is normal mental development and no rise in blood lactate during strenuous exercise. No effective treatment is known but in affected individuals muscle cramps can be reduced with continued exercise, the reason being utilization of other energy sources through other metabolic pathways.

DISORDERS OF STEROID METABOLISM

The products of adrenocortical steroidogenesis are glucocorticoids, mineralocorticoids and sex steroids. Inherited deficiency of various enzymes involved in cortisol and aldosterone synthesis leads to a group of diseases called congenital adrenal hyperplasia. The clinical characteristics of congenital adrenal hyperplasia (CAH) depend on which enzyme in the pathway of cortisol synthesis is deficient. Even for a specific enzyme, variability exists in the severity of disease expression and timing of onset of symptoms. The two most commonly seen defects are 21-hydroxylase deficiency and 11-hydroxylase deficiency.

ADRENOGENITAL SYNDROME (CONGENITAL ADRENAL HYPERPLASIA)

21- hydroxylase Deficiency

Accounts for 90% of cases and are inherited as autosomal recessive traits.

a. Classic salt wasting 21-hydroxylase deficiency: This is a severe deficiency resulting in decreased cortisol and aldosterone secretion, increased ACTH and 17 hydroxyprogesterone. Females infants are born with ambiguous genitalia, (Fig. 10.3) males have no genital abnormalities. Symptoms of salt wasting, vomiting, dehydration and shock develop in the first 2-4 weeks of life. Infants are hyponatremic, hyperkalemic, acidotic and often hypoglycemic.

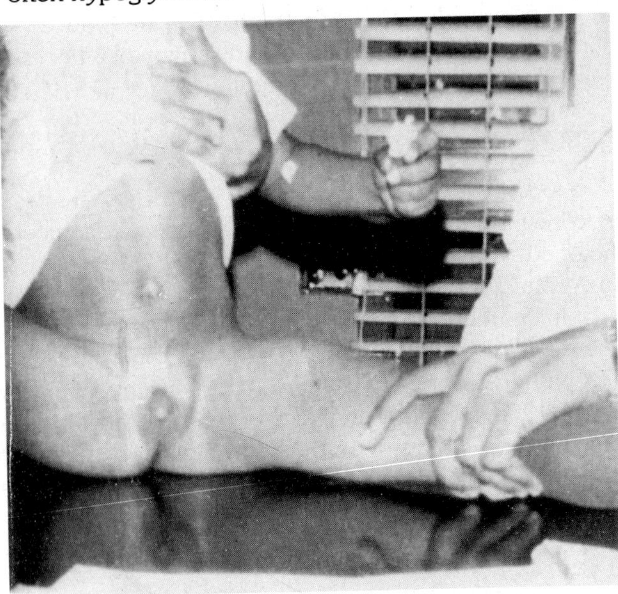

Fig. 10.3: Congenital adrenal hyperplasia
(For color version see Plate 4)

b. Simple virilizing 21-hydroxylase deficiency: Clinical features are caused solely by overproduction of adrenal androgens. Therefore, only female infants with ambiguous genitalia are diagnosed during the neonatal period.
c. Non-classic 21-hydroxylase deficiency (acquired or late onset): This variant is diagnosed in female adolescents or adults and patients manifest signs and symptoms of androgen excess, like menstrual irregularities, hirsutism, acne and advanced bone age.

11-hydroxylase Deficiency

This accounts for about 5% of the cases of congenital adrenal hyperplasia. Patients manifest with hypertension and hypokalemia.

Abnormal sexual differentiation results in a newborn who appears sexually ambiguous, and can be classified as male pseudohermaphroditism, female pseudohermaphroditism, and abnormal gonadal differentiation.

Male Pseudohermaphroditism

Male pseudohermaphroditism refers to infants who are 46XY males and can be caused by a variety of endocrine disorders involving testosterone synthesis, metabolism or action at the cellular level.

1. Defects in testosterone synthesis and metabolism are caused by one of the 5 enzyme deficiencies inherited as autosomal recessive disorders. These include defects in cortisol synthesis and are classified as forms of CAH.
2. Defects in androgen action
   a. 5α reductase deficiency impairs conversion of testosterone to dihydrotestosterone (DHT). Boys are born with ambiguous genitalia because DHT is necessary for masculinization of male external genitalia.

b. Androgen resistance syndromes (Testicular feminisation syndromes) (Fig. 10.4). In complete androgen resistance, an XY male infant with testes appears unambiguously female because of complete resistance to androgen action at the cellular level. In partial androgen resistance, the affected XY individual has ambiguous genitalia.

Female Pseudohermaphroditism

Female pseudohermaphroditism refers to infants who are 46XX females with ovaries, who appear masculinized at birth. This can be caused by CAH (discussed above) or maternal androgen or progestin exposure.

Abnormal Gonadal Differentiation

True hermaphroditism occurs when there is both ovarian and testicular tissue in the gonads. In 80% of the cases the karyotype

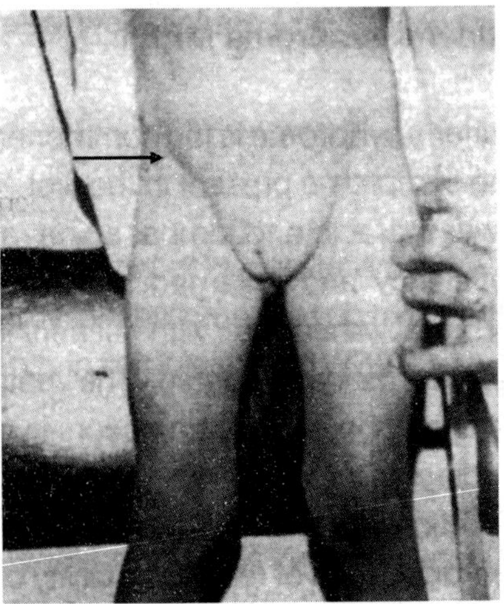

Fig. 10.4: Testicular feminization

is 46XX. Mixed gonadal dysgenesis has a karyotype of 45X/46XY. There is a spectrum in the appearance of the genitalia from completely male to completely female.

MUCOPOLYSACCHARIDOSES

These are hereditary disorders that are clinically progressive and are characterized by accumulation of glycosaminoglycans in various tissues causing skeletal and extracellular matrix deformities. Mucopolysaccharidoses are caused by a deficiency of one of the lysosomal hydrolases normally involved in the degradation of one or more of the glycosaminoglycans. They also result in oligosaccharides in urine due to incomplete degradation of glycosaminoglycans. All the deficiencies are autosomal recessive except Hunters syndrome, which is X-linked. No effective therapy exists, but prenatal diagnosis for these deficiencies is possible by measurement of lysosomal hydrolases.

Hurler's Syndrome (MPS I)

Hurler's syndrome is the commonest type of MPS and is clinically more severe. The symptoms present in the first year of life with corneal clouding, curving of lower thoracic and lumbar spine, and poor growth. Patients develop hearing deficiency and enlarged liver and spleen. During the second year of life, vertebral changes with stiffening of the joints occur. The facies is characteristically coarse. The features start progressing along with mental deterioration, and death occurs in mid teens due to respiratory infections and cardiac failure. Hurler syndrome is diagnosed by a urine test showing excretion of dermatan and heparan sulphate. Confirmation is done by demonstration of reduced activity of the ∝-L iduronidase lysosomal hydrolase. Levels of residual ∝-L iduroindase activities vary and on this basis the disease was separately classified as Scheie's disease (MPS IS) and Hurler / Scheie disease (MPS I H/S), which are allelic disorders.

Hunter's Syndrome (MPS II)

This is inherited as an X-linked disorder and affected males present between 2-5 years of age with hearing loss, diarrhea, recurrent infections and poor growth. Clinical examination reveals coarse features (Fig. 10.5), enlargement of liver and spleen and stiffness of joints. X-rays of the spine show lipping of the vertebral bodies. Both physical and mental retardation are progressive and death occurs before the age of twenty. Confirmation of MPS is by a urine test and further classification by an assay of the enzyme iduronate sulfatase sulphatase in serum or WBCs.

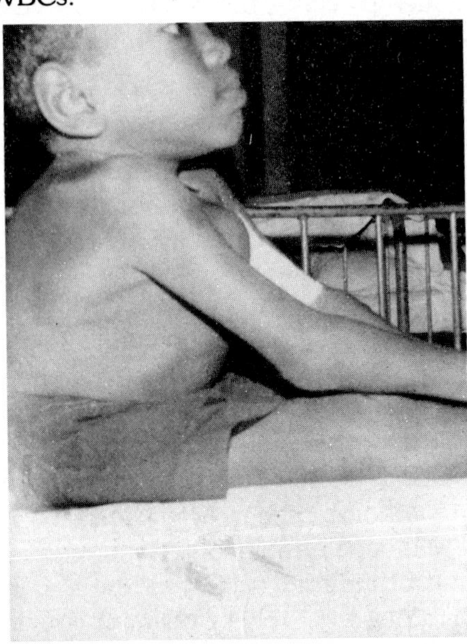

Fig. 10.5: Hunter's syndrome (MPS II)
(For color version see Plate 5)

Sanfilippo Syndrome (MPS III)

This form of MPS is seen commonly. The disease presents itself in the second year of life. The facial features become coarse, and skeletal changes and there is progressive intellectual loss. There may be associated behavioural problems. Convulsions occur often and death results in the twenties or thirties. Four enzymatic steps are necessary and the deficiencies are described below. Type A has heparan sulphaminadase deficiency, Type B has N-acetyl glycosaminadase deficiency, Type C has N-acetyltransferase deficiency and Type D has N-acetyl glucoseamine deficiency. Though the enzymes involved are different, clinical presentation remains the same.

Morquio Syndrome (MPS IV)

Morquio syndrome (MPS IV) is seen in the second or third year of life with skeletal abnormalities. These include short stature, thoracic deformity and kyphoscoliosis. Patients have a normal IQ and the prognosis for long-term survival is good, though there is an increased risk of spinal cord compression. Urinary test is used for screening and confirmation by enzyme assays shows a deficiency of N-acetylgalactosomine sulphate (MPS IV A) or B Galactosidase (MPS IV B)

Martoleaux-Lamy Syndrome (MPS VI)

Patients with Martoleaux-Lamy syndrome (MPS VI) have an expression similar to that of Hurler syndrome. The intelligence is normal. Life expectancy is up to early adulthood but in minor forms, patients may live up to the third decade. The diagnosis is confirmed by deficiency of arylsulphatase B deficiency in fibroblasts and WBCs.

Sly Syndrome (MPS VII)

This syndrome has variability in the severity and involvement of the systems, ranging from mild kyphoscoliosis to coarse facial features. It is caused by a deficiency of b glucuronidase. Corneal clouding, cardiac anomalies, hepatosplenomegaly, and a low IQ are other features, and death occurs in early childhood. There is an increase in urinary glyosaminoglycans. Enzyme assays in white blood cells or in fibroblasts confirms the diagnosis. Treatment by enzyme replacement has been unsuccessful so far. However, bone marrow transplant has met with limited success.

SPHINGOLIPIDOSES

In a normal individual, the synthesis and degradation of sphingolipids are balanced, so the amount of the compounds present in the membranes is constant. If a specific hydrolase required for the degradation process is partially or totally missing, sphingolipids accumulate in the lysosomes and are called sphingolipidoses. These include Tay Sach's disease, GM1 gangliosidosis, Gaucher's disease, metachromatic leukodystrophy, Krabbe's disease, Sandhoff's disease, Fabry's disease, Niemann Pick disease and Farber's disease. All of the above are autosomal recessive diseases except for Fabry's disease, which is X-linked. The incidence of sphingolipidoses is low in most populations except for Gaucher's disease and Tay Sachs disease, which show a high frequency in Ashkenazi Jews. The diagnosis of sphingolipidoses can be made by the presence of enzyme activity and accumulated lipid by analysis of tissue samples, cultured fibroblasts, peripheral leukocytes, plasma and amniotic fluid (for antenatal diagnosis).

Tay-Sachs Disease

It occurs due to increased gangliosides due to a deficiency of b hexosaminidase A. This disorder occurs commonly in

Ashkenazi Jews with an incidence of 1 in 2600 individuals. Affected infants start showing symptoms within a few months after birth with poor feeding, lethargy and floppiness. Developmental regression continues and becomes apparent in the later half of the year. Visual impairment and deafness occur and spasticity increases with rigidity in limbs. Death occurs by the age of 3 years. There have been reports of juvenile and adult forms. Presence of a cherry red spot in the centre of the macula confirms the clinical diagnosis of Tay-Sachs disease. Laboratory confirmation is done by demonstrating reduced hexosaminidase levels in serum, WBCs or cultured fibroblasts.

Gaucher's Disease

It occurs due to increased glucocerebrosides due to a deficiency of b glucosidase. Gaucher's disease is a common type of sphingolipidoses seen in Ashkenazi Jews. The age of onset differs in patients of Gaucher's disease, and based on this they are divided in 2 groups. The adult type or type I is more common and affected persons present with symptoms of with pain in limbs and joints and a tendency to pathologic fractures. Clinically patients are anemic with an enlarged spleen and liver. There are bony changes seen on X-rays in the vertebral bodies and femora. In infantile Gaucher's disease or type II, there is involvement of the central nervous system. The age of onset is 3-6 months. Failure to thrive, neurological deterioration and developmental regression occur together with convulsions and increasing spasticity. Death occurs in the second year of life due to recurrent respiratory infections. The diagnosis is confirmed by reduced levels of β-glucosidase in WBCs and cultured fibroblasts.

Treatment for adult type of Gaucher's disease is symptomatic. Splenectomy is occasionally required which can however cause secondary anemia. The current treatment with enzymes is by modifying β-glucosidase by addition of mannose-6-phosphate. Dramatic improvement in symptoms and regression of spleen is noted.

Niemann-Pick Disease

It occurs due to increased sphingomyelins due to a deficiency of sphingomyelinase. Clinically patients with Niemann-Pick disease present in infancy with failure to thrive, hepatomegaly, developmental regression and presence of a cherry red spot in the macula (also occurs in Tay-Sach's disease). Death occurs by the age of 4 years. Diagnosis is confirmed by presence of deficiency of the enzyme sphingomyelinase. Bone marrow of patients with Niemann-Pick disease show typical foam cells due to sphingomyelin accumulation.

COPPER METABOLISM

Copper homeostasis is maintained by gastrointestinal absorption and biliary excretion. Inherited disorders of copper transport include Wilson's disease, Menkes disease, and aceruloplasminemia.

Wilson Disease

The Wilson disease copper transporting adenosine triphosphatase (ATPase) transports copper into the hepatocyte secretory pathway for incorporation into ceruloplasmin and excretion into the bile. Thus individuals present with signs and symptoms arising from impaired biliary copper excretion. The disorder is inherited in an autosomal recessive manner, and a large number of mutations have been identified in the Wilson disease gene. The impaired copper excretion results in accumulation in the liver. When the capacity for hepatic storage is exceeded, the copper is released into the plasma resulting in haemolysis and deposition of copper in extra-hepatic tissues. Affected individuals may present with chronic hepatitis and cirrhosis or acute liver failure. Copper deposition in the retina is called the Kayser Fleischer ring. Copper accumulation in the basal ganglia and other parts of the brain results in dystonia, tremor, personality changes and cognitive impairment. The diagnosis is confirmed by decreased serum ceruloplasmin, increased urinary copper, and elevated hepatic copper concentration. The treatment is copper chelation using penicillamine.

Menkes Disease

The Menkes disease ATPAse transports copper across the placenta, gastrointestinal tract and blood brain barrier and clinical features of this disorder result from copper deficiency. In the fetus, there is copper deficiency in utero. The clinical features include abnormal hair and pigmentation, laxity of the skin, metaphyseal dysplasia, cerebellar degeneration and failure to thrive. Decreased serum copper and ceruloplasmin confirm the diagnosis. The disorder is inherited in an X-linked manner and mutations found in the gene for Menkes disease are unique to each family.

Aceruloplasminemia

This is an autosomal recessive disorder characterized be absent serum ceruloplasmin due to mutations in the ceruloplasmin gene. It is characterized by progressive neurodegeneration due to iron accumulation in the basal ganglia. Thus ceruloplasmin has an essential role in iron homeostasis. Affected individuals present with dysarthria, dystonia and dementia due to iron accumulation in affected tissues.

PEROXISOMAL DISORDERS

Peroxisomes are single membrane lined organelles present in virtually all eukaryotic cells and range from 100-1000 peroxisomes per cell. Peroxisome biogenesis involves synthesis of the matrix proteins on free cytosolic ribosomes followed by receptor mediated import into the organelle. *PEX* genes encode peroxins, proteins involved in and necessary for peroxisome biogenesis. There are 15 *PEX* genes known in humans. The peroxisome disorders are comprised of at least 12 complementation groups. Defective biogenesis of the organelle leads to two clinical spectra: The Zellweger spectrum, which includes Zellweger syndrome, neonatal adrenoleukodystrophy and infantile Refsum disease. The second spectrum consists of rhizomelic chondrodysplasia punctata. The gene for X-linked adrenoleukodystrophy also codes for a peroxisomal membrane protein, and hence this disorder will also be discussed.

Zellweger Syndrome

This cerebrohepatorenal syndrome has an incidence of approximately 1 per 50,000 births, and affected infants rarely live more than a few months. Patients have multiple congenital anomalies as well as ongoing metabolic disturbances. There are characteristic features including large anterior fontanel, full forehead, hypoplastic supraorbital ridges, epicanthal folds, broad nasal bridge, and a small nose with anteverted nares, cataracts, glaucoma, corneal clouding, Brushfield spots, pigmentary retinopathy, and optic nerve dysplasia, severe hypotonia, weakness and neonatal seizures. Radiologic examination reveals abnormal punctate calcifications (calcific stippling) in the patella and epiphyses of long bones. The cause of Zellweger syndrome is failure to import newly synthesized peroxisomal proteins into peroxisomes. There is plasma and tissue accumulation of very long chain fatty acids (VLCFAs).

Infantile Refsum Disease

Infantile form of Refsum disease can be caused by mutations in the *PEX1* and *PEX2* genes. Patients with the infantile form show both clinical and biochemical differences from patients with the classic form of Refsum disease. Features include early onset, mental retardation, facial dysmorphism, sensorineural hearing loss, hepatomegaly, osteoporosis, failure to thrive, delayed development, mental retardation, hepatomegaly, skeletal changes and retinitis pigmentosa. The biochemical abnormalities include accumulation of very long chain fatty acids (VLCFA). Deficiency of peroxisomes in hepatocytes and cultured skin fibroblasts is demonstrable. Biochemically, IRD patients show accumulation of phytanic acid and defective bile acid metabolism.

Rhizomelic Chondrodysplasia Punctata (RCDP)

RCDP is a rare, multisystem, developmental disorder, characterized by the presence of stippled foci of calcification in hyaline cartilage, coronal vertebral clefting, dwarfing, joint contractures, congenital cataract, ichthyosis, and severe mental retardation. Biochemically, RCDP patients have subnormal levels of red cell plasmalogens and progressive accumulation of phytanic acid starting from normal at birth and increasing to levels more than 10 times normal by age 1 year.

Adrenoleukodystrophy

Two types of adrenoleukodystrophy are known, X-linked adrenoleukodystrophy (X-ALD), and autosomal recessive neonatal adrenoleukodystrophy, which resembles Zellweger syndrome. The gene for X-linked ALD maps to Xq28 and encodes a peroxisomal membrane protein with homology to the ATP-binding cassette (ABC) transporter family of proteins. The incidence of males with X-ALD is between 1-20,000 to 50,000. The disorder causes malfunction of the adrenal cortex and nervous system myelin, and is characterized by abnormally high levels of very long chain fatty acids in tissues and body fluids. The very long chain fatty acid (VLCFA) accumulation is associated with an impaired capacity for their degradation, a reaction that takes place in the peroxisome. Clinically the children with the childhood cerebral form suffer from dementia, adrenal insufficiency and progressive neurologic deficit. Bone marrow transplantation is the most effective therapy in children who show early evidence of cerebral involvement. Dietary therapy to reduce plasma VLCFA levels is using a 4:1 mixture of glyceryl trioleate and glyceryl trierucate known as Lorenzo's Oil.

DISORDERS OF PURINE AND PYRIMIDINE METABOLISM

Defects in the Purine Salvage Pathway

Purines that result from the normal turnover of cellular nucleic acids or those that are obtained from the diet and are not degraded can be reconverted into nucleoside triphosphates and used by the body. This is the salvage pathway for purines, and two enzymes are involved, APRT (adenine phosphoribosyl transferase) and HGPRT (hypoxanthine guanine phosphoribosyl transferase). A deficiency of HGPRT causes Lesch Nyhan syndrome, discussed below.

Lesch Nyhan Syndrome

Defects in the degradation of purine nucleotides

Purine nucleotides are sequentially degraded to form uric acid. Several genetic diseases are associated with deficiencies of specific degradative enzymes in this pathway. Some of these are discussed below.

a. A defect in adenosine deaminase (ADA) deficiency causes severe combined immunodeficiency (SCID) involving T-cell and B-cell dysfunction. dATP is the major nucleotide that accumulates in cells.
b. Purine nucleoside phosphorylase deficiency results in impairment of T-cell function but no apparent effect on B-cell function. This results in decreased uric acid formation combined with increased levels of purine nucleosides and nucleotides. dGTP is the major nucleotide that accumulates in red cells.

Gout

Gout is characterized by hyperuricemia with recurrent attacks of acute arthritic joint inflammation, caused by deposition of uric acid crystals. Primary gout is attributable to an inborn error of metabolism such as overproduction of uric acid. Treatment with allopurinol inhibits xanthine oxidase resulting in the accumulation of hypoxanthine and xanthine, which are compounds that are more soluble than uric acid.

Hereditary Orotic Aciduria

This condition presents in children during first year of life. The children fail to thrive and have megaloblastic anemia and delayed development. The condition is due to deficiency of enzymes orotate phosphribosyl transferase or orotidine-5' phosphate decarboxylase. These enzymes are important in pyrimidine synthesis. Large amounts of orotic acid are excreted in the urine. Therapy is with uridine, which reduces orotic acid excretion and is aimed at correcting growth and anemia.

PRENATAL DIAGNOSIS OF INBORN ERRORS OF METABOLISM

The first criterion in the prenatal diagnosis of an IEM is to have a confirmed laboratory diagnosis in an index case in whom the deficient gene product has been identified. First trimester prenatal diagnosis is possible by cultured chorionic villi and it is not necessary to wait until second trimester for amniotic fluid culture. With the use of recombinant technology, it is possible to use linked DNA sequences or mutations and this is of great value when the biochemical basis has not been established or the enzyme in question is not expressed in chorionic villi.

Some defects, their genetics, deficient enzymes and clinical features are discussed below:

Characteristics of some inborn errors of metabolism (AR and AD = autosomal recessive or dominant. XR and XD = X-linked recessive or dominant

Type of defect	*Genetics*	*Deficient enzyme*	*Main clinical features*
Amino acid metabolism			
Phenylketonuria	AR	Phenylalanine hydroxylase	Mental retardation, fair skin, eczema, epilepsy
Alkaptonuria	AR	Homogentisic acid oxidase	Dark urine on standing, arthritis
Oculocutaneous albinism	AR	Tyrosinase	Lack of skin and hair pigment, eye detects
Homocystinuria	AR	Cystathione β-synthetase	Mental retardation, dislocation of lens, thrombosis, skeletal abnormalities
Maple syrup urine disease	AR	Branched chain α-ketoacid decarboxylase	Mental retardation

Contd...

Contd...

Type of defect	*Genetics*	*Deficient enzyme*	*Main clinical features*
Urea cycle disorders			
Carbamyl synthetase deficiency	AR	Carbamyl synthetase	Hyperammonemia, coma, death
Ornithine carbamyl transferase deficiency	XD	Ornithine carbamyl transferase	Hyperammonemia, death in early infancy
Citrullinemia	AR	Argininosuccinic acid synthetase	Variable clinical course
Argininosuccinic aciduria	AR	Arginino-succinic acid lyase	Hyperammonemia, mild mental retardation, protein intolerance
Hyper-argininemia	AR	Arginase	Hyperammonemia, progressive spasticity, intellectual deterioration
Carbohydrate metabolism			
Monosaccharide metabolism			
Galactosemia	AR	Galactose-1-phosphate uridyl transferase	Cataracts, mental retardation, cirrhosis
Hereditary fructose intolerance	AR	Fructose-1-phosphate aldolase def. type A,B,C	Failure to thrive, vomiting, jaundice, convulsions
Glycogen storage diseases			
Primarily affecting liver			
Von Gierke's disease (GSD I)	AR	Glucose-6-phosphatase	Hepatomegaly, hypoglycemia
Pompe's disease (GSD II)	AR	Lysosomal α-1-4-glucosidase	Heart failure, muscle weakness

Contd...

Contd...

Type of defect	*Genetics*	*Deficient enzyme*	*Main clinical features*
Cori disease (GSD III)	AR	Amylo-1 glucosidase	Hepatomegaly, hypoglycemia
Anderson disease (GSD IV)	AR	Glycogen brancher enzyme	Abnormal liver function/ failure
McArdle's disease (GSD V)	AR	Muscle phosphorylase	Muscle cramps
Hepatic phosphorylase deficiency (GSDVI)	AR/X linked	Hepatic phosphorylase	Hepatomegaly, hypoglycemia, failure to thrive
Pompe's disease (GSD II)	AR	Lysosomal α-1, 4-glucosidase	Heart failure, muscle weakness
Steroid metabolism			
Congenital adrenal hyperplasia	AR	21-hydroxylase, 11 β-hydroxylase, 3β-dehydrogenase	Virilization, salt-losing
Testicular feminisation	XR	Androgen receptor	Female external genitalia, male internal genitalia, male chromosomes
Lipid metabolism			
Familial hyper-cholesterolemia	AD	Low density lipoprotein receptor	Early coronary artery disease
Lysosomal storage diseases			
Mucopolysaccharidoses			
Hurler's syndrome (MPS I)	AR	α-iduronidase	Mental retardation, skeletal abnormalities, hepatosplenomegaly, corneal clouding
Hunter's syndrome (MPS II)	XR	Iduronate sulphate sulphatase	Mental retardation, skeletal abnormalities, hepatosplenomegaly

Contd...

Contd...

Type of defect	*Genetics*	*Deficient enzyme*	*Main clinical features*
Sanfilippo syndrome (MPS III)	AR	Heparan-S-sulphaminidase (MPS III A), N-ac-α-D-glucosaminidase (MPS III B), Ac-CoA-α-glucosaminidase-N-acetyltransferase (MPS III C), N-ac-glucosamine-6-sulphate Sulphate (MPS III D)	Behavioural problems, dementia, fits
Morquio syndrome (MPS IV)	AR	Galactosamine-6-sulphate Sulphate (MPS IV A) β-galactosidase (MPS IV B)	Corneal opacities, short stature, skeletal abnormalities
MPS V (formerly Scheie-now known to be a mild allelic form of MPS I)			
Martoleaux-Lamy syndrome (MPS VI)	AR	Arylsulphatase B N-acetyl-galactosamine α-4-sulphate sulphatase	Corneal clouding, skeletal abnormalities, cardiac abnormalities
Sly syndrome (MPS VII)	AR	β-glucuronidase	Variable presentation, skeletal and cardiac abnormalities, corneal clouding, hepatosplenomegaly, mental retardation

Contd...

Contd...

Type of defect	*Genetics*	*Deficient enzyme*	*Main clinical features*
Sphingolipidoses			
Tay-Sachs disease	AR	Hexosaminidase–A	Developmental regression, blindness, cherry-red spot, deafness
Purine/pyrimidine metabolism			
Lesch-Nyhan disease	XR	Hypoxanthine guanine phosphoribosyl-transferase	Mental retardation, uncontrolled movements, self-mutilation
Adenosine deaminase deficiency	AR	Adenosine deaminase	Severe combined immunodeficiency
Purine nucleoside phosphorylase	AR	Purine nucleoside phosphorylase deficiency	Severe viral infections due to impaired T cell function
Hereditary orotic aciduria	AR	Orotate phosphoribosyl-transferase or orotidine 5'-phosphate decarboxylase	Megaloblastic anemia, failure to thrive, developmental delay
Adenosine deaminase deficiency	AR	Adenosine deaminase	Severe combined immunodeficiency
Purine nucleoside phosphorylase	AR	Purine nucleoside phosphorylase deficiency	Severe viral infections due to impaired T cell function
Hereditary orotic aciduria	AR	Orotate phosphoribosyl transferase, orotidine 5'phosphate decarboxylase	Megaloblastic anaemia, failure to thrive, developmental delay

Contd...

Contd...

Type of defect	*Genetics*	*Deficient enzyme*	*Main clinical features*
Porphyrin metabolism			
Hepatic porphyries			
Acute intermittent porphyria (AIP)	AD	Uroporphyrinogen I synthetase	Abdominal pain, CNS effects
Hereditary coproporphyria	AD	Coproporphyrinogen oxidase	As for AIP, photosensitivity
Porphyria variegata	AD	Protoporphyrinogen oxidase	Photosensitivity, as for AIP
Erythropoietic porphyrias			
Congenital erythropoietic porphyria	AR	Uroporphyrinogen III synthase	Hemolytic anemia, photosensitivity
Erythropoietic protoporphyria	AD	Ferrochelatase	Photosensitivity, liver disease
Organic acid disorders			
Methylmalonic acidemia	AR	Methylmalonyl-CoA mutase	Hypotonia, poor feeding, acidosis, developmental delay
Propionic acidemia	AR	Propionyl-CoA mutase	Hypotonia, poor feeding, failure to thrive, vomiting, acidosis, hypoglycemia
Copper metabolism			
Wilson disease	AR	ATPase membrane copper transport protein	Spasticity, rigidity, dysphagia, cirrhosis
Menkes disease	XR	ATPase membrane copper transport protein	Failure to thrive, neurological deterioration
Peroxisomal disorders			
Peroxisomal biogenesis disorders			
Zellweger syndrome	AR	peroxisomal enzymes	Dysmorphic features, hypotonia, large liver, renal cysts
Adreno-leukodystrophy	XR	Very long chain fatty acid-CoA synthetase	Mental deterioration, behavioural changes, adrenal failure

(AR and AD = Autosomal recessive and dominant
XR and XD = X linked recessive and dominant)

CHAPTER 11

THE HEMOGLOBINOPATHIES

INTRODUCTION

Hemoglobinopathies are classic models for study of molecular diseases as practically all types of mutations are observed in hemoglobin disorders. These are the most common genetic disorders in the world, (approximately 25,000 persons are born each year). They have very high mortality and morbidity thus are of major concern.

STRCTURE OF HEMOGLOBIN

Hemoglobin is found exclusively in red cells where its main function is to transport oxygen from the lungs to the capillaries of tissues. There are three major types of hemoglobin, HbA, HbA_2, and HbF. Each of the different types of hemoglobin is a tetramer composed of two α-globin like peptides and two β-globin like peptides. Each globin chain is associated with a heme group (Fig. 11.1). Heme is the iron-containing compound that combines with oxygen.

1. HbA, Adult hemoglobin ($\alpha_2\beta_2$): HbA forms 90% of the fraction of total hemoglobin, and is the major hemoglobin in adults. It is composed of four polypeptide chains, two α chains and two β chains.
2. HbA_2 ($\alpha_2\beta_2$): HbA_2 forms 2-5% of the fraction of total hemoglobin and is composed of two a chains and two δ chains. It first appears about 12 weeks after birth.

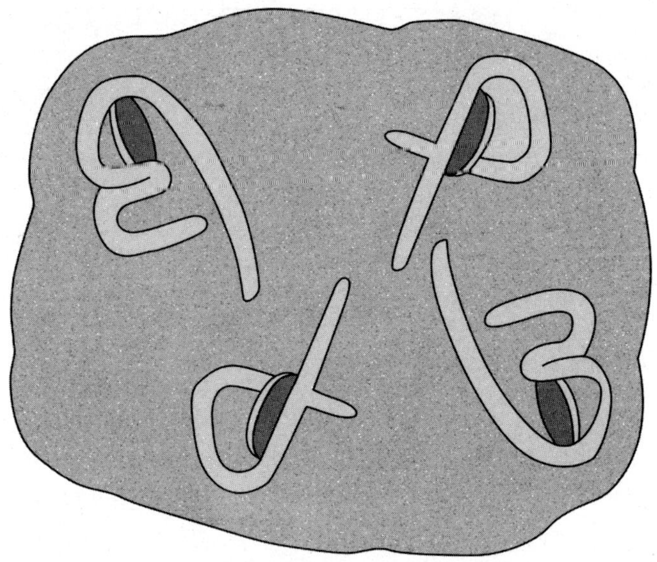

Fig. 11.1: Structure of hemoglobin

3. HbF fetal hemoglobin, ($\alpha_2\gamma_2$): HbF forms less than 2% of the fraction of total hemoglobin. It consists of two a chains identical to those found in HbA, and two γ chains. The γ chains are members of the β-globin gene family. HbF is the major hemoglobin found in the foetus and newborn. During the last months of fetal life, HbF accounts for 60% of the total Hb in the erythrocyte. In the first few weeks after conception, embryonic hemoglobin, ($\sigma_2\varepsilon_2$, Hb Gower 1) is synthesized by the embryonic yolk sac. Within a couple of weeks the fetal liver begins to synthesize HbF, and then the bone marrow takes over. HbA synthesis starts in the first month of pregnancy, and gradually replaces HbF (Fig. 11.2).

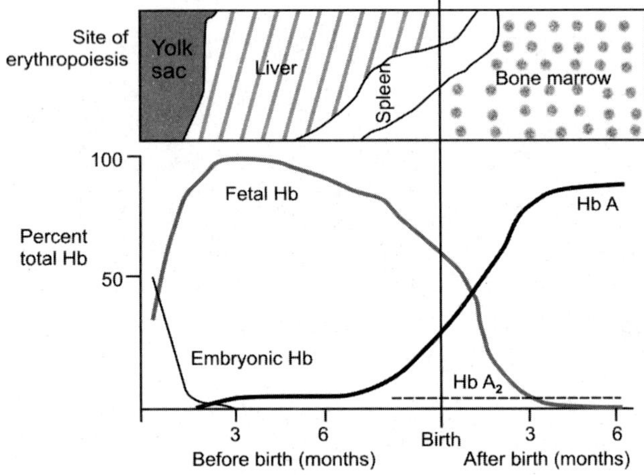

Fig. 11.2: Hemoglobin synthesis during prenatal and postnatal period

Organization of the Globin Genes

1. α globin gene family: The α gene cluster lies on chromosome 16 (Fig. 11.3). It contains two genes for the α-globin chain, the σ gene that is expressed early in development as a component of embryonic hemoglobin, and a number of globin like genes that are not expressed (pseudogenes). The α chain has 141 amino acids.
2. β-globin gene family: A single gene for the β-globin chain is located on chromosome 11, (Fig. 11.3) along with four other β-globin like genes. These include the ε gene (expressed early in embryonic development), two γ genes, Gγ, and Aγ, that are expressed in fetal hemoglobin HbF, and the

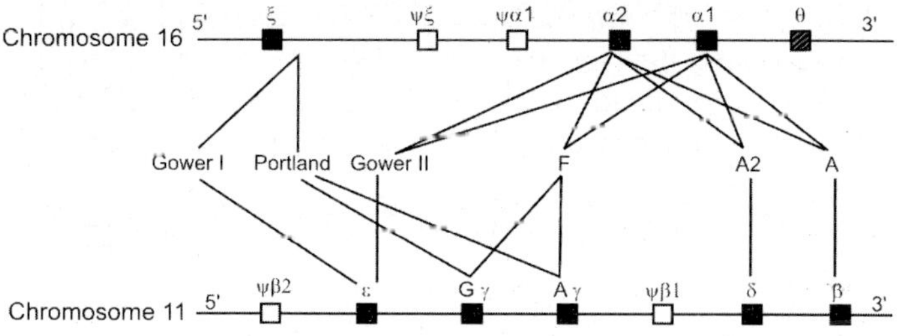

Fig. 11.3: α- and β-globin gene regions on chromosome 16 and 11

δ gene that codes for the globin chain found in the minor HbA_2. The β chain has 146 amino acids.

SYNTHESIS AND CONTROL OF HEMOGLOBIN EXPRESSION

In vitro translation studies with reticulocyte mRNA from normal persons have shown that α- and β-globin chains are synthesized roughly equally. However, studies of globin chain synthesis have also demonstrated that β-globin mRNA is slightly more efficient in protein synthesis than α-globin mRNA and that this difference is compensated for in the red blood cell precursors by a relative excess of α-globin mRNA. From this it seems that the most important level of regulation of expression of the globin genes, like other eukaryotic genes, is likely to occur at the level of transcription.

In addition to the promoter sequences in the 5' flanking regions of the various globin genes, there are sequences 6-20 kb 5' to the ε-globin gene necessary for expression of various β-like globin genes. This region is called the locus control region, lcr, and is involved in the timing and tissue specificity of expression or switching of the β-like globin genes in development.

HEMOGLOBINOPATHIES

Hemoglobinopathies are defined as a family of disorders caused by production of a structurally abnormal hemoglobin molecule, or by synthesis of insufficient quantities of normal hemoglobin. Examples of conditions that result from production of hemoglobin with an altered amino acid sequence include HbS (sickle cell anemia) and HbC (HbC disease). The thalassemia syndromes result due to decreases production of normal hemoglobin.

More than 300 Hb electrophoretic variants have been described. About 200 of these variants are single amino acid substitutions resulting from point mutations. The types of mutations seen include:

Missense mutations are seen in HbS, HbC, and HbE, ***nonsense mutations*** in Hb Constant Spring, ***deletion mutations*** in Hb Freiburg, ***insertion mutations*** in Hb Grady and fusion polypeptides that result due to unequal cross over events in meiosis in Hb Lepore and Hb Kenya. Though some of the hemoglobin variants are associated with disease, many are harmless and do not interfere with normal function, and are identified only in the course of population surveys of Hb electrophoretic variants.

Any mutation on the inside of the globin subunits in close proximity to the hem pockets or at the interchain contact areas, can produce an unstable Hb molecule which by precipitating in the red blood cell, damages the membrane resulting in hemolysis of the red blood cell. In addition, mutations can also interfere with normal oxygen transport, leading either to an enhanced or reduced oxygen affinity, or to an Hb, which is stable in its reduced form, the so-called methemoglobin. It is not possible to detect all structural variants of Hb by electrophoretic techniques. This is because only about one-third of the possible Hb mutations produce an altered charge in the Hb molecule and thereby can be detectable by electrophoresis.

SICKLE CELL ANEMIA

An autosomal recessive disorder characterized by the substitution of valine for glutamic acid at position 6 in the β globin chain (HbS). This results in a solubility problem in the deoxygenated state, and upon deoxygenation, the affected RBC changes from a biconcave disc to a crescent or sickle shaped cell. Sickle cell anemia is the most common cause of hemolytic anemia in the black population. It is also common among Greeks, Italians, Saudi Arabians, and certain communities in India. There is an association between heterozygote status and protection against malaria.

Sickle Cell Trait

This is a heterozygous state where both HbA (55-60%) and HbS (35-40%) are present. Those with the trait are usually asymptomatic unless they are subjected to severe hypoxic stress. Abnormalities include failure to concentrate urine (isosthenuria) and painless hematuria secondary to medullary infarcts. Complications include retinal artery occlusion and splenomegaly.

Sickle Cell Anemia

This is the homozygous state, with two HbS alleles. During the first few months of life, high levels of HbF protect the child and the earliest manifestations occur at 4-6 months of age.

The patient may manifest with symmetrical painful swelling of the dorsal surfaces of the hands and feet (hand foot syndrome). This is due to avascular necrosis of the bone marrow of the metacarpal and metatarsal bones. A vasocclusive crisis can involve the chest, abdomen, back and joints. One fourth are preceded by a viral or bacterial infection. Many factors like dehydration, vascular stasis, acidosis or hypoxia can precipitate episodes. Repeated vasocclusive episodes in the spleen lead to infection and fibrosis and the spleen is not palpable after age 5. Due to the spleen being malfunctional, there is increased susceptibility to infection with encapsulated bacteria. Skin may be involved leading to chronic ulcers in the distal lower extremities. All the patients have isosthenuria and renal failure is common. Hepatic infarcts and cholelithiasis also occur. There is aseptic necrosis of the head of the femur. Biconcave ("fishmouth") vertebrae are pathognomic of sickle cell disease. Osteomyelitis with *Staphylococcus* or *Salmonella* is common. Aplastic crises may be precipitated by infection with parvovirus B19.

The diagnosis is made initially by using metabisulfite (an oxygen-consuming agent), which is added to blood. If HbS is present, cells will sickle. The diagnosis is confirmed by hemoglobin electrophoresis.

Thalassemias

Thalassemia are hereditary hemolytic anomies characterized by decreased or complete absence of one or more of the globin subunits of the hemoglobin molecule.

a. α-thalassemia results from reduced α-globin chain synthesis, usually the result of a gene deletion. Normally there are four α chains.
b. β-thalassemia results from reduced β-globin chain synthesis, usually the result of abnormal DNA sequence due to single base substitutions. Normally there are two β chains.

Normally the synthesis of α and β chains are co-ordinated so that each a globin chain has αβ globin chain partner. In the thalassemias the synthesis of either the α globin chain or the β globin chain is defective. Each thalassemia can be classified as a disorder in which no globin chains are produced, called as α^0 or β^0 thalassemia, or in which some chains are synthesized, but at a reduced rate called α^+ or β^+ thalassemia. The excess unpaired globin chains are a hazard to the RBC because they produce insoluble tetramers that precipitate, causing membrane damage, and susceptibility to destruction within the reticuloendothelial system.

α Thalassemias

These are defects in which the synthesis of the α globin chains is decreased or absent. Because each individual genome contains four copies of the globin gene, two each on each chromosome 16), there are four levels of globin chain deficiency. If one of the four a globin genes is defective, the individual is a silent carrier because no physical manifestations of the disease occur. If two α-globin genes are defective, the individual is designated as α thalassemia trait, or α-thalassemia minor, and the patient has a moderate hypochromic, microcytic anemia. If three α-globin genes are defective, the individual has hemoglobin H disease with mild to moderately severe hemolytic anemia. If all four of the a globin genes are defective, hydrops fetalis and fetal death result, as α-globin chains are required for formation of HbF. The synthesis of unaffected γ, and then β chains continues, resulting in the accumulation of γ tetramers in the newborn (γ_4 or Hb Bart), or β teramers (β_4 or HbH). These variants have a high affinity for oxygen, which is not released to the tissues. The result is severe anemia, heart failure, hepatosplenomegaly, generalized edema and death *in utero*.

Mutational Basis of α Thalassemia

Restriction mapping studies of the α-globin region of chromosome 16 reveal that there are two α-globin structural genes on the short arm of chromosome 16. The various forms of α thalassemia have been shown to be due to deletions of one or more of these structural genes. Deletions of the α-globin genes in a thalassemia are believed to occur as a result of unequal crossover events in meiosis. These events are more likely to occur where genes with homologous sequences are in close proximity. Support for this hypothesis comes from the finding of the other product of such an event, that is persons with three α-globin structural genes located on one chromosome.

β Thalassemias

In the β thalassemias, synthesis of β-globin chains is decreased or absent, whereas β-globin chain synthesis is normal. α globin chains cannot form soluble tetramers, and therefore precipitate causing the premature death of cells destined to become mature red cells. Because there are only two copies of the globin gene, individuals with β gene defects have either the β thalassemia trait or β thalassemia minor if they have one defective gene or β thalassemia major, if both genes are defective. Because the β-globin gene is not expressed until late fetal gestation, the physical manifestations of β thalassemia appear only after birth.

β Thalassemia trait or β thalassemia minor

The growth and development of patients is normal. There is mild anemia and elevation of HbA_2. No treatment is necessary.

β Thalassemia major

Also known as Coolies anemia, or homozygous β thalassemia. Molecular defects range from complete absence of the b globin gene chain synthesis (β^0 β^0), to partial reduction of the gene product at the affected locus. Beginning in the first year of life, the infant develops a progressively severe hemolytic anemia with hepatosplenomegaly and bone marrow hyperplasia. The bone marrow hyperplasia produces features such as tower skull and frontal bossing. Death occurs due to congestive failure unless the patient is supported by blood transfusions. HbA is markedly decreased and HbF forms 30-90% of the total Hb. The treatment includes repeated transfusions and the regular daily use of iron-chelating drugs, such as desferrioxamine.

Mutational basis of β thalassemia

Restriction mapping studies have shown that β thalassemia is rarely due to a deletion, and DNA sequencing has often been necessary to reveal the molecular pathology. A wide variety of different mutations, which include point mutations, insertions and deletions of one or more bases, have been shown to be responsible. These occur at a number of places, both within the coding and the non-coding portions of the β-globin genes as well as in the 5' flanking promoter region, the 5' capping sequences and the 3' polyadenylation sequences (Fig. 11.4). The various types of mutations causing β thalassemia are often unique to certain population groups and can be considered to fall into five main functional types.

Transcription Mutations

Mutations in the 5' flanking TATA box or the promoter region of the β-globin gene can result in reduced transcription level of the β-globin mRNA.

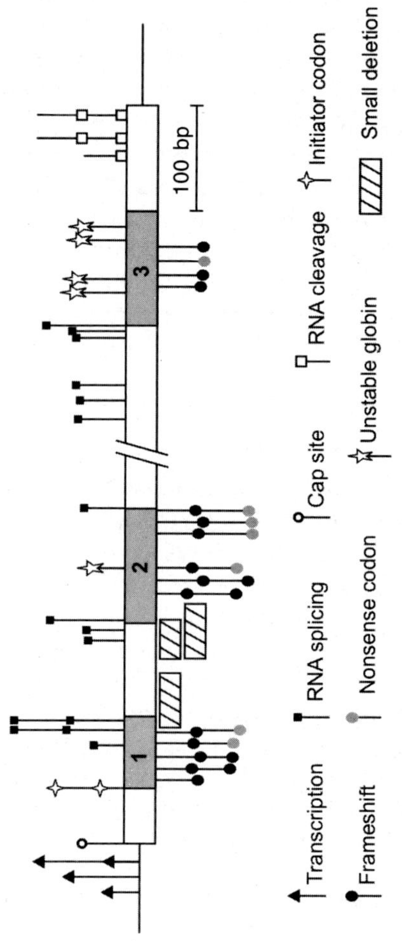

Fig. 11.4: Mutational types of β thalassemia

mRNA Splicing Mutations

Mutations involving the invariant 5' GT or 3' AG dinucleotides of the introns in the β-globin gene or the consensus donor or acceptor sequences result in abnormal splicing with consequent reduced levels of β-globin mRNA. In the commonest β thalassemia mutation in persons from the Mediterranean region, the mutation leads to the creation of a new acceptor AG dinucleotide splice site sequence in the first intron of the β-globin gene creating a so-called cryptic splice site. The cryptic splice site competes with the normal splice site leading to reduced levels of the normal β-globin mRNA. Mutations in the coding regions of the β-globin region can also lead to cryptic splice sites.

RNA Modification Mutations

Mutations in the 5' and 3' DNA sequences, involved respectively in the capping and polyadenylation of the mRNA, can result in abnormal processing and transportation of the β-globin mRNA to the cytoplasm with consequent reduced levels of translation.

Chain Termination Mutations

Insertions, deletions and point mutations can all generate a nonsense or chain termination codon, resulting in the premature termination of translation of the β-globin mRNA. This will result in the majority of instances in a shortened β-globin mRNA, which is often unstable and more rapidly degraded with consequent reduced levels of translation of an abnormal β-globin.

Missense Mutations

Missense mutations, which lead to a β-globin chain, which is highly unstable, rarely result in β thalassemia. An example is Hb Indianapolis.

δβ Thalassemia

In δβthalassemia there is underproduction of both the δ- and β-globin chains. Persons homozygous for δβ thalassemia produce no δ- or β-globin chains. Although one would expect such persons to have a family profound illness, they are only mildly anemic, due to an increased production of γ-globin chains, with Hb F levels being much higher than the mild compensatory increase seen in homozygotes for β thalassemia.

Mutational basis of δβ thalassemia

δβ thalassemia has been shown to be due to extensive deletions in the β-globin region involving the δ- and β-globin structural genes. Some deletions extend to include the $^{A}\gamma$-globin gene so that only the $^{G}\gamma$-globin chain is synthesized.

HEREDITARY PERSISTENCE OF FETAL HEMOGLOBIN

Hereditary persistence of fetal Hb, or HPFH, in which there is persistence of the production of fetal Hb into childhood and adult life is included in the thalassemias. Most forms of HPFH are in fact a form of δβ thalassemia in which continued γ-chain synthesis compensates for the lack of production of δ- and β-globin chains. In persons with hereditary persistence of fetal Hb, the fetal Hb accounts for 20-30% of total Hb in heterozygotes and 100% in homozygotes. This is not associated with any symptoms and was originally considered more of a scientific curiosity than a medical problem.

Mutational basis of HPFH

Some forms of HPFH have been shown to be due to deletions of the δ- and b-globin genes. Analysis of the non-deletion forms of HPFH has shown point mutations in the 5' flanking promoter region of either the $^{G}\gamma$ or $^{A}\gamma$ globin genes near the CAT box sequence involved in the control of expression of the hemoglobin genes.

CHAPTER 12

PHARMACOGENETICS

INTRODUCTION

Pharmacogenetics deals with pharmacological responses and their modification by hereditary influences. Variation of drug metabolising enzymes represents variations within the chemical defense systems between individuals. These variations also affect susceptibility to infectious diseases like tuberculosis and malaria and aid the survival of populations exposed to toxins or infectious agents.

Pharmacogenetics will give clinicians the tools to predetermine response to pharmacotherapy by looking for specific polymorphisms in cytochrome P450 and other enzymes involved in drug metabolism. Pharmacogenetics also will have an important role in determining or predicting patient response to environmental toxins.

Genetic differences can result in considerable variation in the rate of metabolising a drug. The metabolism may take longer than expected, increasing the risk of side effects. In case of high metabolic rates, the therapeutic effect may be diminished or absent. Metabolic rates depend on the cytochrome P450 and N-acetyltransferase enzymes, and patients are classified as fast or slow metabolises depending on the activity of the level of these enzymes. The best known of the cytochrome P450 enzymes is CYP2D6, which plays a role in the metabolism of several drugs including β-blockers and antidepressants. Slow N-acetyltransferase forms are found in a majority of the population. These enzymes play a role in the metabolism of various drugs like isoniazid used in the treatment of tuberculosis.

Pharmacogenetic effects can be caused by differences in enzymatic conversion rates and by inter-individual variation in the proteins to which the drugs are targeted (target proteins). Genetic differences in receptors can mean variation in drug efficacy from patient to patient. Examples of this include the variable efficacy of salbutamol in asthma and treatment with anti-malarial drugs in some patients with malaria resulting in severe anemia.

Pharmacogenetics can help address why some individuals respond to drugs and others do not. It can also help physicians understand why some individuals require higher or lower dosing for optimum response to a drug. It could potentially tell physicians who will respond to a drug and who will have toxic side effects. Systemic drug concentration is the end result of drugs ingestion absorption, metabolism, clearance and excretion. Much of pharmacogenetics has focused on the mechanisms that control the systemic drug concentration.

Drug metabolising enzymes known to be genetically variable include esterases, transferases, dehydrogenases, oxido-reductases, and the cytochrome P450 group of enzymes. Many of the well-defined pharmacogenetic variants represent Mendelian (monogenic traits). Therefore, the rate of occurrence of such a variant in a population can be defined in terms of an allele frequency. These frequencies differ between racially or ethnically defined populations accounting for geographical differences in drug safety. In addition, multifactorial variation accounts for innumerable differences between individuals as well as between populations. The Table 12.1 outlines ethnic variation in some pharmacogenetic disorders.

An example of pharmacogenetic variability is seen in a genetic defect, which affects the function of a specific enzyme of cytochrome P450, CYP2D6. The P450 system is important

Table 12.1: Ethnic variation in some pharmacogenetic disorders

Disorder	*Ethnic group*	*Frequency*
Slow acetylation	Europeans	50
	Orientals	10
Pseudocholinesterase variants	Europeans	<1
	Eskimos	1-2
G6PD deficiency	N Europeans	0
	S Europeans	Up to 25
	Afro-Caribbean	10%
Hypolactasia	Europeans	<20
	Asians	100
Atypical ADH	Europeans	5
	Orientals	85

for the metabolism of many endogenous compounds and for the detoxification of exogenous substances. This polymorphism affects the oxidative biotransformation of debrisoquine and over 60 other therapeutic agents. The CYPD gene cluster is located on chromosome 22q13.1 and is highly polymorphic in the human population. It may contain 2-4 genes, only one of which (CYP2D6) produces functional enzyme in individuals of the extensive metabolizer (EM) phenotype. Poor metabolizers (PM) possess two of the known 60 mutant CYP2D6 mutant alleles. The clinical importance of genetically variable function is for the response of a given drug or chemical. The significance is the role of CYP2D6 in governing the fate of a compound, its therapeutic window and its use in clinical practice.

Pharmacogenetics is the study of the hereditary basis for differences in a populations' response to a drug. The same dose of a drug will result in elevated plasma concentrations for some patients and low concentrations for others. Some patients will respond well to the drugs, while others will not. A drug might be toxic to some patients but not to others.

Researchers can identify candidate genes that might influence the effectiveness of a drug and look for polymorphisms that correlate with a certain clinical outcome. Most polymorphisms simply contribute to individual diversity, including a variable affinity for drugs. High-throughput technologies like DNA chips will allow simultaneous analysis of thousands of genes for thousands of people, providing information that could then be correlated with clinical outcomes data. An interesting polymorphism could then be examined in prospective and/or retrospective clinical trials of a drug.

PHARMACOGENETICS IN CARDIOLOGY

The 2D6 mutation in the group of CYP drug metabolising enzymes is responsible for the metabolism of a large number of cardiac drugs like beta-blockers. Beta-blockers are used for the treatment of both hypertension and congestive heart failure. Poor metabolizers can have two to three-fold higher plasma concentrations and can have a higher rate of side effects like dizziness.

Another example of the importance of pharmacogenetics is the 2C9 enzyme and warfarin. About one percent of Caucasians and Africans are poor metabolizers. Patients that take warfarin and that do not have the particular active gene, 2C9, ought to be on a dose of about five milligrams a week as rather than the normal dose of five milligrams a day.

PHARMACOGENETICS IN NEUROLOGY

Treatment of Alzheimer's Disease

There are two major forms of Alzheimer's disease, familial and sporadic. The sporadic form comprises 85% of all cases worldwide, and 50 to 60% of these cases have been linked to the apolipoprotein gene.

Apolipoprotein E (ApoE) appears to modulate Alzheimer's pathology. There is a clear association with the number of ApoE4 isoforms a person has and the risk of developing the disease, the age of onset, and the accumulation of brain markers of Alzheimer's. Two copes of E-4 are linked to an Alzheimer's disease that starts roughly at 60 years of age. One copy of E-4 produces an Alzheimer's disease that starts around the age of 75 years old. And for those patients with no copies of E-4, the age of onset is normally around 85 years. For example, on looking at genotype and drug response, the non-ApoE4 subjects responded quite well to a drug called Tacrine, while the ApoE4 subjects did not. Those drugs designed to stimulate the cholinergic system tend to work well in the non-E4 patient, whereas those agents that are non-cholinergic will work in the E4 subject.

PHARMACOGENETICS IN ENVIRONMENTAL MEDICINE

Human disease is the consequence of both genetic susceptibility and environmental exposure. By identifying the genes and variants that affect the individual response to environmental toxins, we can better predict health risk. People with a polymorphism that makes them more susceptible, however, will have a much higher risk. People with one kind of p53 polymorphism, for example, will have a higher risk of cervical cancer if they get exposed to human papilloma virus.

Environmental carcinogens are metabolically activated or inactivated by metabolizer enzymes like the variants of Cytochrome P450. Some human population studies have also shown that CYP polymorphisms like CYP2D6 are linked to a higher incidence of various cancers. CYP2E1 is a major CYP enzyme and has several known polymorphisms that have been linked to cancers of the lung, stomach, liver, and nasopharynx.

Normal Drug Metabolism

There is a common sequence of events in the normal metabolism of any drug. The drug after being absorbed from the gastrointestinal tract enters into the blood stream and is distributed to various tissues and tissue fluids. The final step of excretion of the drug takes place through organs like the liver, the kidney or the lungs. The drugs undergo biochemical reactions like conjugation, glucuronidation or acetylation to increase their solubility and facilitate their excretion through different channels. Some are completely oxidized to CO_2, which is exhaled through the lungs; others are excreted via kidneys into the urine, or by the liver into the bile and then into feces.

Pharmacokinetics

The aim of drug therapy is to control, cure or prevent disease. To achieve this goal, therapeutic non-toxic levels need to be delivered to the target tissues. Four pathways of drug modification control the speed of onset, duration and intensity of drug action. These pathways include drug absorption, distribution, metabolisation and elimination of the drug. Pharmacokinetics is defined as the quantitative time dependant changes of both the plasma drug concentration and the total amount of drug in the body.

Pharmacokinetics is the study of the metabolism and effects of a particular drug. It involves giving a standard dose of the drug and monitoring its bioavailability and the response to that particular dosage. Several such studies when conducted earlier showed considerable differences in the bioavailability of the same drug in different patients having same phenotype. This is due to variability in response. Using statistical methods this variability shows a form of continuous or discontinuous distribution.

Target Selection

The pharmaceutical industry is concerned with validation of target data that will predict the tolerance and the effectiveness of the drug in question. Existing data of those drugs, which have proved their efficacy in humans, forms the basis of such a study.

Two broad strategies are involved in the identification and expression of genes through their proteins. Two types of terminologies are used for this study. The first is discovery genetics, where disease related genes are identified from human disease populations. The second is discovery genomics where bases of DNA sequences from families of genes are used for screening purposes.

The information on disease susceptibility genes of patients is very important and is relevant to the patient's genetic contribution to the disease. In order to identify the products of gene expression, it becomes necessary to compare differential metabolisms related to the relevant gene variants with that of a control population. Critical enzymes or receptors associated with the altered metabolism are then used as targets. This helps in the understanding of the role of specific susceptibility gene variants on appropriate cellular metabolisms. With the help of reverse Genetic Engineering, it is again possible to find out the expressed protein sequence from affected tissues or cells from an affected population and compare it with the same data in a healthy population.

With the genomic approach, it becomes necessary not only to validate tissue distribution of the gene, but also correlate the corresponding disease or the clinical indication. On the other hand using the genetic approach, the susceptible gene is automatically validated once the disease related variants are known. Modern research focusing on the relationship of a particular gene with the disease can lead to a greater understanding of pharmacogenetics.

HOW PHARMACOGENETICS CAN HELP IN MEDICAL PRACTICE

Genetic constitution of a person greatly influences the therapeutic responsiveness to drugs. Sometimes a drug or drug combinations may have synergistic effect. Individual and family history is used to indicate susceptibility before subjecting the patient to a drug. Some persons show adverse reaction to a drug, for example anaphylactic shock with penicillin. Some drugs may have a teratogenic effect or malignant type of action or mutagenic effect at a cellular level in certain genotypes.

By applying the results of pharmacogenetic research in clinical practice, physicians will be more confident about the patient's response to a specific medicine by using information from the patient's DNA. Polymorphisms in genes encoding P450 enzymes, N-acetyltransferase and other key enzymes in drug metabolism determine the bio availability of the drug in patient's blood, as a different population shows variation in the metabolism of ethanol, due to polymorphism in the enzyme alcohol dehydrogenase. In future, metabolic screens of genetic variants will be standardized so that it will be possible to have automated read-outs of a persons' predicted response to any medicine. These DNA based screens will not provide disease specific diagnosis but will help the physician in determining an optimum dose and avoid side effects.

SNP Mapping a Tool for Personalized Genetic Profiling

Single Nucleotide Polymorphisms (SNP's) can be defined as differences in a single base pair in the DNA sequence that is observed between individuals in a population. It is the simplest form of DNA polymorphism. SNPs are present throughout the human genome with an average frequency of approximately 1 in 1000 base pairs (bp). A SNP fine map will enable disease and drug response phenotypes to be mapped by linkage disequilibrium, which is the non-random association of susceptible disease gene and genetic markers. Linkage disequilibrium mapping is used to identify candidate genetic markers in the vicinity of the gene of interest. It is also now possible to narrow down the large size of the DNA region containing disease susceptible genes from a millions of base pairs to a few thousands. This fine mapping will help a quicker identification of disease susceptibility genes from a large chunk of DNA. For example, polymorphism of the apolipoprotein E (ApoE) gene is the first example of SNP linkage disequilibrium mapping to find out the locus around a known susceptibility gene for Alzheimer's disease. In 1997, a high-density SNP map for a region of 4 million bases around the ApoE locus on chromosome 19 was constructed. The next goal was to detect a small region of linkage disequilibrium as a susceptible locus associated with Alzheimer's disease. Moreover by using DNA from patients with Alzheimer's disease and controls, it is possible to detect those SNP's in linkage disequilibrium that are associated with the disease.

Today advanced DNA automated systems such as chip-based re-sequencing or microsphere-based analytical methodologies are available. With this it is possible to read out thousands of SNPs automatically. Chip technologies are now available for genotyping hundreds to a few thousand SNP's. Each chip contains profiles of abbreviated SNP linkage disequilibrium for a number of drugs, which are prescribed in similar clinical indications.

The abbreviated SNP linkage disequilibrium profiles predict a patient's response to medicines, but they do not specifically test the patient for the presence or absence of a disease gene-specific mutation. In addition they do not provide any disease predictive information about the patient or family members. In simple terms, medicine response profiles measure phenotypic responses to a medicine based on a pattern of inherited factors detected as small regions of linkage disequilibrium. From this abbreviated SNP linkage disequilibrium profiles, it is possible to find out, which SNP is responding to which drug in a specific disease. Similarly analysis of patients with identical disease phenotypes could be used to determine disease heterogeneity. Different SNP linkage disequilibrium profiles of patients with the same disease phenotype could define patterns of disease heterogeneity without necessarily identifying actual genes and alleles involved. As a result of disease heterogeneity, there can be large definable sub-groups of patients suffering with a common phenotype as in Alzheimer's disease where treatment can be varied. Focusing drug development on such or similar sub-groups with a disease specific diagnosis or a medicine response profile will provide opportunities to develop more medicines for a large proposition of patients with heterogeneous diseases.

Application of SNP mapping technology will help in the development of more effective medicines for clinical use by using abbreviated SNP linkage disequilibrium mapping. Medicine response profile is being identified in the phase II clinical trials. This will further lead to selection of patient groups for drug efficacy in phase III studies. This is likely to make these trials smaller, faster and more efficient. The phase II trials will enable identification of the location of genes contributing to heterogeneous forms of the disease, leading to the discovery of new medicines and additional susceptibility targets.

The application of pharmacogenetics to the delivery of medicines will maximize the value of each medicine. Medicines can then be prescribed to patients in anticipation of therapeutic response and a high probability of efficacy without significant adverse events by considering genetic constitution of patients. Using effective and well-tolerated medicines. The prevention or cure of a disease will be more frequent and it will be treated well in advance before it takes a chronic form. In consequence, the period for hospitalisation will also be reduced leading to a decrease in the costs of hospitalisation and long-term medical care. Thus genetic methods are useful in differentiating those patients who experience good efficacy and lower significant adverse events in response to a medicine from other patients who fail to respond and develop serious adverse effects. In future, pharmacogenetics will have a stronger impact on medicines and medical practice.

PHARMACOGENOMICS

While pharmacogenetics has to do with individuals' response to certain drugs, pharmacogenomics is a broader term used to describe the commercial application of genomic technology in drug development and therapy. Pharmacogenetics is probably the study of known polymorphisms and known metabolic enzyme families of known drug targets. It is the role of polymorphisms and candidate genes and drug therapy and toxicity. It will be the discovery of new drug response genes and development of novel molecules to target these genes. After genes are linked with disease pathogenesis, pharmacogenomics will validate targets as appropriate sites of therapeutic intervention. Then scientists will identify or design therapeutic agents that interact with these targets in a way that achieves positive clinical outcome and minimal toxicity. Genetic tests will be used to predict clinical progression, likeliness of therapeutic response, and environmental influences. This will be coupled with drug development that will be rationally based on our understanding of molecular pathogenesis. The role of genes in determining disease susceptibility, progression, complications, and its response to treatment will be equally important. Pharmacogenomics can identify the patients for whom a drug would be safe and effective and eliminate possible drug toxicity at "normal" doses in non-metabolisers.

By taking into account individual genetic makeup, dosages prescribed for individual patients may be adjusted on the basis of DNA polymorphism analysis, hastening recovery and reducing side effects. As pharmacogenetics develops, new drug development may result in drugs that exhibit less variation in their metabolic conversion rates or drugs for which pre-prescription DNA testing is available. The role of the clinical laboratory should be in applying pharmacogenetics to medical care. One role might be to develop genetic profiling strategies to maximize the sensitivity and specificity of tests in predicting phenotypes. Another role might be to reduce the cost of the test and the technical difficulty of the test.

CHAPTER 13

IMMUNOGENETICS

INTRODUCTION

The main function of immune system is to identify and attack foreign antigens. Knowledge of genes of the immune system is of clinical importance in studying the response to infection, study of autoimmune disease and transplantation technology. Most of the antigens are proteins, but some are polysaccharides and some nucleic acids. In addition to being the causative factor for a number of single gene disorders, the genes of the immune system provide models for study of gene expression. The genes of the immune system have great diversity in a few loci (Fig. 13.1).

There are two components to an immune response cellular and humoral. The thymus is the primary lymphoid organ where cells differentiate into thymus dependent or T cells. Lymphoid stem cells are present in the growing fetus. Lymphocytes in the secondary lymphoid organs like the spleen or in the cortical regions of the lymph nodes differentiate into B cells.

Cellular immunity is produced by T lymphocytes, and is responsible for homograft rejection and delayed hypersensitivity. The T lymphocyte cells have two functions, they act as cytotoxic or helper cells. The cytotoxic or killer lymphocytes are sensitized to destroy cell-bearing antigens produced by viral infections. The other group, helper lymphocytes are necessary for induction of antibody response by B-lymphocytes. A third group is called the suppresser lymphocytes, which suppress immune responses.

Humoral immunity is produced by differentiation of lymphocyte stem cells into plasma cells or B-lymphocytes. They

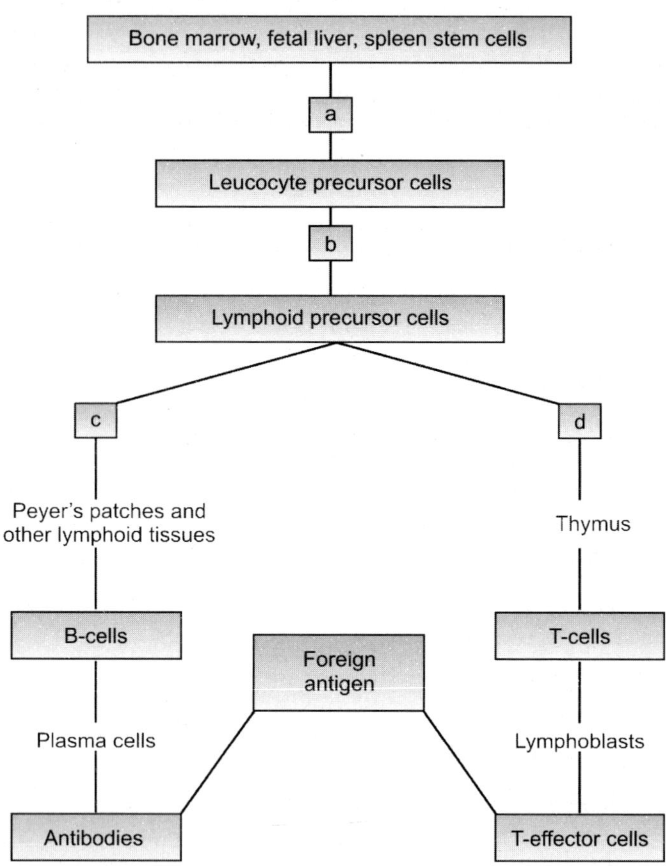

Fig. 13.1: Sites of blocks in the generation of immunodeficiency syndromes. (a) Reticular dysgenesis (b) severe combined immunodeficiency syndrome (c) Bruton's agamaglobulinemia (d) DiGeorge syndrome

are responsible for production of antibodies or immunoglobulins. The differentiation occurs in the fetal liver, spleen and bone marrow. These are the primary lymphoid organ sites where general hematopoiesis occurs. As this initially takes place in the Bursa of Fabricius (fetal equivalent of these tissues), they are known as B cells. Plasma cells are formed in the secondary lymphoid organs, the red pulp of the spleen and medulla of lymphoid nodes.

The T lymphocyte binds with the antigen through its receptor T cell on the surface of the cells, in conjunction with the major histocompatibility complex. A number of lymphokines are released, which promote division of polymorphonuclear leukocytes, macrophages and B-lymphocytes.

IMMUNOGLOBULINS

Immunoglobulins are antibodies, and form one of the important and major classes of serum proteins responsible for the body's defense mechanism against infection by its antigenic properties.

Structure of Immunoglobins

In any individual, an infinite number of different antibodies are encoded on the germline DNA. It is estimated that about 10^8 different antibodies are produced, even though the number of base pairs of DNA is only 3×10^6. This is because a relatively small number of genes in the germline that encode antibodies undergo a process of somatic rearrangement and recombination during B-cell development, which probably allows for the diversity.

The immunoglobulin molecule is made up of four polypeptide chains, two identical heavy chains (H) with 440 amino acids and two identical light chains (L) with 220 amino acids. These are held together in a Y shape by disulphite bonds (Fig. 3.2). A eolytic enzyme, papaine cuts immunoglobulin into three fragments, two of, which are similar, each containing an antibody site that can combine with a specific antigen. This is called antigen binding fragment or Fab. The third

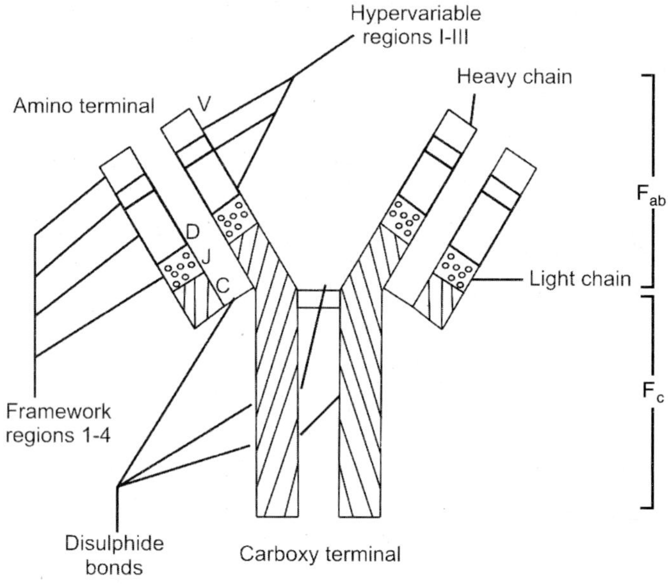

Fig. 13.2: Structure of an antibody molecule V is the variable region, D is the diversity region, J is the joining region, C is the constant region

fragment can be crystallized and is called Fc that binds complement and receptors or cell types involved in immune response.

The 'H' chains are sub divided into five isotopes, on the basis of structural differences at the carboxy terminal portion of the H chains. The Fab fragment is composed of L chains and linked with 'N' terminal portion of the H chains. The L chains are of two types, kappa (κ) or lambda (λ). The heavy chains are of five different classes ϒ, μ, ∝, δ and ε, and each

Table 13.1: Classes of immunoglobulin

Class	*Heavy chain*	*Light chain*	*Molecular weight*	*Property*
IgG	γ	κ or λ	150,000	Antibody activity to bacteria and viruses, only class to placental transfer
IgM	μ	κ or λ	900,000	Antibody activity to blood group and proteins. Placental transfer? Precedes IgG in immune response.
IgA	∝	κ or λ	170,000	Surface immunity (local), placental transfer likely
IgD	δ	κ or λ	185,000	Function not yet known.
IgE	ε	κ or λ	200,000	Allergic response

chain is specific for the five different classes of immunoglobulins IgG, IgM, IgA, IgD, and IgE. All five classes of immunoglobulin have two types of chains, and the molecular formula therefore reads λ_2, or k_2r_2. Table 13.1 gives outline of these immunoglobulin.

All normal individuals have the five classes of immunoglobulins. Their genetically determined variants have also been recognised. Those associated with the heavy chain of IgG are called G*m* systems, and the A*m* System is associated with IgA heavy chain. K*m* and I*nv* systems are associated with kappa light chain. The Oz system is for the λ light chain and the *Em* for IgE heavy chain. The *Gm* and *Km* systems are not interdependent and are polymorphic with frequent variations in different ethnic groups.

Immunoglobulin Diversity

Various combinations of heavy and light chains are responsible for immunoglobulin (antibody) diversity. Several genes would be required for this. In multiple myleoma, study of Bence Jones proteins revealed immunoglobulins have two regions. Variable region V, and constant region C. Region V is further subdivided into four regions. These are further subdivided into three regions, which show great variation, and are called hypervariable region. DNA studies have shown that segments coding for the V and C regions, are separated by a J region, which joins the two. DNA sequencing of heavy chain genes shows that they are coded by four different DNA segments, one each for V, D, C, and J.

Chromosomal Locations of Immunoglobulins

Immunoglobulins have their locations on autosomes 14, 2, and 22. Their synthesis is an exception to the one gene-one polypeptide theory, as V and C regions of each chain are coded differently by different genes.

INHERITED IMMUNOGENETIC DISORDERS

Immunodeficiency disorders can be divided into primary immunodeficiency disorders, which are usually genetically determined and secondary immunodeficiency disorders. Primary immunodeficiency disorders affect specific immunity or non-specific host defense mechanisms mediated by complement proteins and phagocytosis.

Primary immunodeficiencies are divided into several groups:

1. Deficiency of phagocytic cell function
2. Deficiency of a complement protein
3. Deficiency of B cell development or function
4. Deficiency of T cell development or function
5. Combined B and T cell deficiencies

DEFICIENCY OF PHAGOCYTIC CELL FUNCTION

Another mechanism involved in the body's defense system is chemotaxis and phagocytosis responsible for cell mediated killing of micro organisms. The disorders seen include Chronic granulomatous disease, leucocyte adhesion deficiency, glucose 6 phospahte dehydrogenase deficiency (which involves a defect in the hexose monophoshate shunt), myeloperoxidase deficiency (a granule enzyme deficiency), and Chediak Higashi syndrome (a granule structural defect which manifests with recurrent infection with bacteria due to chemotactic and degranulation defects). A few of these are discussed below.

Chronic Granulomatous Disease

The molecular defect is deficiency of NADPH oxidase. Chronic granulomatous disease (CGD) is inherited as an X-linked or autosomal recessive disorder. Due to a disorder of phagocytic function patients get recurrent catalase positive bacterial or fungal infections. There is high childhood mortality, unless supportive treatment with prophylactic antibiotics is used. CGD is diagnosed by an abnormal nitroblue tetrazolium test (NBT). The test is based on the increase in metabolic activity of normal granulocytes after phagocytosis, and the absence of such an increase in CGD.

Leucocyte Adhesion Deficiency

Individuals with leucocyte adhesion deficiency have an increased susceptibility to bacterial infections of skin and mucous membranes, which can be life threatening. The cause of increased susceptibility is due to inability of phagocytosed cells to migrate, as a result of adhesion related functions like chemotaxis and phagocytosis, and absence of the B_2 integrin receptor. Bone marrow transplant is the treatment of choice;

however antibiotics are required prophylactically until this can be done.

DEFICIENCY OF A COMPLEMENT PROTEIN

The complement system is a complex system of nine distinct serum proteins designated C_1 through C_9 that require serial activation through the classical or alternative pathways. The interaction of various components of complement often called as Complement Cascade results in increased inflammation and vascular permeability. Patients with complement protein deficiencies are susceptible to different diseases depending on which component is missing, since different complement proteins have different biological functions. Frequent modes of presentation for complement component deficiencies are collagen vascular diseases for C_1 through C_4, disseminated infections with pyogenic bacteria for C_3, and disseminated Neisserial infections for C_5 through C_8. The most common deficiency is that of the C_1 esterase inhibitor of the complement system. This causes hereditary angioneurotic edema, described below.

Angioneurotic Edema

Angioneurotic edema is inherited as an autosomal dominant disorder. This is a severe condition and is characterized by recurrent episodes of edema of the skin, throat or gut which is life threatening and poses a challenge for treatment. The condition occurs due to deficiency of an inhibitor of the first component of complement C_1. The deficiency lies either in the total amount of inhibitor, or lack of functional activity in the normal amounts of inhibitor. The treatment consists of infusion with normal fresh-frozen plasma during an acute attack. The androgenic drug Danazol and E-dminocaproic acid can be used to prevent the attacks.

DEFICIENCY OF B CELL DEVELOPMENT OR FUNCTION

These include transient neonatal hypogammaglobulinemia, common variable immunodeficiency, selective IgA deficiency, and Bruton's agammaglobulinemia, discussed below.

Bruton type Agammaglobulinemia

This is an X-linked immunodeficiency syndrome, due to failure of pre-B cells to differentiate into B cells. Clinically, the affected babies have multiple bacterial infections of the skin and respiratory system. There is some protection in first few months of life due to placental transfer of maternal IgG. Prognosis is fair with antibiotics and intravenous immunoglobulins, but children can die due to repeated lung infections leading to respiratory failure. Diagnosis is confirmed by the absence of B lymphocytes. The genetic defect is a mutation is in the tyrosine kinase gene (*btk*).

DEFICIENCY OF T CELL DEVELOPMENT OR FUNCTION

DiGeorge Syndrome

In this syndrome children present with recurrent viral infections due to an abnormality in cellular immunity, characterized by reduced or absent T lymphocytes as a result of absence of the thymus gland. There are other congenital malformations noted in these children, like congenital heart disease and absent parathyroids. Individuals have tetany due to low serum calcium levels. Embryologically there are abnormalities of the third and fourth pharyngeal arches as a result of a deletion on chromosome 22 at 22q11.2. Routine chromosomal studies do not reveal this abnormality and fluorescent *in situ* hybridization technique is necessary for visualization of this defect.

COMBINED B AND T CELL DEFICIENCIES

Severe Combined Immunodeficiency (SCID)

SCID occurs due to a severe abnormality in cellular and humoral immunity, leading to increased susceptibility to bacterial and viral infections in infancy. SCID can be inherited as an X-linked form or autosomal recessive form due to adenosine deaminase or purine nucleoside phosphorylase deficiency.

The X-linked form occurs due to mutation in the lambda chain and the interleukin IL-2 receptor. In the autosomal recessive form, there is a deficiency of the enzyme adenosine deaminase or purine nucleoside phosphorylase. This deficiency occurs in more than 2/3 of the individuals. Other types of autosomal recessive forms of SCID occur due to mutations in the lymphocyte cytokine receptor or the T cell receptor. The class II genes of major histocompatibility complex are also associated with it. Children with the autosomal recessive form of SCID have cellular and humoral immunity with deficiency of granulocytes. Death occurs in the first year of life. Until recently the only available treatment was bone marrow transplant. However, today the treatment of choice is gene therapy and the first successful gene therapy recipient now being 9 yr of age.

Wiskott-Aldrich Syndrome

This is an X-linked disorder, and has several associated immunodeficiencies, in which T cells remain nonresponsive to antigens. Lymphocyte numbers are near normal, but the antibody is catabolized rapidly, showing abnormal substances. Affected males have eczema, diarrhea, repeated infections, thrombocytopenia and low Serum IgM levels bone marrow transplants are helpful in these cases, however death due to hemorrhage or B cell malignancies is common, especially in untreated cases.

Ataxia Telangectasia

This is a neurological disease associated with immunodeficiency. Children with ataxia telangectasia present with cerebellar ataxia (difficulty in control of movements and balance), dilated blood vessels of the face and conjunctiva, and pulmonary infections with a hypoplastic thymus. IgA levels are low.

Laboratory diagnosis is made by demonstration of low or absent serum IgA and IgG. Cytogenetic studies show characteristic abnormalities called chromosomal instability (Fig. 13.3). Individuals suffering from ataxia telangectasia have an increased risk of developing leukemia or lymphoid malignancies.

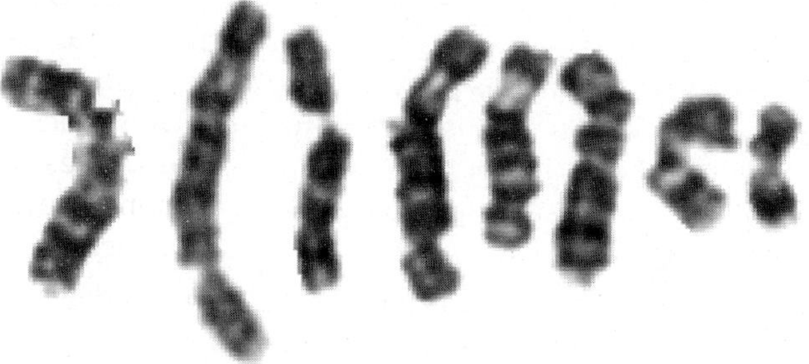

Fig. 13.3: Breaks observed in ataxia telangectasia

Blood Groups

Red cells have antigenic factors on their cell surface, and the significance of this led to safe blood transfusions, as well as prevention of Rhesus hemolytic disease of the newborn. So far about 400 blood group antigens have been described, and of these the best known are the ABO and Rhesus blood group systems.

ABO BLOOD GROUPS

Landsteiner in 1900 discovered ABO blood groups, when it was observed that sometimes transfusion of red blood cells from some persons to other leads to rapid hemolysis suggesting their blood was incompatible.

Four major blood groups have been identified A, B, AB and O. Individuals with A blood group have antigen A on the surface, B with have antigen B, AB have A and B antigens, while individuals with blood group O have neither. This means individuals with A blood group have anti B antibodies, B will have anti A and with O have both anti A and anti B antibodies in their blood.

ABO blood groups are an example of co-dominance. This means that alleles at the ABO blood group locus for antigens A and B are inherited in a co-dominant manner, but are dominant to the gene for the O antigen. Blood groups thus have genotypes which are homo and heterozygous for A and B which means we can have AA, AO, BB, BO.

Individuals with blood group AB will not produce A or B antibodies and therefore can receive blood transfusion from individuals of all ABO blood groups. They are therefore called universal recipients. Similarly individuals with O blood group do not express A or B antigens on red cells and are referred to as universal donors.

Molecular Aspects of ABO Blood Groups

Basic blood groups A, B and AB have enzymes with glycosyltransferase activity, which converts a basic blood group known an antigen H, into A or B antigen. A and B blood groups have a difference of seven single base substitutions which result in different A and B transferase activities. The A allele is associated with the addition of an N acetyl galactoseaminyl group and the B allele with a D galactosyl group. The O allele results from single base pair deletion resulting in an inactive protein, which cannot alter the H antigen.

Most people secrete the ABO blood group into body fluids like saliva ,sweat, plasma and semen. This is due to a secretor locus on the short arm of chromosome 19.There are two alleles, Se, and se, hence three genotypes are possible. SeSe, Sese, and sese. The recessive homozygotes are unable to secrete their blood group substances into body fluids. This is thus determined as an autosomal dominant trait.

RHESUS BLOOD GROUP

The Rhesus (Rh) system is of importance in clinical practice because of its role in hemolytic disease of the newborn, as well as incompatibility arising in blood transfusion. The system was discovered by conducting experiments on Rhesus monkeys, thus the name Rh. Phenotypically there are two main rhesus blood groups, Rhesus positive and Rhesus negative. Rhesus positive individuals possess Rhesus antigen on their red cells and other tissues. Rhesus negative persons do not possess the same. The location of the rhesus group gene complex is on chromosome 1. Rh alleles are closely linked, and each allele has a specific polypeptide chain with multiple antigenic sites. Rh alleles have approximately eight antigenic combinations.

In clinical practice, the main significance of the Rh system is that Rh negative persons form anti Rh antibodies against Rh positive red blood cells. One has to remember that Rh negative females must be given Rh negative blood. If an Rh negative woman is pregnant and the father of the child is Rh positive, she can develop antibodies which in turn can produce hemolysis of the fetal red blood cells. This risk can be minimized by giving Rh immunogolulin injections during pregnancy, delivery, and after fetal tissue sampling, especially when the placenta is intervened, as in chorionic villus sampling and fetal blood sampling or in termination of the pregnancy.

Hemolytic Disease of the Newborn (HDN)

This disorder, once considered to be the most common genetic disease, has now become rare, as Rh immunoglobulin injections are readily available. During pregnancy, small volumes of fetal blood crosses the placental barrier to reach maternal blood stream ,stimulating the maternal cells to form antibodies. In HDN, due to these antibodies produced by maternal blood, fetal red blood cells are damaged, resulting in serious consequences. HDN can occur due to either Rh incompatibility where mother is Rh negative and the fetus Rh positive, or ABO incompatibility where mother is O and the fetus is type A or B. This is much milder and no treatment is required.

Transplantation Genetics

Organ transplantation has an become an integral part of clinical medicine. Corneal grafts and bone grafts are easily accepted by the body, but for other organ transplants, it is essential to have antigenic similarity between the donor and the recipient, otherwise there is rejection of the graft. Immune rejection remains the major barrier to successful tissue and organ transplantation. The basis for this is that the major histocompatibility complex (MHC) molecules, which all T cells must recognize in order to respond to foreign or abnormal peptide antigens are highly polymorphic in the human population. These are described below.

THE MAJOR HISTOCOMPATIBILITY COMPLEX (MHC)

The major histocompatibility complex is a highly polymorphic gene cluster on the short arm of chromosome 6 (6p21.3), which is responsible for regulating immune response. The genes for this cluster are 70 closely linked loci, and are called the HLA system. These code for the human leukocyte or HLA antigens.

These are divided into class I (A B C E F and G), class II (DR, DQ, and DP) and class III genes.

HUMAN LEUKOCYTE ANTIGEN (HLA) SYSTEM

The HLA system consists of highly polymorphic sites, hence phenotypic variation is high. The HLA phenotype of two unrelated individuals is highly unlikely to be exact. Various serological methods are used to define HLA patterns of an individual. Currently to this group of tests, DNA diagnostic tests have been added. As the HLA loci are closely linked they are inherited *en block*. HLA alleles of an individual are called haplotypes, and will be present on both the number 6 chromosomes. Due to segregation at meiosis each will have a 25% chance of sharing the same gene with a sib thus antigenically have more similarity than the parents, and therefore preferred for organ transplantations.

HLA AND DISEASE

Due to the extensive polymorphism of MHC molecules, they can serve as markers for disease susceptibility, if a disease gene were linked to the MHC. The different antigen presenting abilities of different individual MHC molecules might protect some individuals from disease while making others highly susceptible.

Certain HLA antigens show striking associations with certain diseases Table 13.2. The best known is the association of ankylosing spondylitis with HLAB27. While only 7% of the population has B27, the frequency in patients with ankylosing spondylitis is 95%. Other significant associations include HLADR3 and HLADR4 in insulin dependant diabetes mellitus, HLADR2 in multiple sclerosis, HLADR7 in psoriasis, HLAB27 in Reiter disease, HLADR7 in Rheumatoid arthritis and HLADR3 and HLAB8 in systemic lupus erythematosus.

Table 13.2: HLA associated diseases and symptoms

Disease	*Symptoms*	*Antigen*
Ankylosing spondylitis	Inflammation and ossification of ligaments causing fusion of sacroiliac joint.	HLAB27
Insulin dependent diabetes mellitus	Raised blood sugar due to insulin deficiency	HLADR3, HLADR4
Multiple sclerosis	Chronic inflammatory demyelinating disease of the central nervous system	HLADR7
Myasthenia gravis	Neuromuscular junction disease	DR2/DR3
Systemic lupus Erythematous	Multiorgan connective tissue disorder	HLADR3, HLAB8
Reiters syndrome	Conjunctivitis, urethritis, arthritis	HLAB27
Rheumatoid arthritis	Collagen disease affecting small joints in children or adults	HLADR7

CHAPTER 14

CANCER GENETICS

INTRODUCTION

A neoplasm is an abnormal tissue, which grows when normal cellular control mechanisms fail. A neoplasm can involve any tissue of the body and may be benign or malignant. The etiology of most neoplasms is multifactorial. Both inherited and non-inherited factors are involved in the pathogenesis. Non-inherited factors are genetic somatic mutations, which act as the main components in the development of a neoplastic process. Some malignant neoplasms have predisposing factors, which are inherited as Mendelian traits. In these cases neoplasms have an earlier age of onset. The specific abnormalities are characteristic of specific Mendelian patterns, suggesting that some predisposing factors responsible for neoplasm are heritable.

MENDELIAN TRAITS

a. Autosomal dominant traits include conditions such as neurofibromatosis type I, multiple endocrine neoplasia, inherited breast cancer, familial polyposis coli, and hereditary non-polyposis colon cancer (HNPCC).
b. Autosomal recessive traits are seen in abnormalities of DNA or chromosome repair. Affected individuals show an increased frequency of abnormal DNA repair or increased chromosomal breakage. Some examples of these are xeroderma pigmentosum, Fanconi's anemia, and ataxia telangectasia.

c. Sex linked traits include the immunodeficiency syndromes. In this group affected individuals have congenital abnormalities of immunologic function and traits, which are inherited as autosomal or sex linked. Examples include X-linked agammaglobulinemia, and Wiskott–Aldrich syndrome.

Some examples of single gene disorders with cancer as a complication include skin carcinomas in xeroderma pigmentosum, lymphomas in ataxia telangiectasia, acute leukemia's in Down syndrome, renal embryonic tumors in Wilm's tumor, colonic adenocarcinomas in familial adenomatosis polyposis, breast carcinomas in hereditary breast cancer, cerebellar hemangioblastomas and renal carcinomas in Von Hippel Lindau disease, fibrosarcomas and optic gliomas in neurofibromatosis type 1, acoustic neuromas, schwannomas and meningiomas in neurofibromatosis type 2, retinal embryonic tumors in retinoblastoma, renal angiomyolipomas, cardiac rhabdomyomata and giant cell astrocytomas in tuberous sclerosis, pheochromocytoma and medullary thyroid carcinoma in multiple endocrine neoplasia type IIa and IIb.

CHROMOSOME ABNORMALITIES AND NEOPLASIA

Constitutional Chromosomal Abnormalities

Some constitutional chromosome abnormalities (i.e. inherited abnormalities that are present in every cell of the body) show an increased frequency of certain kind of malignancies in a proportion of patients. Examples of these include leukemia in patients with Down syndrome, retinoblastomas in patients with a, deletion of chromosome 13 (13q14.1) (Fig. 14.1) and Wilms tumor in patients with a deletion of chromosome 11p13.

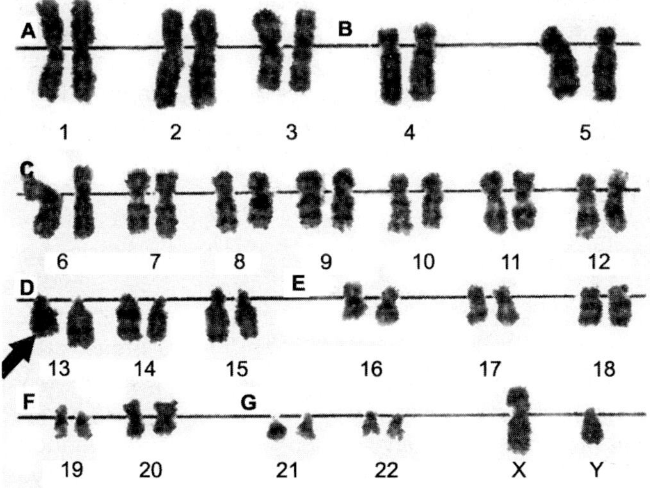

Fig. 14.1: Karyotype of a patient with retinoblastoma. The arrow shows short chromosome 13 due to interstitial deletion of 13q 14

Acquired Chromosome Abnormalities

Each tumor results from one or more mutations of cellular DNA. These are seen in most malignant neoplasms. Patients do not have a constitutional chromosomal abnormality; instead, the tumor tissue acquires mutations. An example of this is chronic myelogenous leukaemia (CML). The chromosome abnormalities noted is a translocation between chromosomes 9 and 22, der(22)t(9;22),(Fig. 14.2) commonly known as Philadelphia chromosome.

Certain cells exhibit different karyotypic abnormalities in a single neoplasm, but the progenitor may be the same. As the neoplasm progresses, the karyotype tends to become more

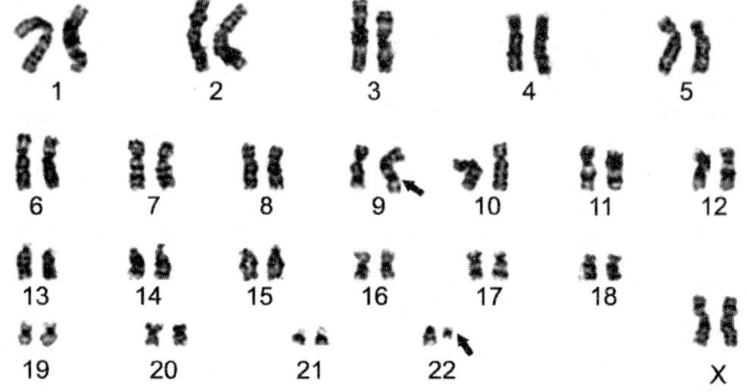

Fig. 14.2: Karyotype of a patient with chronic myeloid leukaemia. A part of chromosome 22 is translocated on to the long arm of chromosome number 9

abnormal. Karyotype abnormalities usually precede clinical sign of relapse.

Clonal Origin

The majority of malignant neoplasms are of clonal origin. That means all of the neoplastic cells originate from a single progenitor, which is abnormal. Malignancies occur as a multistep neoplastic process.

Telomeres and Cancer

After a fixed number of cell divisions, normal cells become arrested in a terminally non-dividing state known as cellular senescence. With each cell division, there is shortening of the telomeres at the ends of chromosomes. Once the chromosomes are shortened beyond a certain point, the loss of telomere function leads to end-to-end chromosome fusion and cell death. In germ cells, telomere shortening is prevented by the sustained function of the enzyme telomerase, thus explaining the ability of these cells to self-replicate extensively. Telomerase is absent from most somatic cells and hence they suffer progressive loss of telomeres. In cancer cells, telomerase activity has been detected in a vast majority of human tumors.

THE ROLE OF THE ENVIRONMENT AND GENES IN CANCER

Molecular studies have confirmed the genetic basis of both sporadic and heritable cancer.

The role of the environment in the development of cancer has also been clearly established. The role of factors such as chemical carcinogens, radiation energy, chronic irritation, hormones, parasites and oncogenic viruses in the development of cancer has also been established. Environmental predisposing factors leading to cancer may be occupational, like prolonged exposure to carcinogenic chemicals. Examples include bladder cancer in aniline dye workers, lung cancer in asbestos workers or skin cancer in tar workers. Genetic predisposition such as heredity, age, pigmentation, sex, and tumor immunity are also responsible factors. Cancers like those of the breast, ovary and colon are known to have a strong familial predisposition.

PREDISPOSING GENETIC FACTORS IN CANCER

Carcinogenesis is a multistep process, at both the phenotypic and genetic levels. Phenotypically, a malignant neoplasm shows excessive growth, local invasiveness and ability to metastasise. At the molecular level, accumulation of mutations in genes and chromosomes result in tumor progression.

In cancer genetics, genes acting as predisposing factors for carcinogenesis are grouped into four main classes. These groups are growth-promoting oncogenes, tumor suppressor genes, genes that regulate programmed cell death or apoptosis and DNA repair genes.

ONCOGENES

Oncogenes are derived from proto-oncogenes, which are cellular genes that promote normal growth and differentiation. They were first recognised, as genes of tumor causing viruses that are responsible for the process of transformation. *v-onc* denotes viral oncogene and *c-onc* denotes cellular counterpart of a viral oncogene. Proto-oncogene conversion to oncogenes commonly occurs at the somatic level and causes sporadic cancers. A known germline mutation in the *ret* oncogene is responsible for multiple endocrine neoplasia type IIa, which is inherited as a dominant pattern.

Oncogene products can be grouped into five classes:

1. Protein tyrosine kinases such as *abl* (Abelson murine leukemia virus) and *src* (Rous/avian sarcoma virus)
2. Growth factors such as *sis* (simian sarcoma virus)
3. Growth factor receptors such as *erbB* (avian erythroblastosis virus)
4. Guanyl nucleotide binding proteins or G proteins such as *H-ras* (Harvey murine sarcoma virus) and *K-ras* (Kirsten murine sarcoma virus)
5. Transcription factors/DNA binding proteins such as *myc* (avian myelocytomatosis virus) and *fos* (FBJ osteosarcoma virus).

In tumor cells, oncogenes act in a dominant fashion. Mechanisms by which proto-oncogenes become oncogenes include:

1. *Point mutations:* A large number of human tumors carry point mutations in the *ras* group of oncogenes.
2. *Chromosomal rearrangements including translocations:* Alteration in chromosome number and structure is well

documented in leukemia's lymphomas, and solid tumors. Certain chromosomes are more involved and are specific to the type of malignancy. Chromosomal translocations result in rearrangements in the vicinity of the region of proto-oncogenes. These rearrangements lead to chimeric fusion and alteration in biochemical functions. Over 100 translocations are associated with carcinogenesis. An example of translocation is in Burkitt's lymphoma, where there is a translocation of the *c-myc* gene from chromosome 8 to chromosome 14 next to the immunoglobulin heavy chain gene. Another example of an oncogene activated by translocation is in chronic myeloid leukemia, where there is formation of the Philadelphia chromosome. This is a reciprocal translocation between chromosomes 9 and 22 where a portion of the *c-abl* oncogene from chromosome 9 is translocated to *bcr* on chromosome 22.

3. *Gene amplification:* Activation of proto-oncogenes may result in amplification of their DNA sequences. In some cases the amplified genes produce cytogenetic changes that can be seen microscopically, called *double minutes* (*dms*) or *homogenous staining regions* (*HSRs*). Examples of gene amplification include the *n-myc* gene in neuroblastoma and the *c-erbB2* gene in breast cancers.

TUMOR SUPPRESSOR GENES

Normal cells contain genes with tumor suppressor activity, which when lost or inactivated can lead to malignancy.

Tumor suppressor genes include the following categories:

1. Molecules that regulate nuclear transcription and the cell cycle. These include the retinoblastoma gene (*Rb*), and the *p53* gene.
2. Molecules that regulate signal transduction. These include the products of the gene for neurofibromatosis type-1 (*NF1*) and the gene for familial adenomatosis coli (*APC*)

3. Other tumor suppressor genes. These include genes for neurofibromatosis type 2 (*NF2*), the gene for von Hippel Lindau disease (*VHL*), and the gene for Wilms' tumor (*WT-1*).

Some of the disorders caused by these genes are discussed in more detail below.

Retinoblastoma (Rb)

This is a rare highly malignant disorder of the retinal cells and leads to blindness and death if undetected. It affects approximately 1 in 20,000 children. Unilateral tumors are mostly sporadic while bilateral tumors are hereditary, in which mutation or loss of both normal copies of *Rb* genes are required to produce retinoblastoma. Bilateral tumors, which are hereditary, follow Knudsen's two hit hypothesis. This hypothesis states, that in bilateral tumors, the first mutation is non functional and present in all the cells while a second gene at the same locus becomes inactivated somatically in the developing retina. This suggests that the retinoblastoma gene acts recessively as a tumor suppressor gene. The mode of inheritance for retinoblastoma is autosomal dominant with incomplete penetrance. 80-90% of children who inherit the autosomal gene develop retinoblastoma. 5% of children with retinoblastoma have some associated physical abnormalities. Cytogenetic analyses of affected children show an interstitial deletion of the long arm of one of the pair of chromosome 13 at 13q14.

Wilms Tumor

Wilms' tumor commonly occurs unilaterally and its occurrence is sporadic. 20% of bilateral tumors show hereditary occurrence in at least 1% of the cases. The clinical features include aniridia, genitourinary abnormalities and mental retardation in a few cases. Some cases show identification of an interstitial deletion of chromosome 11 (11p13) and the gene *WT1* acts as a tumor suppressor gene.

von Hippel Lindau Disease (VHL)

It is inherited as a multisystem disorder characterized by abnormal growth of blood vessels. This results in the development of hemangioblastomas throughout the brain, especially in the cerebellum, retina and spinal cord. Renal, hepatic, adrenal and pancreatic cysts are known to occur. The *VHL* gene on chromosome 3 is a tumor suppressor gene and is inherited in an autosomal dominant fashion. If the gene is lost or mutated then its inhibitory effect on cell growth is lost or diminished which in combination with defects in other regulatory proteins can lead to cancerous growths.

Colorectal Cancer

Colorectal tumors progress through a series of stages ranging from benign adenomatous polyps to malignant carcinomas. This progression is the result of a series of genetic changes that involve activation of oncogenes and inactivation of tumor suppressor genes. Colorectal cancer typifies the multistep nature of the biology and pathogenesis of cancers in general. In general, colorectal carcinoma is thought to originate mainly from adenomas. A combination of at least six genetic events are involved in the pathogenesis of colorectal cancer. The initial event is a germline or somatic mutation in the *APC* gene, a tumor suppressor gene located on 5q21. The next stage involves loss of heterozygosity (LOH) of the second *APC* gene. Activation of two recessive oncogenes (*Ras* genes, *KRAS1* on chromosome 6p12-11 and *KRAS2* on chromosome 12p12) has been associated with this transformation. Loss of the *DCC* (deleted in colorectal carcinoma) tumor suppressor genes, located at 18q21.3, and mutation in the DNA sequences at 5q21-22

(*MCC*, mutated in colorectal carcinoma) are also seen. The final step into a cancerous state is the result of mutations in the tumor suppressor gene, *p53* located on chromosome 17p12-13. The transition to metastatic carcinoma involves mutations in the two RAS genes, *KRAS1* and *KRAS2*. The exact order of genetic changes described above varies, although some mutations occur more frequently as an early event, while other mutations typically happen later in the process. It is the accumulation of genetic mutations, which is important in colorectal cancer development.

Of all colon cancers that are diagnosed in the United States, most are sporadic, with no family history of colon cancer. However, up to 10% of colon cancers are thought to be due to an inherited gene mutation that may be passed directly from generation to generation. Familial adenomatosis polyposis (FAP) and hereditary non-polyposis coli (HNPCC) are types of inherited colon cancer.

FAP is inherited as an autosomal dominant disorder and carries a high risk of malignancy. Patients with FAP develop hundreds of benign colorectal tumors, some of which will progress to carcinomas. FAP is associated with germline mutations of the *APC* gene on chromosome 5q. In addition, the *APC* gene mutations also occur somatically in over 60% sporadic colorectal tumors. Mutations in the *APC* gene can be identified in tumors as small as 0.5 cm in diameter.

HNPCC is also inherited in an autosomal dominant manner. The genes implicated in the genetic susceptibility to HNPCC are called mismatch repair genes or *MMR* genes. These genes act as spellcheckers to ensure that the sequence of DNA is correct as genes are duplicated during the cell cycle. The *MMR* genes are responsible for repairing mistakes in the DNA sequence so that each new cell receives a correct set of genes. Within HNPCC families, mutations in four different *MMR* genes have been identified. Mutation in the gene, *hMSH2*, located on chromosome 2, accounts for 31% of HNPCC families. Mutation in the gene, *hMLH1*, located on chromosome 3, account for 33% of HNPCC families. Mutations in the *hPMS1* (chromosome 2) and *hPMS2* (chromosome 7) genes appear to account for 2% and 4% of HNPCC families, respectively.

Breast Cancer

Breast cancer is the most frequently diagnosed cancer in Western women. Numerous risk factors for the development of breast cancer have been identified. 20% of women with breast cancer have a family history of the disease, and 5% of these are attributable to mutations in two genes. Mutations in the *BRCA1* or *BRCA2* genes increase susceptibility to develop breast and/or ovarian cancer. The *BRCA1* gene is on chromosome 17q21 and families with germ-line mutations in *BRCA1* have an autosomal dominant inheritance in the pattern of breast cancer as well an increased incidence of ovarian cancer. Mutations in *BRCA1* account for 20-30% of the inherited breast cancers. The *BRCA2* gene is located on chromosome 13q12-13. Families with germ-line mutations in *BRCA2* account for 10-20% of inherited breast cancers. The pattern of breast cancer inheritance for *BRCA2* is autosomal dominant, an increased incidence of ovarian cancer that is less striking than that with *BRCA1* and an increased incidence of male breast cancer.

Many somatic mutations are believed to be responsible for the development of breast cancer. Oncogenes *erbB1*, *erbB2*, *myc* and *int2* are responsible for the malignancy. Loss of heterozygosity for a number of chromosomes for example 1q, 3p, 11p, and 13q is also seen.

Neurofibromatosis Types 1 and 2

Neurofibromatosis type 1 (NF1) also known as von Recklinghausen's disease and has an incidence of 1:3000. It is commonly inherited in an autosomal dominant manner. Patients present with café au lait patches, cutaneous neurofibromas, Lisch nodules of the iris, axillary freckling and optic gliomas. 5% of the affected people show malignancies including neurofibrosarcomas and embryonal tumors. The gene for *NF1* is cloned and is localized to chromosome 17q11.2.

Neurofibromatosis type 2 (NF2) is also a dominantly inherited condition. Patients have bilateral acoustic neuromas (vestibular schwannomas). 40% of the patients have spinal and intracranial tumors. The prognosis of NF2 is poor as surgical removal of the VIII th nerve tumor is difficult. The *NF2* gene is located on chromosome 22. Presymptomatic screening and prenatal diagnosis in affected families is possible.

GENES THAT REGULATE APOPTOSIS

Genes that prevent or induce programmed cell death or apoptosis also play a role in cancer. Examples of genes that regulate apoptosis include the *bcl-2* gene, which inhibits apoptosis and the bax, and *bad* genes that favour programmed cell death. Two other cancer-associated genes that are also connected with apoptosis are the *p53* gene and the *c-myc* proto oncogene.

GENES THAT REGULATE DNA REPAIR

DNA repair genes themselves are not oncogenic but allow mutations in other genes during the process of normal cell division. Individuals born with inherited mutations of DNA repair proteins are at greatly increased risk of developing cancer.

Examples of such diseases are Hereditary non-polyposis coli (HNPCC), in which of the various DNA mismatch repair genes, mutations in *hMSH2* on chromosome 2 account for tumor development in 50% of families. Microsatellite instability is the hallmark of defective mismatch repair. Other examples include xeroderma pigmentosum, Bloom's syndrome, ataxia telangiectasia and Fanconi's anemia (These are discussed in detail in the chapter on chromosomal syndromes).

Ovarian Cancer

Ovarian cancer is a potentially lethal neoplasm of the female reproductive system. It is observed that 80% of malignant tumors of the ovary originate from the surface epithelium. Several molecular events such as loss of heterozygosity (LOH) at different sites on chromosomes 6, 11,13 and 17, mutations in tumor suppressor genes (such as *p53*, *BRCA1*, *BRCA2*), and mutation of proto-oncogenes (*RAS*, *FOS* and *MYC*) are responsible for development of ovarian tumors. Majority of ovarian cancers are of sporadic in origin. Diagnosing ovarian cancer at on early stage is difficult due to the large space available for the ovaries to grow, as a result patients are asymptomatic in the early stages and by the time it is detected it reaches incurable stage. Transvaginal sonography and colour Doppler is recommended annually in high-risk cases.

SCREENING FOR FAMILIAL CANCER

As of today the standard management for cancer is prevention and early detection. Prevention aspects include diet, change in life style, drugs, prophylactic surgery or screening. Screening is carried out at early stage, before any phenotypic expression occurs. For example, in individuals at risk for familial adenomatous polyposis screening is by endoscopic examination. Retinal examination for congenital hypertrophy of the retinal pigment epithelium in family with a history of retinoblastoma is worthwhile. Presymptomatic screening should be considered in high-risk families.

The test should be sensitive and specific enough to pick a malignant or pre-malignant condition prior to producing symptoms. Screened persons should benefit, due to early detection resulting in improved prognosis. Benefits from the test should be more than the potential dangers. It should be non-invasive whenever possible. Appropriate pre-screening counselling and facilities for follow up of the cases should be available. In colorectal cancer endoscopy provides a sensitive test that can be offered to at risk patient. In breast cancer regular mammography after the age of 40 years at intervals of five years in women who are at risk for breast cancer is ideal and is a national program in the United Kingdom. Breast self examination or clinical examination should be encouraged as a preventive early screening.

RECENT DEVELOPMENTS IN BIOTECHNOLOGY IN CANCER THERAPEUTICS

Some of the Techniques Used in the Treatment of Cancer Biotechnology are Discussed

Antisense Technology

Antisense methods involve the disruption of gene expression using short, sequence specific DNA molecules called oligonucleotides. These synthesized oligonucleotides bind complementary DNA molecules in the double helix of the genome, and form triplexes that prevent ribosomal protein synthesis by prohibiting the translation process of mRNA.

Recombinant Retroviral Vectors

Retroviral mediated gene transfer has also been used to incorporate antisense vectors into cancerous cells. The vector will produce complementary RNA sequences that combine with the target RNA sequence, resulting in a double strand of RNA, which will be degraded by intracellular enzymes, instead of being expressed through ribozymes.

Gene Therapy

In this technique, recombinant vectors are used so that they will infect specific cells of interest. There are many viruses with different predilection sites in body, which affect only specific cells. These vectors will transfect specific cells and express genes, which will induce an immune response to malignant cells. There are several mechanisms involved by which cancer cells are able to escape from immune surveillance. Recombinant retrovirus mediated gene transfer of vectors expressing interferon γ can boost the expression of MHC I and II proteins which induce strong cytotoxic T cell immune response and inhibit the growth of cancer cells.

Drug Resistance Genes

In chemotherapy, the main hurdle is side effects such as hemotoxicity. Recombinant-mediated gene transfer of drug resistance genes such as multi-drug resistance gene (*MDR1*), mutant dihydrofolate reductase genes, and methyl-transferase genes to the bone marrow stem cells have the potential to produce drug tolerance to toxic drugs. This may permit an increased dose of the drugs.

Gene Chip Technology

The gene chip is also referred to as DNA chip array technology. The gene chip is a glass wafer, which is approximately 2cm^2 in size. On top of this glass, several arrays of known nucleotide sequences of oligonucleotide probes are arranged. This glass chip is encased into black plastic cartridges in which the reaction takes place. The main principle of this technology is the ability of nucleic acids to hybridise with complementary DNA sequences with high stringency. For example, DNA with sequence TTGGCAT will hybridise with AACCGTA nucleotide sequence.

If there is single nucleotide, which is not complementary, then it will reduce the binding affinity with a low signal of fluorescence. This technology can be exploited to detect well-characterized mutations in cancer. A person with one type of cancer showing a similar phenotype may show different mutations in candidate genes. It may be a point mutation, deletion, insertion or base substitution. (Based on types of mutations in candidate genes, it may be possible to design effective drugs) Using the gene chip technology, it is possible to test more than 600 mutations of the CFTR gene responsible for cystic fibrosis, on a single chip. Routine genetic techniques to detect mutations are difficult, laborious, time consuming and at times may be inconclusive. This DNA chip technology will also be used for clinical surveillance of presence of cancer genes or cancer associated mutations in affected tissues at an early age, in patients who are predisposed for developing specific cancers before it gets expressed in later life. Accordingly, preventive or prophylactic therapeutic strategies can be recommended for the high-risk patient.

CHAPTER 15

GENETICS OF COMMON DISEASES

INTRODUCTION

The study of medical genetics mainly involves the study of chromosomal and single gene disorders that are rare, when compared to other more common diseases occurring in population, which also have a genetic component. For example, diabetes mellitus, cancer, and cardiovascular diseases not only have a have high degree of morbidity and mortality, but the number of individuals suffering from them far out number those affected by classical genetic diseases. There are chances that a percentage of these diseases will increase due to an increased life span of humans. These diseases are characterized by not having a known pattern of inheritance. Multiple genetic factors interact with each other and get enhanced or triggered by environmental factors.

GENETIC SUSCEPTIBILITY

These common diseases, which occur due to interaction of gene and environment are said to have polygenic inheritance. In familial hypercholesteremia, the FH gene is mutated and the development of coronary artery disease is triggered off by conditions like obesity, smoking and lack of physical exercise. Similarly, smoking or exposure to dust, very often an occupational hazard, is responsible for pulmonary emphysema. Patients with α-1 antitrypsin deficiency manifest with a severe form of emphysema, which gets worse on smoking. Such examples suggest that a single gene mutation couples with the environment contributes to these disorders. The mechanism of genetic susceptibility may not be always clear, as genetic polymorphism leads to variation in the susceptibility of a disease. An example of this is the correlation between alcoholism and acetaldehyde dehydrogenase enzyme activity. In order to demonstrate that a particular disease has a genetic susceptibility different approaches are can be used. Some of these are: Family studies, twin studies, study of adopted children, and population studies.

APPROACHES FOR STUDY

Family Studies

If a disease shows a higher frequency in a particular family as compared to the general population, it can be assumed as being of familial origin. Familial aggregation may not necessarily prove genetic susceptibility, especially if the environmental circumstances are similar. A control study could examine the respective spouses. If they too have a similar problem the condition has more of an environmental factor than genetic, as both the partners will have different genetic make-ups.

Study of Twins

Identical twins showing similar traits could be explained by heredity, but the fact that identical twins may share the same environment needs to be considered. Members of a pair of twins are called concordant when either both are affected or not affected. They are termed discordant when only one member is affected. If a disease is purely environmental, identical and non-identical twins will have the same concordance. Non-identical twins sharing a similar environment but not sharing the same genes will not be similarly affected unless it is a single gene disorder or a chromosomal translocation. The ideal way to study this is the study of identical twins brought up in different environments. In such cases, if a similar disease exists in them one can assume a genetic component in the disorder.

Adoption Studies

Studying adopted children can be a different approach in studying genetic and environmental factors. Adopted individuals will have their genes from their biological parents, thus predisposition to some disease – if a disease is more similar to that in adopted parents the environmental factors are more likely the cause of disease.

Population Studies

A majority of genetic diseases in a population occur irrespective of race and social status of an individual. However, differences in the incidence of some diseases in some specific populations is known. For example, there is a high incidence of thalassaemia in the Mediterranean region. Specific mutations occur in a particular community, for example in India, Kachhi lohanas, Punjabis, Bhatias have a high incidence thalassaemia.

There are situations where an incidence of a particular genetic disease with low occurrence increases in an immigrant population, suggesting the influence of environmental factors. If a low incidence of disease is maintained in the immigrant population, genetic factors would play a role.

THE GENETIC COMPONENTS OF SOME COMMONLY SEEN DISEASES

Diabetes Mellitus

Diabetes mellitus is a syndrome characterized by elevated levels of glucose in the serum. The criteria for the diagnosis of diabetes according to the American Diabetes Association are:

1. A fasting plasma glucose level of greater than 126 mg/dl or,
2. A random plasma glucose level of greater than 200 mg/dl or,
3. A plasma glucose level greater than 200 mg/dl at 2 hours after the ingestion of oral glucose (75 g).

Diabetes is a heterogeneous clinical syndrome with multiple etiologies.

Type I Diabetes

The frequency in the Caucasian population is estimated to be 1 in 400. The mode of inheritance is polygenic. Type I diabetes (also known as insulin dependant diabetes mellitus, or IDDM) is caused by destruction of pancreatic beta cells, most often by autoimmune mechanisms. IDDM is associated with specific HLA antigens, where over 95% of the individuals with IDDM have HLA DR3 or DR4 or both antigens, and these persons develop pancreatic islet cell antibodies. Infections like occurrence of mumps, cytomegalovirus or Coxsackie B in autumn or winter with autoimmune disorders are common in IDDM persons, suggesting a possible viral etiology. The immune mediated form of type-I diabetes (IMD) is present when autoantibodies to islet cells and or insulin are detected in the presence of diabetes. The pathogenesis involves multiple genetic lesions affecting immunoregulation against self, coupled with strong influences from the environment affecting penetrance. There is increased propensity to develop multiple organ-specific autoimmune diseases such as Addison disease, Hashimoto's thyroiditis pernicious anemia, vitiligo and celiac disease. The long natural history and relatively low concordance of IMD in twin pairs affected by the disease provides an opportunity for disease prevention. The mutant gene product is the HLADQβ1 on 6p21.3, the most common being a substitution at codon 57. The mutant gene product is presumed to predispose to autoimmunity directed against pancreatic β cells.

Type II Diabetes

Type II diabetes which is the most common form of diabetes accounting for greater than 90% of patients is caused by two defects: a resistance to the action of insulin combined with a deficiency in insulin secretion. Although the primary causes of insulin resistance have not yet been elucidated in most patients with type 2 diabetes, mutations in the insulin receptor gene have been demonstrated to cause several rare syndromes associated with insulin resistance. Some factors are known to contribute to the pathogenesis of insulin resistance. Most patients with type 2 diabetes are obese, and the increase in adiposity is believed to be an important causal factor in the development of insulin resistance. Obesity is the major factor that unmasks diabetes. First-degree relatives of a patient with NIDDM are at risk for diabetes and prevention is to be attempted by keeping optimal body weight. The role of genetic factors in NIDDM is suggested, and preservation of beta islet function, resistance to insulin, lipid abnormalities, obesity and maternal transmission support this.

MODY (Maturity Onset Diabetes of the Young)

The incidence of MODY is 1 in 400. It is inherited in an autosomal dominant fashion. In 60% of cases have mutations in the glucokinase gene on chromosome 7p13. Other families have been mapped to a locus on chromosome 20. Mutations in the glucokinase gene predispose to impaired glucose sensors in pancreatic β cells leading to decreased insulin secretion.

Gestational Diabetes

Diabetes is also seen in pregnant women. It is called gestational diabetes and occurs in 1-3% of all pregnant women. Their abnormal glucose tolerance returns to normal after pregnancy; however half of them develop diabetes in later life. Gestational diabetes was once thought to be type 2 or NIDDM, but it is genetically heterogeneous, as it shows association with HLA antigens DR3 and DR4, pancreatic islet cell antibodies and autoimmune diseases.

Diabetes can also be due to other genetic syndromes and non-genetic diseases. In myotonic dystrophy, diabetes is inherited in an autosomal dominant manner. Various studies on animal models and twin studies have shown enough evidence to suggest that in identical twins 96% of them are concordant while only 3 to 37% of non-identical are concordant. Family studies show about 25 to 50% diabetics have family history of diabetes as compared to 15% in general population. Various family studies have shown that incidence of diabetes in other family members of diabetics is higher up to 30% while in non-diabetics up to 6%.

Genetic Basis for Predisposition to Diabetes and its Complications

Common complications of diabetes are renal, retinal, coronary artery disease and peripheral vascular disease. It was once believed that, complications of diabetes are related to the control and duration of diabetes. However, it is now believed that this too has a genetic predisposition. Individuals with IDDM homozygous for the I (insertion) allele in angiotensin I converting enzyme (ACE) are at a lower risk of developing renal complications, while presence of the D (deletion) allele in persons with NIDDM have a high risk for coronary disease.

HYPERTENSION

Introduction

Determinants of blood pressure variation include genetics and environmental factors as well as factors such as age, gender and ethnicity. Monozygotic twins who share 100% of their genes show significantly greater concordance in blood pressure than do dizygotic twins who only share 50% of their genes.

The incidence of hypertension in the general population is as high as 10 to 25%. By convention, any young adult with a persistently high blood pressure of 140/190 is to be considered hypertensive. Systolic blood pressure tends to increase with age but is medically significant. The main complications of hypertension are stroke, coronary artery disease and renal disease. They can be prevented by therapy.

Hypertensive patients fall into two groups the first one where onset is usually in early adult life and is secondary to renal disease or endocrine and the second one beginning at a later age with no apparent cause. This group is called essential hypertension.

Environmental factors responsible for developing hypertension are a high salt intake, reduced physical exercise, obesity and alcohol consumption. The role of environment has been studied in surveys of migrant populations. Moving from a low prevalence group to a high prevalence group shows that a migrant population suffers from hypertension with an increase in incidence in 1-2 generations, thus supporting the idea that environmental factors play a role in the aetiology of hypertension.

Genetic factors are important and biochemical studies indicate there is a possibility of an autosomal dominant gene responsible for hypertension. In some hypertensives, an extrusion of sodium from the red cells because of abnormal enzymatic controlled sodium potassium co-transport in the cell membrane has been detected. This leads to an increase in intra cellular sodium. Twin and family studies support that genes are also important for deciding the choice of hypertensive therapy for example, African races respond better to beta-blockers than Caucasians.

Regulation of blood pressure is a highly complex process and depends on many physiological factors. These include kidney and heart function, cellular ion transport. Components which influence blood pressure variation are angiotensin, angiotensinogen, urinary kallikerin, sodium and lithium counter transport. These factors appear to be under control of few genes. Studies have implicated gene for angiotensinogen in developing hypertension and pre-eclmpsia.

Genetic studies confirm that mutations underlying all mendelian forms of high and low blood pressure converge on a final common pathway: Mutations that cause an increase in salt reabsorption result in hypertension, whereas mutations that cause salt wasting produce hypotension.

Mendelian forms of hypertension include glucocorticoid remediable aldosteronism, Liddle syndrome, and hypertensive forms of congenital adrenal hyperplasia due to deficiencies in the steroid synthesis pathways.

Efforts to identify genetic variants that underlie blood pressure variation in the general population have revealed an interval on human chromosome 17, which is a blood pressure locus in rat, and shows evidence for linkage in both Mendelian and essential hypertension in humans.

CORONARY ARTERY DISEASE

The main cause of coronary artery disease is atherosclerosis, in which lipid is deposited in the intima of the arteries resulting in narrowing of the coronary arteries. The constituents of the blood attack the endothelial surface of the arteries that are lined with lipid deposits, where after entering they proliferate and differentiate into macrophages. These macrophages engulf the lipids and produce fatty acid streaks. They are responsible for proliferation of smooth muscles and for atherosclerotic plaques. The plaques rupture and lead to the occurrence of thrombotic events resulting in myocardial ischemia and infarction. Coronary artery disease can occur secondary to other diseases like diabetes mellitus and hypertension. The sex ratio tends to be predominantly male, while females after menopauses have an increased risk due to hormonal charges. Familial and twin studies have confirmed the genetic background and the risk is about 7 times more for a person with family history.

Although coronary heart disease is of multifactorial etiology, about 5% of subjects with premature myocardial infarctions are heterozygotes for familial hypercholesterolemia, a single gene disorder that produces atherosclerosis in the absence of an extraordinary environmental factor. However even in this disorder, other loci such as genes for apolipoprotein B, apolipoprotein (a) lipoprotein lipase, and apolipoprotein E could influence the phenotype, and non-genetic factors such as diet and smoking can modify the risk. Therefore it is clear that numerous interrelated biochemical, genetic and non-genetic factors modify the risk for coronary artery disease.

EPILEPSY

Epilepsies are a heterogeneous set of neurologic disorders defined by repeated clinical seizure episodes due to aberrant electrical synchronization of the brain. Epilepsy affects approximately 1% of the population. Heredity represents the single largest aetiology of the epilepsies. Genetic transmission patterns of epilepsy are both Mendelian and complex. Over 180 known

Mendelian variants share epilepsy as one expression of the inherited gene error. Most cases are sporadic. Currently recognized monogenic syndromes represent a small subset of all epilepsies. Twelve forms of epilepsy have been demonstrated to possess some genetic basis. Epileptic seizures are categorized by the extent of their cerebral involvement (partial or generalized), by the sparing or impairment of consciousness (simple or complex) and by the pattern of associated motor activity (tonic, clonic, atonic, arrest). Clinical epilepsy syndromes are defined by the seizure type, natural history, precipitating factors, drug sensitivity, and presence of associated neurological deficits. In benign epilepsy syndromes, seizures resolve over time. Benign or familial convulsions are inherited as an autosomal dominant trait. They begin during first neonatal week of life and resolve by 6 months of age. Grand mal epilepsy has a 1 in 25 recurrence risk to first-degree relatives, rising to 1 in 10 if two relatives are affected. Petit mal epilepsy has 7% recurrence in siblings. Numerous gene loci have been identified for common seizure patterns and syndromes. The genes involved include a broad range of molecules regulating brain assembly, activity and cell death.

ALZHEIMER DISEASE

Alzheimer disease (AD) is an adult onset neurodegenerative dementia characterized by the intracellular and extracellular accumulation of proteins, which assemble into β-pleated sheet fibrils. Alzheimer disease is a common cause of dementia in persons of less than 55 years (early onset) or more than 55 years (late onset). The disease presents with a constellation of symptoms that reflect dysfunction and degeneration of neural cells in the cerebral cortex and other selected brain regions. The dementia in AD is irreversible and progressive. The characteristics are impaired memory, intelligence, social skills and loss of control over emotions. Risk to the first-degree relatives, of an affected individual is approximately 10%, and variation is likely because of age dependence and heterogeneity.

Missense mutations in the β amyloid precursor protein (βAPP) gene on chromosome 21, in the presenillin 1 gene (PS1) on chromosome 14, and the presenillin 2 (PS2) gene on chromosome 1 are associated with early-onset forms of familial Alzheimer disease.

The late onset form may be linked to chromosome 19, which has a gene for apolipoprotein E (APOE). The ε4 (Cys112Arg) variant of apolipoprotein E (APOE) is associated in a dose-dependant fashion with increased risk for late-onset Alzheimer disease (after age 55). The inheritance of one or more APOE ε4 alleles is not deterministic for AD, and the mechanism by which inheritance of one or more ε4 alleles causes AD is unclear.

OBESITY

Obesity is the presence of an excess amount of adipose tissue. The excessive adipose tissue causes increased blood pressure, hepatic lipid synthesis, insulin resistance and susceptibility to certain cancers. Studies of concordance rates for adiposity among mono and dizygotic twins and among adoptive children and their family members, and segregation and linkage analysis point to a contribution of genes to the determination of body composition in humans. Human obesity is complex and multigenic, with the penetrance of responsible genes showing strong dependence on environmental circumstance. More recently rare mutations of human orthologs of some of the rodent single gene obesity mutations have been identified (*LEP*, *LEPR*), as well as in other genes that play a role in the control of body fat. The hormone leptin produced by adipocytes was initially discovered in mice. Leptin is a 146 amino acid peptide and has structural homology to the cytokine family. Deficiency of leptin action, due either to an absence of the peptide (as in the *ob* mutation), or inability to detect the signal (as in the *db* mutation of the receptor), results in extreme obesity and infertility.

ASTHMA

Asthma is a chronic inflammatory disorder of the airways characterized by coughing, shortness of breath and chest tightness, caused by narrowing of the airways due to edema and an influx of inflammatory cells. A variety of triggers may initiate or worsen an asthma attack, including viral respiratory infections, exercise and exposure to irritants such as tobacco smoke. There are a number of genes that contribute toward a person's susceptibility to asthma, and genes on chromosomes 5, 6, 11, 14, and 12 have been implicated. The region on chromosome 5 is rich in genes coding for key molecules in the inflammatory response seen in asthma, including cytokines, growth factors, and growth factor receptors.

CHAPTER 16

GENETICS AND CONGENITAL ABNORMALITIES (DYSMORPHOLOGY AND TERATOGENESIS)

INTRODUCTION

The development of a human fetus is an extremely complex process and is dependent on genetic as well as environmental factors. Genetic factors contribute to malformations from birth, though they can be expressed anytime during life. The effect of environmental factors or teratogens leading to congenital malformations is dependent on the developmental stage at the time of exposure, the duration of exposure and the dose. The mechanism of the abnormality leading to a structural defect can be studied in animal models. Though diagnosis of congenital malformations may be difficult at times, it is important for genetic counseling for recurrence risk estimation, and for preventive reproductive options.

INCIDENCE

Spontaneous Abortions and Genetics

A large number of conceptuses are lost before implantation at 5-6 days, before a woman realizes that she is pregnant.

Amongst recognizable pregnancies, 15% end in the first trimester, of which 80% have abnormalities either in the form of a blighted ovum or a specific abnormality of a chromosome, namely aneuploidy, trisomy, monosomy or triploidy. It has been observed that genetic diseases and environmental teratogens significantly contribute to the fetal loss rate and malformations. With the extensive use of ultrasound in obstetric care, the term spontaneous abortion is used synonymously with missed abortions. This is because most pregnancy losses are picked up by an ultrasound examination before they are spontaneously aborted. Analysis of abortuses has shown that 50% of early fetal losses are due to chromosomal errors. Evaluation of causes of fetal loss is becoming more important for two reasons. Firstly, a decrease in the average family size and secondly, a delay in maternal age at first conception. This causes an increased emotional focus on each individual pregnancy.

In a fetus as young as 10 weeks gestation, certain morphological abnormalities can be visualized, therefore the fetus should be examined for morphological abnormalities and a co-relation between gestational and developmental age should be made. For example, at 10 weeks gestation the presence of intestines in the umbilical cord is a normal finding (Fig.16.1A). If the same condition is observed at a later gestational age, it is classified as omphalocele and could be associated with chromosomal defect like trisomy 18. Another example is coloboma of the iris (Fig.16.1B), which is a normal finding up to the age of 45 days, or cleft lip and palate, (Fig. 16.1C) which is normally seen up to 10 weeks of development. If these are seen after the above mentioned specific periods, these are labeled as developmental defects.

Many a times in early pregnancy, fetal demise could have occurred several weeks before an actual miscarriage. In such cases, fetal tissue may not be available or may not be suitable

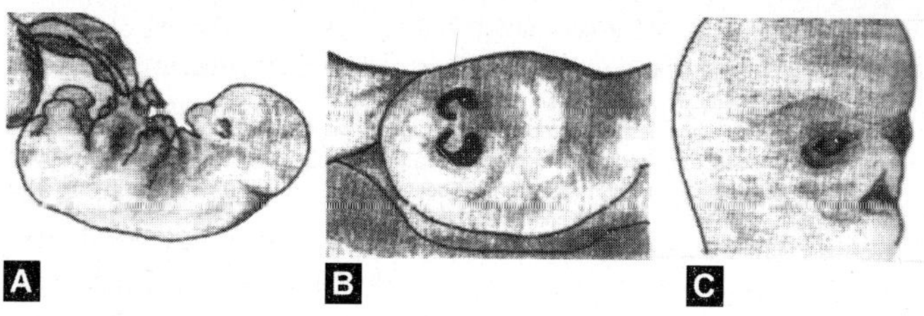

Figs 16.1A to C: (A) Physiological hernia in a fetus at 9 weeks, (B) Coloboma iris. (C) Cleft lip and palate at 10 weeks

for karyotyping. Histopathological studies in early abortions may be of value in early losses. On histopathological examination, markedly hydropic villi with cistern formation indicate a molar gestation. Hydropic villi intermingled with small normal villi are diagnostic of partial mole. Trisomies have slightly hydropic avascular villi. In monosomies chorionic villi differ greatly in shape and are irregular.

In older fetuses it is possible to achieve at a diagnosis by studying the photographs, autopsy reports and X-rays. Such an evaluation is of extreme importance in estimating the recurrence risks and planning a more precise pre-natal diagnosis for future pregnancies.

Perinatal Mortality and Congenital Malformations

Pregnancy losses between 28 weeks and the first week of life fall into this group. 25 to 30% of perinatal mortality is due to a serious structural abnormality, and 80% of these are of genetic origin. Recurrence risk is more than 1%. Many biochemical disorders like amino acidopathies, urea cycle defects and carbohydrate metabolism disorders can prove to be fatal in newborn period and fetal tissues need to be cultured for enzyme assays. A precise diagnosis is necessary for future pregnancy planning.

Ten percent of newborn babies have one to two minor abnormalities. About 2 to 3% of all newborns have some major anomaly presenting at birth and the incidence is about 5% in those which present in later in life. 25% of all deaths in childhood occur due to major structural anomalies. The quality of life in patients with major malformations depends on the nature of the defect and its possible correction. Nearly 25% of the patients with birth defects die in early life and 25% are physically and mentally handicapped.

CLASSIFICATION OF BIRTH DEFECTS

Birth defects are classified into malformations, disruptions, deformities and dysplasias according to the mechanism that has caused the defect. Sequences and syndromes are also identifiable types of birth defects.

Malformations

Malformations are primary structural defects that occur during development of a tissue or an organ. A malformation develops from an abnormality during the course of development. Examples of malformations are cleft lip and palate, congenital heart disease, pyloric stenosis and meningomyelocele. Most of the single gene malformations are polygenic/multifactorial, in origin with a low risk of recurrence. Surgical treatment is recommended for correction. Multiple malformation syndromes comprise of defects in two or more systems and are associated with mental retardation (Fig. 16.2). The recurrence risk depends on the cause, whether it is chromosomal, teratogenic or a single gene defect or unknown.

Disruption

The term disruption is applied to a condition where the fetus has otherwise developed normally, and a disruption in development occurs due to external factors. For example, in

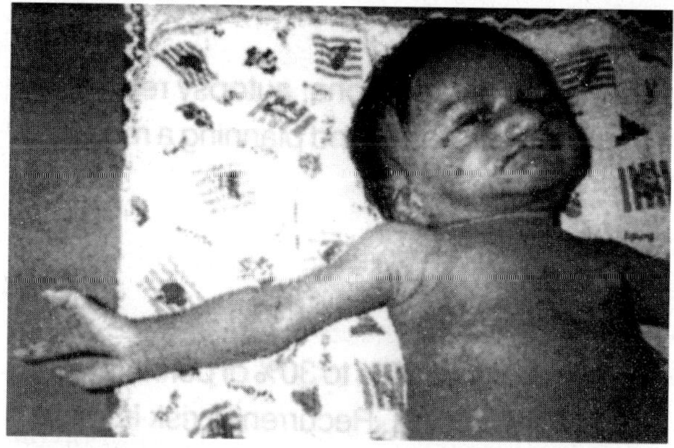

Fig. 16.2: Multiple congenital anomalies

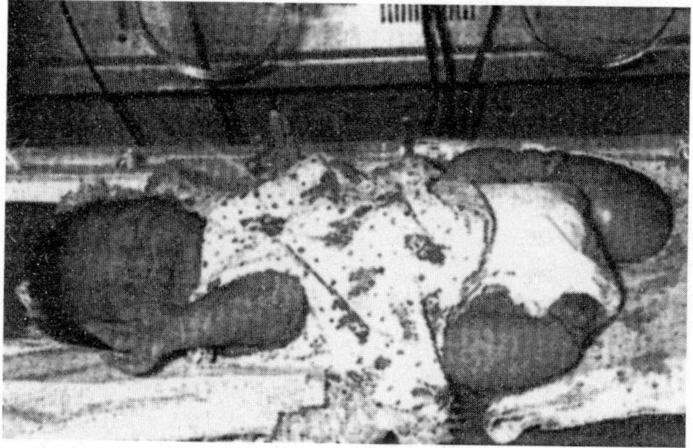

Fig. 16.3: An example of a disruption is the amniotic band syndrome. Here constriction defects seen in the lower limbs due to amniotic bands

amniotic band syndrome, an amniotic band is formed due to early rupture of the amnion and can disrupt a limb, and cause a constriction leading to limb deficiency, classically known as a limb reduction defect (Fig. 16.3). Interference with blood supply to a developing part leading to infarction or infection can also lead to the defect. Association of limb reduction defects with chorionic villous sampling (CVS) has been reported. Although the occurrence of limb reduction defects after CVS are yet to be investigated, in order to reduce the risk, it is safer to do sampling after 9 ½ weeks of pregnancy.

Deformations

Deformities due to abnormal intrauterine moulding can arise because of maternal or fetal conditions. Dislocation of the hip joint, and clubfoot result from oligohydramnios. Fetuses with abnormalities of the musculoskeletal system may have positional deformities. Multiple pregnancies or breech presentation can also result in deformities. A well renal recognized syndrome, Potter syndrome (Figs 16.4A and B) is associated with renal agenesis leading to oligohydramnios, which in turn can cause fetal deformation and pulmonary hypoplasia.

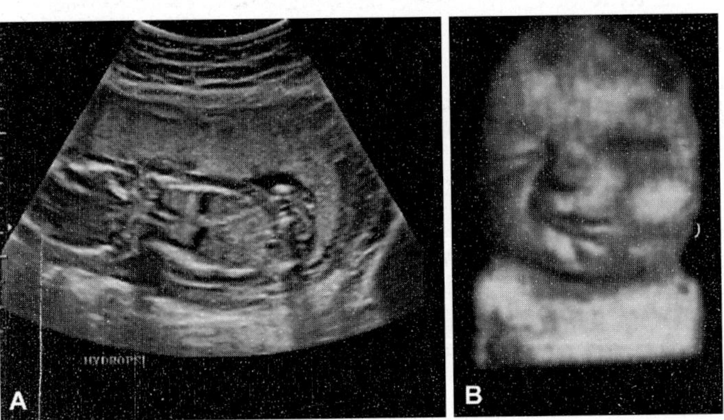

Figs 16.4A and B: An example of a deformation is the potter syndrome. Note the severe oligohydramnios seen on ultrasound (A) and (B) a fetus with Potter syndrome

Dysplasia

The term dysplasia is applied to an abnormal organization of cells in a tissue and usually affects all parts of the body where that particular tissue is present. An example is thanatophoric dysplasia, which is a type of skeletal dysplasia, which occurs due to mutations in FGFR3 gene (Figs 16.5A and B). Here all parts of the skeleton are affected. In ectodermal dysplasia, tissues of ectodermal origin like hair, teeth and nails are involved. Most dysplasias occur as a result of single gene defect, and have a high recurrence risk for siblings and children.

Sequence

Sequence is where a single site defect results in apparently unrelated anomalies due to a developmental cascade. For example, in Potters syndrome due to chronic leakage of amniotic fluid or renal agenesis, oligohydramnios occurs which leads to fetal compression resulting in dysmorphic facial features, dislocation of hips, pulmonary hypoplasia and

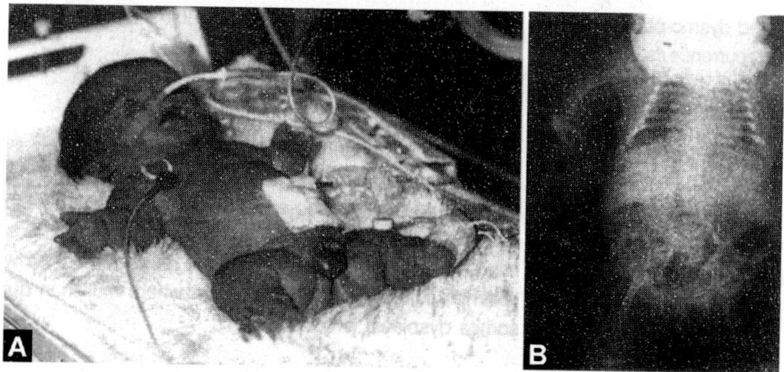

Figs 16.5A and B: (A) Skeletal dysplasia in a new born (B) X-rays of the same infant showing shortening of the long bones and narrow thoracic cavity

talipus. The condition is invariably fatal. Similarly in spina bifida, blockage in the normal CSF flow can result in hydocephalus (Figs 16.6A and B).

Syndrome

The term syndrome is applied to conditions where consistent patterns of abnormalities are seen due to an underlying cause. Syndrome is a combination of birth defects that is consistent in unrelated individuals. Many syndromes show some phenotypic variation both in individuals throughout life and between different individuals. This could be due to chromosomal abnormalities as in Down's syndrome or without any chromosomal abnormality as in Pierre Robin syndrome. Several multiple malformation syndromes are recognized and a computerized dysmorphology data base is now available, which is of great help in evaluating prognosis and estimating recurrence risk.

Association

Association is the non-random association of groups of congenital anomalies but in a relatively inconsistent manner. The recognized malformations have acronyms of the abnormalities, e.g. VATER association comprises of vertebral anomalies, anal atresia, tracheoesophageal fistula and radial defects. The acronym VACTERL is the VATER association but includes cardiac defects and hydrocephalus. CHARGE association includes (coloboma, heart defects, atresia of the choana, retardation of growth, genital anomalies, ear anomalies). Another example is the MURCS association where mullerian duct aplasia, renal aplasia and cervicothoracic somite dysplasia is observed.

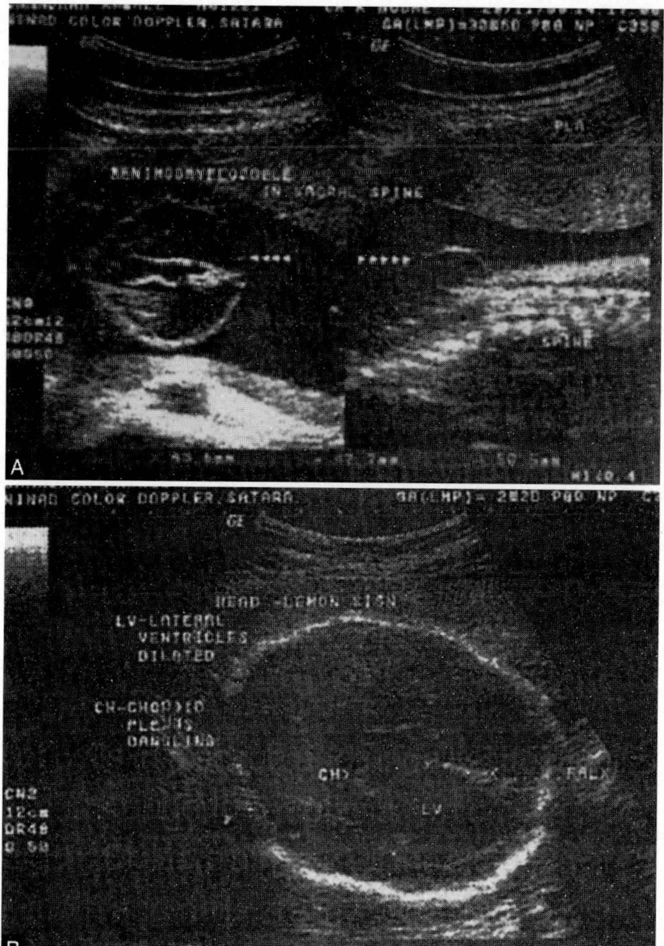

Figs 16.6A and B: Ultrasound showing. (A) Meningomyelocele and (B) Hydrocephalus occurring secondary to obstruction of the flow of cerebrospinal fluid,an example of a sequence

TWINNING AND MULTIPLE BIRTHS

Approximately 7.6% of the pregnancies result in twins, of which 6% vanish and only 1.6% go to term. The rate of malformations is higher in twins. Twins are divided in to two groups - monozygotic (MZ) where twins are identical and are developed from the fertilization of one egg and one sperm (single zygote) within 3-8 days of fertilization. If the division occurs more than two weeks after conception there is a great possibility of conjoined twins. MZ twins usually do not have a family history, have the same genetic composition, are of the same sex though phenotypically they may not be identical. Monozygotic twins sometimes can be discordant for genetic disorders and congenital malformations. MZ female twins can show discrepancy in X-chromosomal inactivation. Dizygotic twins (DZ) are formed when fertilization occurs between two eggs and two sperms in the same ovulatory cycle. They are like sibs and may be of the same or of different sexes. Multiple births occur in a similar fashion. MZ twining is a chance occurrence while DZ twining is familial and has three times increased risk of recurrence. Multiple births like triplets or quadruplets, can be identical or non-identical. Twin studies are of importance in medical genetics. MZ and DZ twins are excellent models for comparative studies of the effects of genes and environment.

GENETIC CAUSES OF MALFORMATIONS

Many genetic causes of congenital malformations are known and are classified as chromosomal, single gene, and multifactorial.

Chromosomal Abnormalities

Chromosomal abnormalities occur in 6% of all recognized congenital malformation.

Single Gene Defects

7.5% of congenital anomalies occur due to a single gene defect. They can present as isolated defects or can involve multiple systems, and have no embryological relationship. An appropriate classification and mode of inheritance is essential to estimate recurrence risk.

Multifactorial Inheritance

A majority of congenital malformations fall into this group where genetic and environmental factors are responsible. Most isolated malformations of the heart, central nervous system and kidneys are due to multifactorial inheritance. The empiric risks need to be calculated before counseling can be offered for recurrence risk estimation. An example of genetic and environmental components for a defect is described below.

Neural Tube Defects

One of the common developmental defects occurs due to a failure of closure of the neural tube. When the defect lies at the upper end of the tube it leads to anencephaly, and when it lies in the lower region it leads to spina bifida and meningomyelocele. Environmental factors play a great role in the causation of a neural tube defect. Most defects have serious implications leading to incompatibility with life due to anencephaly or paralysis of the lower limbs and loss of bowel and bladder control in spina bifida. Recurrence in patients increases in subsequent pregnancies and is also higher in close relatives. Prenatal diagnosis is by estimating serum a fetoprotein levels in maternal blood. Mothers carrying a fetus with open neural tube defects show a high level of serum alfafetoprotein levels in their blood. Ultrasonography can diagnose the condition in 90% of cases. Prevention in a large number of cases is possible by periconceptional high doses of folic acid. If a neural tube defect is associated with other congenital malformation or part of any other syndrome, the underlying cause has to be evaluated and if suspected to be chromosomal, a chromosomal diagnosis should be offered. Socio-economic factors, multiparity and valproic acid embryopathy also contribute to neural tube defects. Therefore folic acid supplement is recommended for all pregnant women, not only to those with a past history or a positive family history.

ENVIRONMENTAL TERATOGENS

An agent which causes a defect in the natural process of development is called a teratogen. The teratogen can be in the form of drugs, chemicals or infections. Organ involvement depends on the nature of teratogens, and the severity of the problem depends on the dose and developmental stage of the fetus.

DRUGS AND CHEMICALS

Overall 2% of all congenital malformations fall in this group. Various drugs are known to be teratogens, for example anti-cancer drugs like methotrexate and chlorambucil and anticonvulsants such as carbamazepine and primidone. Minamata disease a disease caused in children who are born to mothers who had ingested organic mercurials through contaminated fish. This is an example of industrial pollution. The babies have a cerebral palsy like syndrome.

Thalidomide was a drug used as a sedative in Europe during 1958-1962 and caused severe limb anomalies in babies whose mothers were exposed to the drug between the 25th to 35th day of conception. This deformity with severe limb defects is known as phocomelia. In a short span, about 10,000 babies were reportedly born. The limb defects consisted of absence of fore or hind limbs, with retention of digits. Other external anomalies like ear, eye cleft lip and palate are also known to occur. 40% of thalidomide babies died in early infancy due to severe internal anomalies of heart, kidneys and gastrointestinal tract.

Fetal Alcohol Syndrome (FAS)

Ethanol ingestion during pregnancy causes congenital malformations and delayed psychomotor development. The clinical features include mental retardation, microcephaly, hypotonia, poor coordination, hyperactivity and impaired growth. The children tend to show a characteristic facial appearance. This includes short palpebral fissures, short upturned nose, hypoplastic philtrum, micrognathia and hypoplastic maxillae. The risk of alcohol-induced birth defects is established above 3 oz. of absolute alcohol daily.

MATERNAL INFECTIONS

The process of embryogenesis is affected by maternal infections, and these can interfere with fetal development. The most susceptible organs are brain eyes and ears. A group of infections, seen commonly is called the TORCH group of infections, which stands for toxoplasma, rubella, cytomegalovirus and herpes.

Rubella

Infection with the rubella virus causes malformations in 15% to 25% of pregnancies. Infection in the first trimester causes cardiovascular malformations, cataracts and a hearing defect. Prevention of rubella is possible by immunization of all young women independently or as measles mumps and rubella vaccination together (MMR) and should be included in routine health care and obstetric care programs.

Cytomegalovirus

The cytomegalovirus infection in the first trimester leads to occurrence of congenital malformations in 5% of the infected pregnancies.

Toxoplasmosis

This parasitic infection in pregnancy has a 20% risk of fetuses getting infected in the first trimester, which rises to 75% in the second and third trimester. The diagnosis can be confirmed by looking for specific IgM antibodies in the fetal blood. The blood can also be analysed for abnormal liver functions and for thrombocytopenia.

Others

Infections like listeriosis can lead to miscarriage or neonatal meningitis. Parvovirus B-19 infections can cause severe anemia and hydrops fetalis resulting in fetal loss.

PHYSICAL AGENTS

Ionizing Radiations

Heavy doses of ionizing radiation can lead to microcephaly and eye defects. They can have mutagenic and carcinogenic effects. The most critical period is 2-5 weeks post conception. Irrespective of the dose ionizing radiations should be avoided in pregnancy.

Hyperthermia

Prolonged hyperthermia occuring in early pregnancy can cause microcephaly and microphthalmia in the fetus. Nerve migration defects are also reported. Hot baths and saunas should be avoided in first trimester.

MATERNAL ILLNESS

Maternal disease in pregnancy poses a two-fold problem. The effects could be due to the disease itself, or to the drugs administered for the disease. Improvements in neonatal and pediatric care have given an opportunity to individuals with genetic disorders to reach a reproductive age group. Thus clinicians caring for a pregnant women should not only be familiar with routinely seen medical disorders such as hypertension and diabetes or infectious diseases like HIV or syphilis but genetic diseases like cystic fibrosis.

Diabetes Mellitus

Incidence of birth defects in mothers with diabetes is increased two to three fold as compared with the population. Commonly known malformations are congenital heart disease, neural tube defects, sacral agenesis, and sirenomelia. Monitoring of blood glucose levels and glucose and glycosylated hemoglobin level in the mothers is recommended. Gestational diabetes does not increase the risk of malformations.

Epilepsy

Maternal epilepsy by itself does not pose a threat to pregnancy as regards congenital malformations. It may lead to a depletion in placental circulation during an attack. Anticonvulsant drugs are known to have teratogenic effects. Phenytoin has an increased risk for cleft lip and palate, and sodium valproate has an increased risk for anencephaly and spinabifida. A combination of drugs is more teratogenic. However, the risks of withholding drugs and of recurrence of seizures has to be weighed appropriately during care of the pregnant mother.

Phenylketonuria

Untreated maternal PKU leads to mental retardation in the child. In addition microcephaly and congenital heart defects are known. A low phenylalanine diet before and during pregnancy is necessary.

CHAPTER 17

GENETIC COUNSELING

INTRODUCTION

Genetic counseling is an important step in the process of genetic consultation. It is the step, which offers various options available to an individual or the family of an individual affected with a genetic disorder. Counseling is also required at every step in a diagnostic procedure and thus may require several specialists under one roof. For example, in a prenatal diagnostic procedure one requires a counsellor to give an overall idea of the procedure involved till the final results are obtained, and follow-up advice further on the basis of the results obtained. The obstetrician involved in the procedure should counsel before sampling is done. An expert in cytomolecular or biochemical genetics is consulted to interpret the results and a paediatric surgeon may be required if postnatal surgery is planned.

Any couple with a child or a family member with a genetic problem or a history of congenital defect will be keen to know more about the disorder, the risk of recurrence of the disorder, and remedial measures if any (Table 17.1). The aim of the genetic counsellor is to provide these individuals seeking information with an understanding of the disease in question and its implications, as well as the options available. A good counseling process helps families with their problems, allows informed decision-making, reduces possible anguish and is a step towards the final adjustment in dealing with the disorder.

Accurate diagnosis is of paramount importance for meaningful genetic counseling and counseling needs to include all aspects of the condition.

WHO NEEDS GENETIC COUNSELING

People who seek genetic counseling often have the following questions: (1) Do they have any type of genetic disease and or are they carriers (2) Do they run the risk of having another child affected with the particular genetic disease (3) what are the implications of the genetic disease already diagnosed as existing in one or both parents who are planning parenthood, and what is the prognosis and treatment (4) Referral to the appropriate source if they are seeking artificial insemination by donor or adoption (5) What kind of help is available for their already affected child and where they can find it.

Table 17.1: Indications for genetic counseling

- Women with bad obsteric history in the form of repeated abortions, malformations Couple having H/o previous child with mental retardation or any of the above family H/o abnormal births
- Maternal age above 35 years
- Consanguine marriage, maternal diseases, anxiety
- Exposure to X-rays, drugs and infections in pregnancy
- Abnormal ultrasound findings
- Communities at risk for genetic disorder, e.g. thalassemia

WHAT IS GENETIC COUNSELING

The American College of Medical Genetics defines genetic counseling as a communication process, which deals with the human problem associated with occurrence or risk of occurrence of a genetic disorder in a family. This process involves an attempt by one or more appropriate trained persons to help the individual or the family to:

1. Comprehend the medical facts, including the diagnosis, probable course of the disorder and available management.
2. Appreciate the way heredity contributes to disorders and the risk of recurrence in specified relatives.
3. Understand the options for dealing with the risk of recurrence.
4. Choose the course of action, which seems appropriate to them in view of their risk and their family goals, and act in accordance with that decision.
5. Make the possible adjustment to the disorder in affected members and /or to the risk of recurrence of the disorder.

The counsellor should keep all the facts and the available options in front of the patients and let them choose the path.

STAGES IN COMMUNICATION PROCESSES

Five stages can be identified in this communication process:

- History taking and pedigree construction.
- Clinical examination and diagnosis
- Recurrence risk estimation
- Counseling.
- Follow-up.

History Taking and Pedigree Construction

The affected individual who seeks advice is called the PROBAND. Often the proband is a child but he or she may also be interviewed along with relatives. A standard medical history is required for the proband and for any other affected persons in the family. Next, the pedigree is constructed with standardized symbols. Pedigree construction gives a clue to the possible mode of inheritance.

Clinical Examination and Diagnosis

A complete physical examination of the proband is essential. At times it may be necessary to seek an opinion from an expert in a related specialty to confirm the clinical diagnosis. In conditions like mental retardation or hearing impairment where predisposing factors could be purely genetic, or genetic and environmental, a history and clinical examination, and further investigations may be needed. A variety of investigations may be required reflecting the various types of genetic disorders. Occasionally the affected individuals will be otherwise unavailable for assessment and an attempt should be made to obtain hospital or other records, which might aid definitive diagnosis. Both parents should be counselled and all aspects of the condition must be clearly and thoroughly explained.

RECURRENCE RISK ESTIMATION

Counseling in genetic disorders that follows a Mendelian pattern is straightforward, however patient or parents need to understand this. For example, a risk of 1 in 4 may be misunderstood as to when one affected child is present parent's may consider future pregnancies safe. The risk of occurrence of 1 in 4 for every pregnancy should be clearly explained.

Counseling is very often sought in a pregnancy, where information about the affected child is incomplete. In chromosomal disorders prenatal diagnosis can be made successfully without a confirmed laboratory diagnosis of an index case. For example, if a pediatrician has made a confirmed clinical diagnosis, foetal tissue sampling such as amniocentesis or chorion villous biopsy for chromosomal studies can be undertaken. However, in case of a biochemical disorder, precise laboratory diagnosis in an index case as well as carrier status of the parents need to be established. A similar situation arises in some conditions where molecular diagnosis is required. For example, in a recessive disorder such as thalassemia mutation analysis can be applied in the absence of an affected child, however, the carrier status of the couple has to be initially confirmed by mutation analysis. However, in an X-linked disorder such as Duchenne muscular dystrophy unless mutation in the index case is confirmed, no carrier detection test or prenatal diagnostic test in the mother can be planned.

DIRECTIVE AND NON-DIRECTIVE COUNSELING

Patients seeking counseling should be given as accurate information as possible about the disease and all possible options. They should be left to choose a path. Genetic counseling offered to a patient should always be non-directive. Patients often will ask the counsellor what would he or she do if they were in a similar situation. Giving an opinion in this matter is a form of directive counseling which should always be avoided.

In the United Kingdom under congenital disabilities act of 1976, legal action can be taken against a person whose breach of duty to the parents, results in a child being born disabled, abnormal or unhealthy. Failure to give correct advice by the consultant for the risk of fetal abnormality in a future pregnancy, and possibility of prenatal diagnosis may constitute medical negligence.

PROBLEMS IN GENETIC COUNSELING

Genetic Heterogeneity

Counseling is difficult in cases where disease has genetic heterogeneity. Genetic heterogeneity is seen in conditions like

Charcot-Marie-Tooth disease or retinitis pigmentosa, which can be inherited as an autosomal dominant, autosomal recessive or X-linked recessive disorder. However, with molecular diagnostic tests for these disorders it has become possible to diagnose and therefore provide counseling for these disorders.

Consanguinity

Most marriages are non-consanguinous, however in certain Indian communities marriages between blood relatives is a custom. Mortality and morbidity may be higher in conceptions occurring from consanguinous marriages due to the increased chances of inherited a recessive trait that manifests in disease. Incidence of congenital malformations, hearing deficiency and mental retardation may be higher. If the family history is otherwise negative, the risk of major congenital malformation is 5% as compared with the 3% general population risk, and the added risk of autosomal recessive conditions is 1%.

ADOPTION AND GENETIC DISORDER

Parents who are at high risk for a genetic disorder in their offspring often consider adoption as an option. The geneticist may be called upon in such a situation to find out the risk of genetic disease in the child to be adopted. If no family history or obstetric history of the mother is available, routine karyotyping and metabolic screening for certain disorders may be carried out. However, the possibility of an untested genetic disorder can never be ruled out.

PATERNITY TESTING

A geneticist may be consulted to opine in issues of paternity. Until recently, disputed paternity was tested using a series

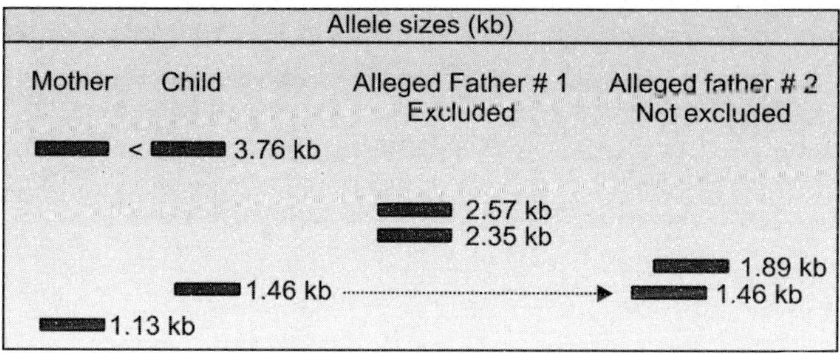

Fig. 17.1: Paternity testing

of polymorphic blood groups and enzymes. If a child possesses a blood group or other polymorphic gene which is absent in both the partners, paternity can be possibly excluded. For example if both the partners lack blood group B but it is present in the child the putative father can be possibly excluded. If a child lacked a marker, which could have come from putative father, again paternity is possibly excluded. For example, a father with a blood group AB will not have a child with group 0. However, paternity in these cases can be excluded in 95% of cases but could never be proven. Testing for paternity has now been transformed by the use of DNA fingerprinting. The probes used identify multiple dispersed sequences of variable size called VNTRs (variable number of tandem repeats). The pattern produced is characteristic for an individual. A child's fragment pattern is a combination of some of the fragments from each parent and a putative father can be either excluded or positively identified (Fig. 17.1). DNA fingerprinting can also be used for forensic testing of DNA from semen or dried blood spots.

CHAPTER 18

CHROMOSOMAL SYNDROMES

INTRODUCTION

In this chapter we will discuss selected chromosomal syndromes. These include autosomal trisomy syndromes of chromosome 21 (Down syndrome), 18 (Edward syndrome) and 13 (Patau syndrome) (Table 18.1) and disorders of the sex chromosomes. In addition we will also discuss the molecular cytogenetics of contiguous gene syndromes. Finally we will discuss chromosomal instability syndromes including ataxia telangiectasia, Bloom syndrome and Fanconi anemia and nucleotide excision repair (NER) syndromes including xeroderma pigmentosum, Cockayne syndrome and trichothiodystrophy.

AUTOSOMAL TRISOMIES

Down Syndrome (Trisomy 21)

Down syndrome (DS) is the first chromosomal disorder to have been clinically defined and is the most commonly recognized genetic cause of mental retardation.

Clinical Features

The physical characteristics of Down syndrome include upslanting palpebral fissures, loose skin on the nape of the neck, narrow palate, brachycephaly, hyperflexibility, flat nasal bridge, gap between first and second toe (sandal foot

Table 18.1: Clinical features of common autosomal trisomies

Syndrome	*Down Trisomy 21*	*Edward Trisomy 18*	*Patau Trisomy 13*
Incidence	1 in 1200	1 in 8000	1 in 10,000
Lost in utero	30%	60%	60%
Life expectancy	30-50	0-1	0-1
CNS	MR,hypotonia	MR, Hypertonia, choroids plexus cyst	MR, seizures
Head, Face, Neck	Brachycephaly, epicanthal folds, hypertelorism, flat facies, excessive skin at the back of neck	Micrognathia, small mouth, redundant skin	Microcephaly, cleft lip/palate facies, abnormal scalp defects
Hands	Short metacarpals and phalanges,transverse palmar crease	Clenched hands, clinodactyly	Polydactyly, compactodactyly, transverse palmar crease
Feet	Plantar crease	Rocker bottom feet, club feet	Polydactyly, rocker bottom feet
Heart	40% VSD, ASD, common atrium, PDA	40% VSD, ASD, PDA	80% VSD, ASD, PDA dextrocardia
GIT	Duodenal atresia, TOF	Umbilical hernia, omphalocele	Inguinal/umbilical/ hernia/horse shoe kidney
Urogenital	Hypogonadism, infertility (specially in males)	Cryptorchidism, horse shoe kidney, single umbilical artery	Polycystic/ectopic kidney Bicornuate uterus

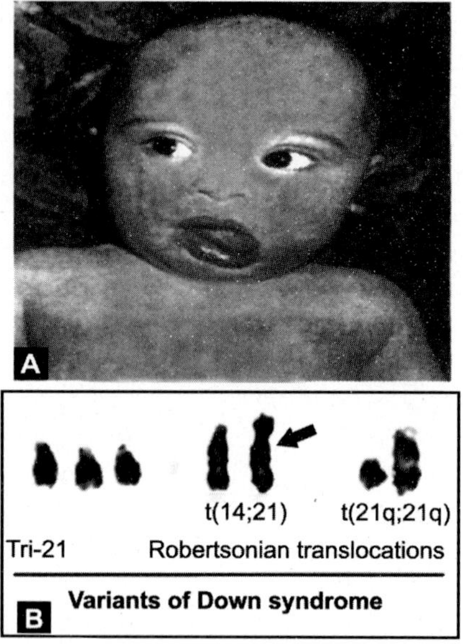

Figs 18.1A and B: (A) Clinical features of Down syndrome (B) Various chromosomal patterns observed in Down syndrome: trisomy 21,t (14; 21) and t (21; 21)

deformity), short broad hands, short neck, abnormal teeth, epicanthic folds, short/incurved fifth finger, open mouth and protruding tongue, Brushfield spots of the iris, furrowed tongue and a transverse palmar crease (Fig. 18.1A).

Mental retardation (IQ varying between 25 and 70) and hypotonia are virtually always present. Congenital heart disease occurs in 40% of individuals, particularly endocardial cushion defects. Heart defects include atrioventricular septal defects, ventricular septal defects and atrial septal defects. Gastrointestinal anomalies like duodenal atresia (double bubble appearance on ultrasound) and Hirschsprung disease are found in 5% of individuals. There is a fifteen to twenty fold increase in the incidence of leukemia in children with Down syndrome, with acute megakaryoblastic leukemia being frequent in cases of acute nonlymphocytic leukemia. Brains of individuals with Down syndrome after the age of 30 show the pathologic, metabolic, and neurochemical changes of Alzheimer disease, and these individuals have a progressive loss in cognitive function.

There is an increased frequency of thyroid dysfunction in newborns and of thyroid autoantibodies throughout life. There is increased susceptibility to infection, due to abnormalities of the immune system, particularly in the maturation and function of T lymphocytes. Males with Down syndrome are invariably infertile, whereas females have decreased fertility but may be capable of reproduction. The principal cause of death in Down syndrome is infection, congenital heart disease and malignancy.

In most cases, trisomy 21 results from an extra chromosome or as part of a Robertsonian translocation or isochromosome. Occasional cases result from a trisomy 21/ diploid mosaicism (Fig. 18.1B). Maternal age plays a role in the incidence of trisomy 21 (Table 18.2). In 86% of cases, the non disjunction event occurs in the mother, with the error occuring at meiosis I, 75% of the time.

Prenatal diagnosis by amniocentesis or chorionic villus sampling can detect a fetus with Down syndrome. In addition maternal triple test screening and fetal ultrasound can detect fetuses with Down syndrome.

Table 18.2: Co-relation between maternal age and Down syndrome

Maternal age	*Risk of Down syndrome in live borns*
25	1 in 1500
25	1 in 400
38	1 in 180
40	1 in 100
45	1 in 40

Edward Syndrome (Trisomy 18)

The incidence of this autosomal trisomy in live births is about 1 in 8,000. Most fetuses with trisomy 18 are aborted spontaneously. Life expectancy is very low, postnatal survival being very rare. The female to male ratio is seen to be higher, probably due to preferential survival. Primary meiotic nondisjunction is suggested as a cause for this type of trisomy. As with other trisomies maternal age is an important association. The effects are more severe than those of trisomy 21. Features include mental retardation, malformations of the heart, kidney and digestive system, skeletal defects, and failure to thrive. Rocker bottom feet with prominent calcanei and tightly clenched hands with incurved little finger are a characteristic feature (Figs 18.2A to C). Single palmar crease can be observed along with distinctive dermal patterns on all digits and hypoplastic nails. Either an entire chromosome 18 in addition to the normal complement or a partial trisomy may be observed. Mosaic trisomy may be seen in some cases, which present with milder expression.

Patau's Syndrome (Trisomy 13)

This is the least frequent of the three common autosomal trisomies with an incidence of 1:10000. The effects are more

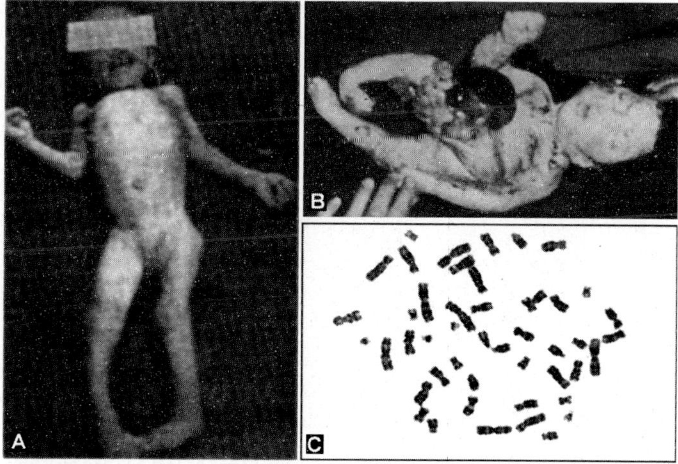

Figs 18.2A to C: Edward syndrome (Trisomy18). (A) Rocker bottom feet and clenched fist. (B) Exomphalos. (C) Metaphase spread showing trisomy 18 *(Figure 18.2B for color version see Plate 5)*

severe. Trisomy 13 results from a nondisjunction in meiosis I. An unbalanced translocation may be seen in some cases. Severe retardation in physical as well as mental development, along with central nervous system malformations such as arrhinencephaly and holoprosencephaly are associated. The characteristic features are a sloping forehead, ocular hypertelorism, micropthalmia, and coloboma of the iris. The most obvious problems are midline defects such as cleft lip and palate. Figures 18.3A to C polydactyly and defects in the scalp may be seen. Heart, kidney and digestive tract anomalies are also seen as a common finding. About half the trisomy 13 individuals die within the first month. Survival beyond 3 years is rare.

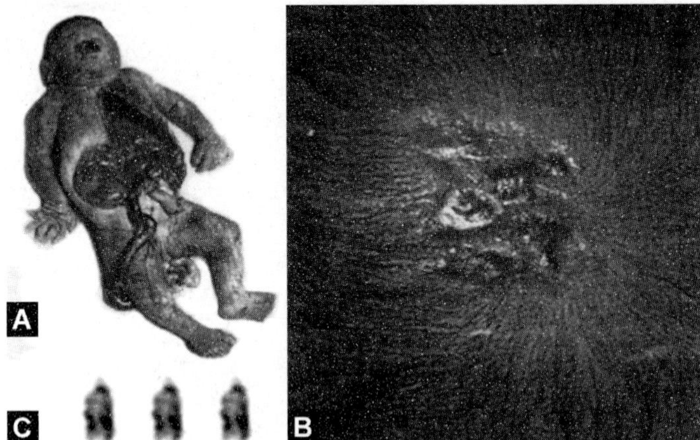

Figs 18.3A to C: Patau Syndrome (trisomy13) (A) Microcephaly, microphthalmus, bilateral cleft lip and palate, polydactyly, enlarged kidneys, (B) Scalp defect, (C) Partial karyotype showing trisomy 13

DISORDERS OF SEX CHROMOSOMES

Cytogenetic abnormalities of the X and Y chromosome occur at a frequency of 1 in 500 live births. Many of the sex chromosomal variations are compatible with life and are among the most commonly seen chromosomal abnormalities. Each has its own set of phenotypic expression, but primarily they involve premature gonadal failure, infertility or abnormal development. The four well-defined syndromes due to numerical abnormalities of the sex chromosomes are are Turner Syndrome (45XO) Klinefelter's Syndrome (47XXY), 47XXX female and 47XYY male. The structural abnormalities include abnormalities of the X and the Y chromosome and are discussed below after the numerical abnormalities.

Turner Syndrome (45XO)

Turner syndrome (monosomy X) occurs in an estimated 1 to 2% of all clinically recognized pregnancies, although fewer than 1% of these survive to birth. 45,XO is the most common sex chromosomal abnormality.

The typical abnormalities seen in Turner's syndrome are short stature, gonadal dysgenesis, webbing of the neck, broad chest with widely spaced nipples, and a low posterior hair line (Figs 18.4A to C). Many a times the condition is not

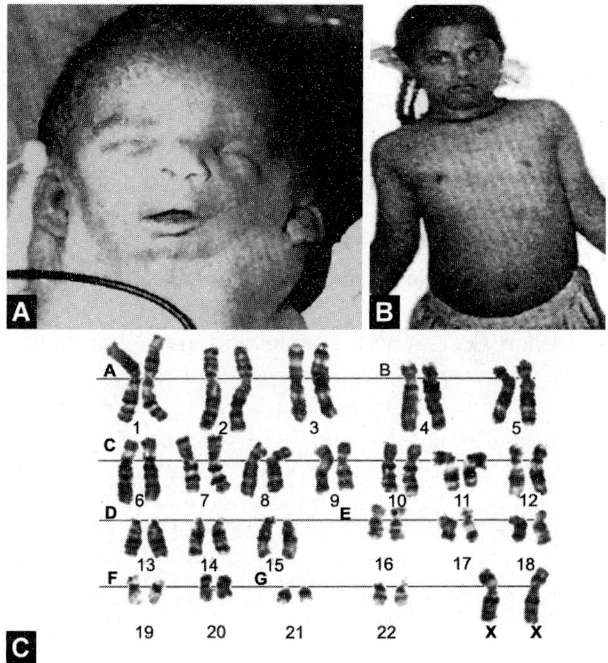

Figs 18.4A to C: Turner Syndrome (45X) (A) Webbing of neck, (B) webbing of neck, shield shaped chest,cubitas valgus, (C) karyotype showing 45X

diagnosed until puberty where patients are referred for primary amenorrhea or short stature. These patients have a higher frequency of cardiovascular and renal abnormalities. Coarctation of the aorta may be seen in some cases. Postnatal webbing of the neck may be due to cystic hygroma as a result of lymphedema in fetal life. Mental retardation is not a necessary manifestation. Variants of Turner syndrome may be seen, such as those with an isochromosome or a deleted form of chromosome X. They are less commonly seen than monosomy. Cases of this syndrome with a deleted Y have also been observed. Mosaic form of this syndrome along with Klinefelter's syndrome or with 47,XXX may be seen in some cases. Ultrasound examination particularly of the genital region is suggested in 45,XO chromosomal anomaly (Table 18.3).

Klinefelter's Syndrome (47XXY)

The incidence of this syndrome is approximately 2:1000 male live births. The main features are increased height with relatively long thin legs. Signs of hypogonadism are seen only when puberty is reached. Gynaecomastia is common, and the penis and testis are smaller than normal (Figs 18.5A and B). Feminization of the hip may be seen. Patients with this syndrome are usually sterile. Dyslexia is a common manifestation leading to learning difficulties. Variants of Klinefelter's syndrome are seen, who have more than two X-chromosomes. 48,XXXY or 49,XXXXY (Figs 18.6A and B) patterns may be seen. Though inactive, these additional X chromosomes are usually associated with mental retardation. The phenotype in 49XXXXY is similar to that in Down syndrome. These chromosomal patterns may be observed as mosaics in a normal male or a normal female chromosomal complement. Patients with Klinefelter's syndrome with

Table 18.3: Various phenotypes in Turner syndrome variants

Karyotype pattern	*Phenotype*
45,X	Features of Classical Turner syndrome
46, Xdel (Xp11)	Persistence of scanty functional ovarian tissue noted, spontaneous menstruation can occur
46, X, del (Xp21)	Menstruate spontaneously, secondary amenorrhea, but are infertile.
Isochromosome (Xq) total deletion of Xp	Streak gonads, short stature and Turner stigmata, occasional menstruation, poor breast development.
46, X, del (Xq13)	(Most important region for ovarian maintenance) Primary amenorrhea, lack of breast development, complete ovarian failure.
46, X, del (Xq21)	Menstruate spontaneously, secondary amenorrhea, 50% are infertile
46, X, del (X) (q25- 27)	Premature ovarian failure
46, X, i (Xp)	Normal stature, primary amenorrhea
Translocation between Autosome and X-chromosome	Ovarian dysgenesis
If long arm of X is involved	Ovarian failure, familial gonadal dysgenesis
Mosaicism	Presentation will depend on the number of cells involved, typical Turner, normal or premature menopause

azoospermia may benefit by newer technologies in the treatment of infertility like intracytoplasmic sperm transfer technique (ICSI). They need to be counseled and offered prenatal diagnosis, as their progeny will be at risk for a chromosomal disorder.

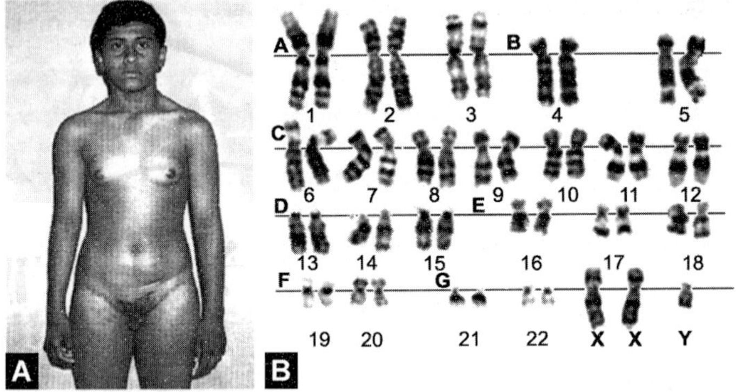

Figs 18.5A and B: Klinefelter syndrome (47,XXY), (A) Gynecomastia, smooth face, female fat distribution and hypogonadism. (B) Karyotype of the same patient showing 47,XXY

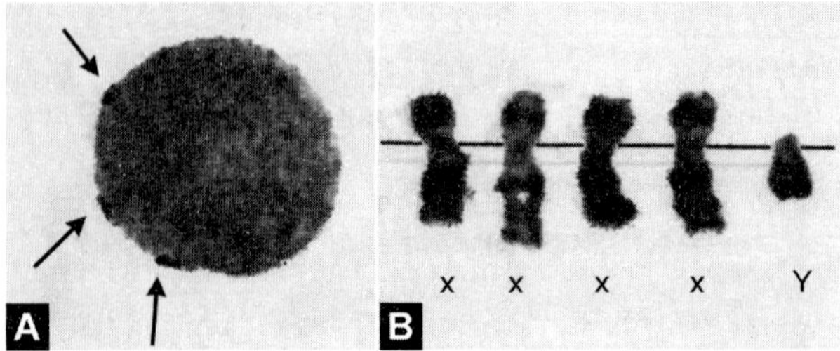

Figs 18.6A and B: (A) Partial karyotype from a patient with Klinefelter variant showing XXXY pattern. (B) Buccal smear from the same patient showing 3 Barr bodies

47, XXX Female

They are the female counterparts of Klinefelter's syndrome seen in males. Rarely tetrasomy X or pentasomy X may be seen. They are phenotypically normal with a taller stature. Patients may develop pubertal changes at an inappropriate age. They are fertile and can bear chromosomally normal children, though there is a greater risk of a meiotic nondisjunction. Patients often have history of repeated fetal wastage. This may lead to the birth of children with other sex chromosomal trisomies. A significant decrease in IQ may be seen. Some have serious learning problems. There may be an effect of late maternal age in some cases. Tetrasomy is associated with serious physical and mental retardation, while pentasomy includes severe developmental retardation and multiple physical defects similar to Down syndrome.

47,XYY Male

This chromosomal constitution is not associated with any observable phenotypic abnormalities. XYY males are very tall and often show behavioral problems such as an excessively violent nature. The intelligence is normal and features are not dysmorphic. The patients are fertile and have nearly no risk of having children with chromosomal abnormalities.

STRUCTURAL ABNORMALITIES OF THE X CHROMOSOME

Deletion Xp Syndromes
Glycerol Kinase Deficiency

This is caused by a deletion of the short arm of the X chromosome at Xp21 (Fig. 18.7). This is characterized by adrenocortical insufficiency, feeding difficulties and hypogonadotropism. In Glycerol kinase deficiency growth and mental retardation are noted. Patients have elevated urinary glycerol.

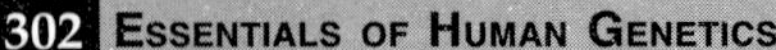

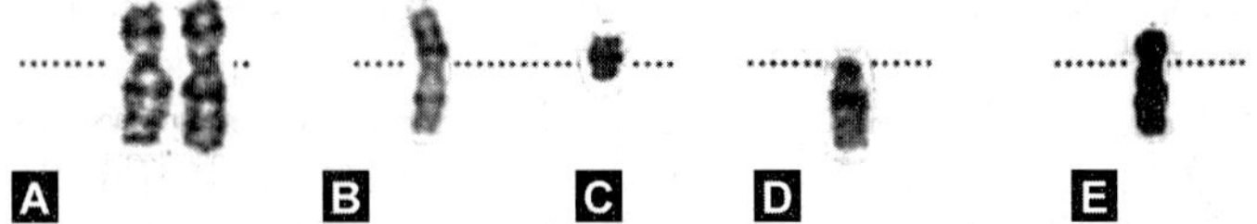

Figs 18.7A to E: Structural anomalies of the X chromosome, (A) XX, (B) i(Xq), (C) deletion Xq, (D) deletion Xp, (E) Translocation t(14;Xq)

Steroid Sulfatase Deficiency/Kallmann Syndrome

The incidence is 1 in 10-15000. It is inherited in an X-linked recessive form. This syndrome is caused by a deletion of chromosome Xp at 22.3. The defects include mutations in the *Kal* gene, which causes a neuronal migration defect. This is characterized by hypogonadotropic hypogonadism and anosmia. The syndrome may be associated with ichthyosis, sparse hair and conical teeth.

Monosomy Xp

The clinical features are same as that of Turner's Syndrome. Most patients menstruate spontaneously but menstruation is rarely normal. Patients with del(X)(p21) though menstruate spontaneously half are infertile.

Monosomy Xq

Region of Xq13 or Xq21 is the single most important region for ovarian maintenance. Deletions involving Xq25→27 are less harmful and patient show premature ovarian failure. In this the secondary sexual characters are well developed, the patients have streak ovaries and patient is sterile. Height is not affected in patients with Xq deletion.

Isochromosome 46,X,i(Xp) These patients have normal stature and primary amenorrhea.

46,XX Males

These patients usually present as infertility cases. Phenotypically they are males with gynaecomastia and testicular atrophy. The majority of these sex reversed XX males have inherited a small fragment of the Y chromosome, which includes the *SRY* gene, transferred to the short arm of one of their X chromosomes.

Structural Abnormalities of Y Chromosome

Structural abnormalities of Y chromosome do not lead to any syndrome but are of great significance in male fertility. The distal portion of Yq shows bright fluorescence with quinacrine stain, and is inherited as a familial marker from father to son. Deletion, isochromosome and elongation of Yp and q, dicentric Y, pericentric Y, ring Y and translocation of Y on an autosome can lead to reproductive loss in a female partner (Figs 18.8A to C). Relationship between optimal length of Y and reproductive fitness is suggested. Y chromosome micro-deletions occur in 10 to 20% of men with oligoazoospermia. Gene localization is at Yq11 this can be transmitted to male offspring.

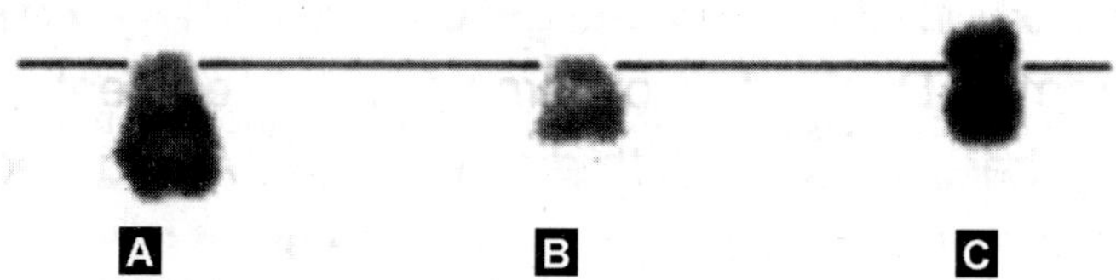

Figs 18.8A to C: Structural abnormalities of Y chromosome. (A) Normal Y, (B) del Yq 12, (C) inv (Y)

SEX CHROMOSOMAL ABNORMALITIES: INTERSEX STATES

These cases are characterized by ambiguous internal and external genitalia. The classification between true and pseudo hermaphroditism is based on the nature of gonads. In true hermaphroditism patients have presence of both male and female gonadal tissue, as mixed gonad (ovo testis) or alternatively an ovary on one side and a testicle on the other side. In pseudohermaphrodism the gonad is either male, (male pseudohermaphrodism) or female (female pseudohermaphrodism). The ambiguity of the genitalia can vary from male to female. Newborns with cryptorchidism or hypospadias are labeled as males. By adulthood, boys may develop gynecomastia or hematuria. Girls present with amenorrhea and hypertrophy of the clitoris. The internal genitalia show persistent Mullerian and Wolfian structures. Cytogenetic studies in true hermaphrodism may show 50% with 46,XX karyotype, 20% with 46,XY karyotype, 20% with XXXY karyotype and remaining 10% with mosaic cell line with one or more additional sex chromosome in one cell line. For example, 47,XXX/46,XX or 49,XXYYY/46,XX.

Male Pseudohermaphrotidism

This is rarely due to chromosomal aberrations. Most of the cases have 46,XY /45,X mosaic cell line. At birth newborns are recognized as male. By puberty axillary and pubic hair develop and a deepening of voice is noted. The built is masculine but genitalia show poor masculinization. A urogenital sinus is always present. The choice of sex rearing must be determined early in life. Male pseudohermaphroditism is also known to occur due to single gene mutation (autosomal recessive or sex linked recessive). The occurrence is usually familial.

Testicular Feminization Syndrome

Earlier known as testicular feminization syndrome, this is not due to a chromosomal rearrangement but due to androgen receptor insensitivity. The phenotype of the individual is female but the karyotype is 46,XY or a mosaic cell line of 46,XY/45,X. It occurs due to androgen insensitivity. The molecular defect is in the *SRY* gene. The inheritance is X-linked recessive and there is a risk to normal female relatives of having an XY female child.

Mixed Gonadal Dysgenesis

This is characterized by a female karyotype with ambiguous external genitalia and hypertrophied clitoris. The gonads and intraabdominal structures are asymmetric. The development of the ducts Mullerian or Wolffian depends on the gonads present on either side.

Female Pseudohermaphrotidism

In a majority of the cases, this occurs due to virilization of a female fetus due to congential adrenal hyperplasia or virilizing hormonal therapy in pregnancy. It is also observed in cases of masculinizing ovarian tumor in the mother.

CONTIGUOUS GENE SYNDROMES

Contiguous gene syndromes (CGS) are defined as a group of clinically recognizable disorders characterized by a deletion or duplication of a chromosomal segment spanning multiple disease genes, each potentially contributing to the phenotype independently. These genes may be interspersed among other genes whose dosage imbalance has no effect on the phenotype. These syndromes were described before their chromosomal etiology was discovered. Cytogenetic abnormalities are sometimes detectable only by high resolution chromosome analysis or submicroscopic deletions or duplications detectable by molecular methods.

For most autosomal loci, deletion causes a reduction of gene dosage to structural and functional monosomy. Haploinsufficiency for specific genes is implicated for Williams syndrome, Miller-Dieker syndrome and DiGeorge syndrome. Some human genes show exclusive expression from a single parental homologue and no expression from the other homologue, known as genomic imprinting. An example of these is seen in the Prader-Willi and Angelman syndromes. Duplication of chromosomal segments causes increased dosage and gene expression. This is seen in Charcot Marie Tooth disease type 1A and Beckwith-Wiedemann syndrome. Some of the syndromes described above are discussed in more detail below.

Williams' Syndrome

The chromosomal anomaly in Williams' syndrome is a deletion of chromosome 7q11.23 including the *elastin* gene and the *LIM kinase* gene. The syndrome is characterized by mental retardation, growth deficiency, elfin facies, gregarious personality, infantile hypercalcemia dental and kidney abnormalities, hyperacusis, musculoskeletal and cardiovascular abnormalities. Mutation or deletion of the *elastin* gene leads to vascular disease. Deletion of *LIM kinase* gene is thought to account for the impaired visuospatial cognition in William's syndrome.

Miller-Dieker Syndrome

The chromosomal anomaly in Miller-Dieker syndrome is a deletion of chromosome 17p13.3. It is a multiple malformation syndrome characterized by lissencephaly and a characteristic facial appearance which which includes a prominent forehead, bitemporal hollowing, a short nose with upturned nares, protuberant upper lip and small jaw (Fig. 18.9). All affected individuals have profound mental retardation, and about half of them acieve no developmental skills. The *LIS1* gene has been identified, and lies within the critical deletion region.

DiGeorge Syndrome/Velocardiofacial Syndrome

These syndromes are caused by a deletion on chromosome 22 at 22q11.21-q11.23. Symptoms vary greatly between

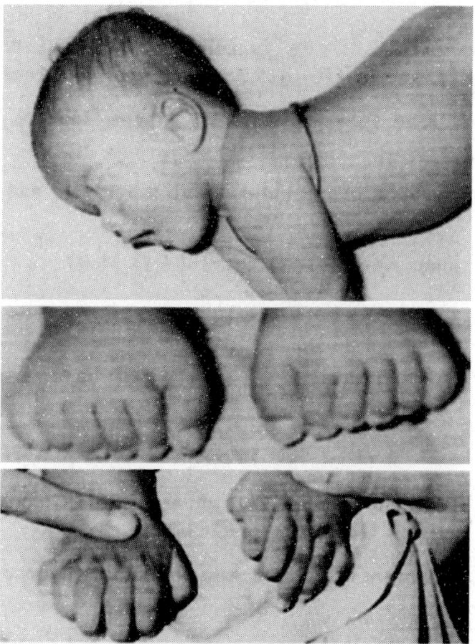

Fig. 18.9: Miller-Dieker syndrome: Showing dysmorphic features, hypotonia, polydactyly

individuals but commonly include a history of recurrent infection, heart defects and characteristic facial features. The patients present with thymic aplasia or hypoplasia, hypocalcemia, hypotonia, developmental delay, sub-mucus cleft palate, dysmorphic facies and cardiac defects of the conotruncal region.

Prader Willi and Angelman Syndromes

These syndromes are due to deletion of 15q11- q13. Prader Willi syndrome occurs due to lack of paternal genes at 15q11-q13, while Angelman syndrome occurs due to lack of maternal genes at 15q11-q13. Normal banded cytogenetic preparations do not show this deletion but is demonstrated by using fluorescent *in situ* hybridisation. In Prader Willi syndrome, patients present with hypotonia and polyphagia. The children are short statured and obese (Fig. 18.10). In Angelman syndrome patients present with inappropriate laughter, convulsions, severe mental retardation, seizures, ataxic gait, and absent speech.

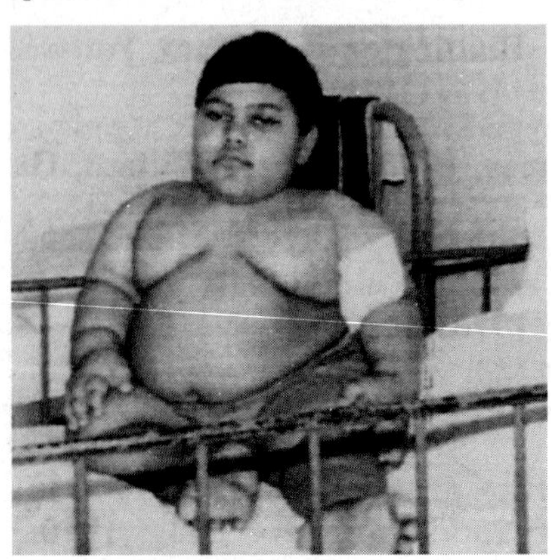

Fig. 18.10: Prader Willi syndrome; Marked obesity and hypogonadism

Charcot-Marie-Tooth Disease (Type 1A)

The chromosomal anomaly is a duplication of chromosome 17 at 17p12. This region contains the PMP22 gene (peripheral myelin protein gene). This is inherited as a peripheral neuropathy. Patients have weakness, decreased nerve conduction velocities and distal muscle wasting.

Beckwith-Wiedemann Syndrome

The chromosomal anomaly is the duplication of 11p15.5. The syndrome manifests with multiple growth anomalies including hemihypertrophy, macroglossia, exomphalos, visceromegaly, umbilical hernia, gigantism and neonatal hypoglycemia. There is an increased predisposition to several malignancies including Wilm's tumor, adrenocortical carcinoma, hepatoblastoma and rhabdomyosarcoma.

Some other chromosomal syndromes due to autosomal deletions are described below.

Smith-Magenis Syndrome

The chromosomal anomaly in Smith Magenis syndrome is a deletion of chromosome 17p11.2. Patients have midfacial hypoplasia, brachycephaly, mental retardation, short broad hands, and self-abusive behavior.

Cri du chat Syndrome

The chromosomal anomaly in Cri du chat syndrome is a deletion of chromosome 5p15.2-p15.3. It is characterized in a newborn by a shrill cry resembling the mewing of a kitten. The disorder occurs 1 in 50,000 live births. Clinically patients have hypotonia, microcephaly, moon shaped face, hypertelorism, and micrognathia. Cerebral anomalies, congenital heart defects and renal malformations are

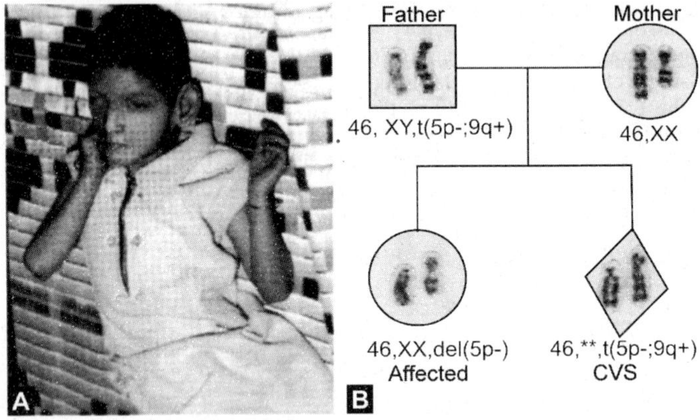

Figs 18.11A and B: (A) Cri du chat syndrome, (B) Pedigree showing partial karyotype from the child with 5p-, normal mother (46XX), father with 46XY t(5p-;9q+). CVS from the mother showed the fetus had the same karyotype as the carrier father

sometimes associated. Most cases occur *de novo* but a chromosomal rearrangement in parents should be investigated (Figs 18.11A and B).

Wolf-Hirschorn Syndrome

The chromosomal anomaly in Wolf-Hirschorn syndrome is a deletion of chromosome 4p16.3. Occurrence is relatively rare and is usually *de novo*, though familial translocations have been seen. Clinically cleft lip and palate, microcephaly, small chin and mental retardation are noted.

CHROMOSOME INSTABILITY SYNDROMES

These are rare inborn disorders inherited in an autosomal recessive fashion. They have hallmarks characteristic for repair defects or inadequate response to DNA damage. The chromosomes in these conditions show morphological abnormalities in culture. The best-studied syndromes are ataxia-telangiectasia (AT), Bloom syndrome (BS) and Fanconi Anemia (FA). All three disorders display different manifestations of cancer proneness and increased susceptibility to specific mutagens.

Ataxia Telangiectasia (AT)

This occurs in 1:40 000 live births in the United States. The carrier frequency is estimated to be 1%. The major clinical features are progressive cerebellar ataxia and telangiectasias of the skin and conjunctiva. There is predisposition to lymphoid malignancies. It is a progressive degenerative disease characterized by cerebellar degeneration, immunodeficiency, and radiosensitivity. Serum alfa-fetoprotein is elevated in 95% of patients. Chromosomal breakage is a feature. Karyotyping reveals characteristic translocations involving chromosomes 14 and 7.

The ATM gene maps to chromsome 11q22-q23. The ATM gene belongs to a large molecular weight family of protein kinases, and the ATM gene product senses double-stranded DNA breaks. When the ATM protein is defective, the signal to arrest the cell cycle is not given, and DNA damage does not get appropriately repaired.

Bloom Syndrome (BS)

Bloom syndrome is an autosomal recessive disorder characterized by proportionate growth deficiency, sun-sensitive, telangiectatic hypo- and hyper-pigmented skin, predisposition to malignancy and chromosomal instability. Patients also have a characteristic facies and head configuration and immunodeficiency, often associated with otitis media and pneumonia. The three major complications are chronic lung disease, diabetes mellitus and cancer. The diagnosis of BS is based on clinical observation. Laboratory confirmation is by cytogenetic demonstration of increased frequency of sister chromatid exchange (SCE) (Fig. 18.12). The gene for BS has been cloned, and is called the *BLM* gene on 15q26.1. The protein shows motifs characteristic of DNA and RNA helicases, specifically the RecQ subfamily of DNA helicases.

Fanconi Anemia (FA)

Fanconi anemia is an autosomal recessive disorder with a predisposition to bone marrow failure and malignancy, particularly acute myelogenous leukemia (AML). FA patients exhibit extreme heterogeneity and may have abnormalities in any organ system. FA is found in all races and has a carrier frequency of 1 in 300. The diagnostic criterion used is the hypersensitivity of FA cells to the chromosome breaking effect of cross-linking agents such as diepoxybutane (DEB). The hypersensitivity of FA cells to cross-linking agents has been

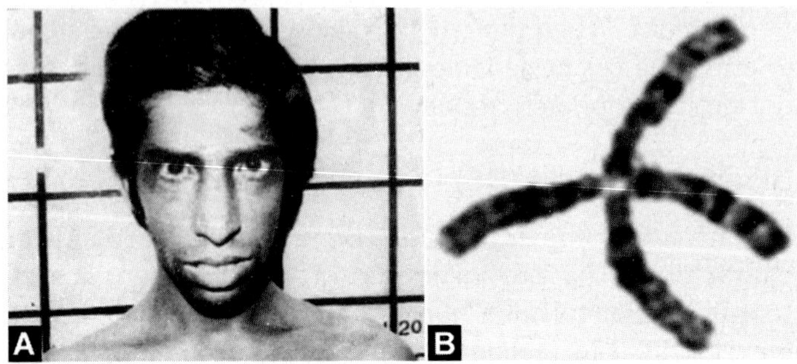

Figs 18.12A and B: (A Blooms syndrome, (B) Quadrilateral chromosome observed in Bloom syndrome

used to assess complementation groups. Complementation groups usually are considered to represent distinct disease genes and for FA four groups represent disease genes namely groups A, C, D and G. The *FAC* gene (formerly *FANCC*) maps to 9q22, the *FAA* gene (formerly *FANCA*) to 16q24, the *FAD* gene (formerly *FANCD*) to 3p22 and the *FAG* gene (formerly *FANCG*) gene maps to 9p13. The only cure for the bone marrow failure in FA is transplantation from hematopoetic stem cells from bone marrow or umbilical cord blood.

Nucleotide Excision Repair Syndromes

Three autosomal recessive syndromes are associated with nucleotide excision repair (NER) defect: Xeroderma pigmentosum (XP), Cockayne syndrome (CS), and the photosensitive form of trichothiodystrophy (TTD). In all three conditions, patients have extreme sensitivity to sunlight.

Xeroderma Pigmentosum (XP)

Affected patients (homozygotes) have sun sensitivity resulting in progressive degenerative changes of sun exposed portions of the skin often leading to neoplasia.

All seven NER genes involved in XP (named *XP-A* through *X-PG*) have been cloned and their defect analyzed in patients.

Cockayne's Syndrome (CS)

Patients with Cockayne's syndrome have a combination of sun sensitivity, short stature, severe neurologic abnormalities due to dysmyelination, cataracts, dental caries, and a bird like facies. Patients do not display a cancer predisposition. After exposure to UV radiation, patients can no longer perform a certain type of DNA repair called transcription coupled repair. Cockayne's syndrome spans a spectrum that includes CS type I, the classical form, CS type II also known as cerebro-oculo-facial syndrome, CS type III a milder form and the above which includes DNA repair defects. Two genes responsible for Cockayne syndrome have been identified, ERCC6 (10q11) CKN1 on chromosome 5. Mutations in the excision repair cross complementing group 6 (ERCC6) cause CSB which accounts for 75% of cases and mutations in the CKN1 gene cause CSA which accounts for 25% of cases. Both genes code for for proteins that interact with components of the transcriptional machinery and the DNA repair proteins.

Trichothiodystrophy: Affected individuals are short, microcephalic, have sparse, short, thin and brittle hair; a receding chin and small nose giving a peculiar facial appearance. Mental impairment is non-progressive. The hallmark of TTD is sulfur defcient brittle hair and nails, and icthyosis. About half of TTD patients are hypersensitive to UV light, and they have a nucleotide excision repair defect. There are no indications for an increased risk of cancer. Three of the NER genes involved in TTD are *XP-B*, *XP-D* and *TTD-A*.

CHAPTER 19

GENETIC AND POPULATION SCREENING

Genetic testing is defined at the use of specific assays to determine the genetic status of individuals already suspected to be a high risk for a particular inherited condition. Genetic screening uses the same assays to screen a target population. Screening can be defined as the systematic search of populations for persons with latent, early or asymptomatic disease. Screening separates apparently healthy individuals into groups with either a high or low probability of developing the disease for which the screening test is being used. Screening is carried out at various levels. These include maternal prenatal screening, newborn screening, screening for heterozygotes and screening of presymptomatic individuals for specific types of cancer.

REQUIREMENTS FOR POPULATION SCREENING

A genetic population screening program is a systematic attempt to identify and counsel as many people at genetic risk in a population as possible. Genetic population screening requires the highest standards of diagnosis, quality control, information, information and counseling.

The general requirements can be summarised as follows:

- A common and potentially serious condition
- A clear diagnosis
- A knowledge of the natural history of the conditions which will permit correct prediction of outcome

- An effective and acceptable solution in the form of treatment of prevention
- Affordable tests for screening
- The program should be socially and ethically acceptable
- The tests must have a high sensitivity and specificity

SENSITIVITY AND SPECIFICITY

The sensitivity and specificity of a test can be measured as follows:

	Affected	*Not affected*
Positive test	a	b
Negative test	c	d

Sensitivity = a/a+c
Specificity = d/b+d

a = the number of individuals with disease whose screening tests are positive (true positives).

c = the number of individuals with disease whose screening test are negative (false negatives).

d = the number of individuals without disease whose screening tests are negative (true negatives).

b = number of individuals without disease whose screening tests are positive (false positives).

Sensitivity is defined as the ability of the screening test to correctly identify individuals who truly have disease. Specificity is the ability of the screening test to correctly identify individuals who truly do not have disease.

Positive Predictive Value (PPV) is the test's ability to identify those individuals who truly have disease (true positives) among all those individuals whose screening tests are positive. PPV = a/a+b

Negative Predictive Value (NPVividuals whos) is the test's ability to identify those individuals who truly do not have the disease (true negatives) among all inde screening tests are negative. NPV = d/c+d

ETHICS OF SCREENING

1. The program must be voluntary with subjects being offered the screening. If they wish to be screened, informed consent should be taken.
2. Individuals who have positive results on screening should not be pressured into a particular course of action such as prenatal diagnosis or termination of affected pregnancies.
3. The privacy of the individual should be respected and information should be confidential. Countries with insurance based health care systems may have a problem about confidentially of data and the access of such information to their insurance companies providing healthcare insurance.

MATERIAL SERUM SCREENING

Alpha Feto Protein Estimation (AFP) and Triple Test

Maternal serum AFP (MSAFP) levels are raised above the base line in pregnancy due to transfer of AFP across the placenta and amniotic membrane. The concentration of MSAFP rises continuously throughout pregnancy, reaching a peak level at 20 weeks and then decreases. There is an association between elevated amniotic fluid AFP (AF-AFP) and open neural tube defects. However, it would not be feasible to perform AF-AFP as a screening test for NTD. Estimation of AFP in maternal serum was a more practical method. (MSAFP) levels more than twice the median value (>2 MOM) at 16-18 weeks of pregnancy can be used to detect

90% of the affected fetuses. This allowed the development of an effective screening program in UK since mid 1972. Prenatal screening by MSAFP can also provide information on other fetal abnormalities or pregnancy complications (Table 19.1), which may be associated with elevated MSAFR The significance of low MSAFP along with raised levels of beta hCG and low estriol has been reported to be more predictive with reference to Down's syndrome and is now routinely used as a screening method to pick up high risk pregnancies for Down's syndrome. For calculating the risk maternal age, weight, diabetic status and exact gestational age is taken in to account. A combination of Triple Test with increased nuchal thickness on ultrasound can pick up to 85% of at risk babies for Down's syndrome. Thus, a single specimen of blood taken at 16 -18 weeks can be used to screen for Down's syndrome and open neural tube defects.

Table 19.1: Conditions associated with high levels of MSAFP

- Underestimated gestation
- Missed or threatened abortion
- Multiple pregnancy
- Anencephaly
- Open spina bifida
- Anterior abdominal wall defects
- Chromosomal syndromes
- Teratoma
- Congenital nephrosis
- Hemangioma of cord/placenta
- Hereditary persistence of AFP
- Intrauterine diagnostic procedures
- Fetal infection

OBSTETRIC ULTRASOUND

Ultrasound examination in pregnancy is offered as a routine test in pregnancy in most centres, deally done at 18 weeks gestation, is valuable in picking up some markers of fetal chromosomal disease. The diagnosis needs to be confirmed by invasive foetal tissue sampling procedure, And is described in details in chapter on prenatal diagnosis.

NEWBORN SCREENING

Newborn screening involves the analysis of blood or tissue samples taken in early infancy in order to detect genetic diseases for which early intervention can avert serious health problems or death.

PRINCIPLES OF NEWBORN SCREENING

1. The disorders screened for are those in which symptoms would not be clinically present until irreversible damage occurred and for which there is an effective treatment.
2. There is a prevalence of the disorder in the population.
3. Collection of the sample is by a simple collection method.
4. The results are reproducible with few false positives and negatives.
5. There is a high benefit-to-cost ratio.
6. Abnormal results can be followed up.

Specimen Collection

The specimens used are usually dried filter paper blood spots, and the infant is < 72 hours of age and preferably after 24 hours of protein feeding.

In the United States, newborn screening is carried out for the following disorders: PKU, congenital hypothyroidism, galactosemia, maple syrup urine disease, homocystinuria, biotinidase deficiency, sickle cell disease, tyrosinemia, congenital toxoplasmosis, congenital adrenal hyperplasia, and cystic fibrosis. Some of these are discussed below.

PKU

The enzyme deficiency in PKU is phenylalanine hydroxylase, causing failure in conversion of phenylalanine to tyrosine. The incidence is 1:12,000 live births in USA. Accumulation of phenylalanine in classic PKU is > 20 mg/dL with normal or reduced level of tyrosine. Atypical PKU is 12-20 mg/dl, and mild persistent hyperphenylalaninemia has levels of 2-12 mg/dl. Treatment is a phenylalanine restricted diet instituted by 3 weeks of age, and frequent monitoring of blood levels and diet adjustments. Early treatment prevents mental retardation and neurologic abnormalities, although learning disabilities are still present. Continuation of diet indefinitely is recommended to prevent decreases in IQ and maternal PKU, which results in fetal microcephaly, congenital heart disease, and IUGR.

Congenital Hypothyroidism

The incidence in the USA is 1:3,600-5,000 live births. Screening is by measurement of T4/TSH. Symptoms include mental retardation, neurologic abnormalities and metabolic symptoms of hypothyroidism. Treatment involves administration of L-thyroxine to maintain T4 levels in the upper half of the normal range. Treatment within the first 3 months of life is associated with prevention of mental retardation and complications of the disease

Galactosemia

The prevalence is 1:40,000 live births. Caused by deficiency of galactose-1-phosphate uridyl transferase. Screening is by measurement of galactose and galactose-1-phosphate, and confirmation is by measurement of the enzyme in erythrocytes. Treatment includes dietary lactose restriction at time of diagnosis, evaluation for sepsis, and immediate treatment to prevent complications of mental retardation, cataracts, and cirrhosis.

Sickle Cell Disease and other Hemoglobinopathies

These include hemoglobin SS disease, hemoglobin SC, and sickle-thalassemia, all of which result from abnormal β-chains of hemoglobin. The incidence in the black population is approximately 1:400. Screening is by hemoglobin electrophoresis by using cord blood or dried filter paper blood spot.

Glucose-6-phosphate Dehydrogenase Deficiency

The incidence is 1:100-1:10 for Mediterraneans, Africans and American Blacks, and 1:50-1:33 for Southeast Asian individuals. This is a sex-linked disorder primarily affecting males, although females may be variably affected. It is a hemolytic disorder, where enzyme deficient RBCs are unable to protect against oxidative effects of infection or certain drugs resulting in severe haemolysis and hyperbilirubinemia. Screening is by a fluorescent spot test, which measures the absence of the enzyme. The diagnosis is confirmed by quantitative analysis.

Congenital Adrenal Hyperplasia

This is an autosomal recessive disorder of the biosynthesis of adrenal corticoids due to a deficiency of one of several enzymatic systems required for complete steroid biogenesis. Most common form of CAH is due to 21-hydroxylase deficiency (90% of cases), in 2/3 there is increased androgen production. The incidence is 1:10000-1:15000 live births. The screening test measures level of 17-hydroxyprogesterone in the dried filter paper blood spot. Early treatment will prevent complications seen in undiagnosed affected newborns, and incorrect sex assignment in females.

Maple Syrup Urine Disease

This disorder is due to deficiency of branched-chain ketoacid dehydrogenase that results in the accumulations of the branched-chain amino acids leucine, isoleucine and valine and their respective ketoacids. The incidence is 1:200,000 live births. The screening tests for leucine by the bacterial inhibition assay on dried blood filter paper. Treatment consists of diet restriction.

Homocystinuria

This is due to deficiency of cystathionine synthase that catalyses the conversion of homocysteine to cystathionine, and results in accumulation of toxic levels in blood or urine. The incidence is 1:100,000-1:200,000. The screening test measures methionine in dried filter paper specimen. Treatment includes a methionine-restricted diet.

Cystic Fibrosis

The incidence is 1:2000 in the Caucasian population. Screening is by measurement of immunoreactive trypsin (IRT) in the dried filter paper blood spot. Affected newborns have elevated levels. A second test is usually requested in 2 weeks if first is positive. If the second test is positive, infant referred for sweat test for definitive diagnosis.

POPULATION SCREENING FOR HETEROZYGOTES

Carrier screening identifies individuals with a gene or chromosome abnormality that may cause problems either for the offspring or person screened the testing of blood can indicate the existence of a particular trait that is associate with inherited disease in asymptomatic individuals.

The following aspects need to be considered before population screening for heterozygotes:

1. Information about the frequency, etiology, symptoms, course and therapeutic possibilities for the disease for which heterozygosity is determined should be known and available. Upon obtaining complete information the individual to be tested should provide informed consent.
2. If heterozygosity is demonstrated comprehensive counseling of the significance of results is required. This is necessary to prevent false judgements leading to discrimination and stigmatisation.
3. If two partners are heterozygotes they should be informed about the risks of their offspring inheriting the disease. They should be offered all options including accepting the genetic risk and offspring with the disorder, prenatal diagnosis, termination of the affected pregnancy of adoption and the couple should be allowed to make an informed unpressured decision.

An example for implementation of carrier screening includes the hemoglobin disorders (Fig. 19.1). Between 3-20% of most populations carry the sickle cell trait or thalassemia. Carriers can be identified by simple methods and carrier screening is accurate. Prevention programs are treatable and cost effective. An example of such as effective screening program involves the control of thalassemia in Cyprus. Each year 5000-8000 children are born with Thalassemia major. Epidemiological studies have shown that

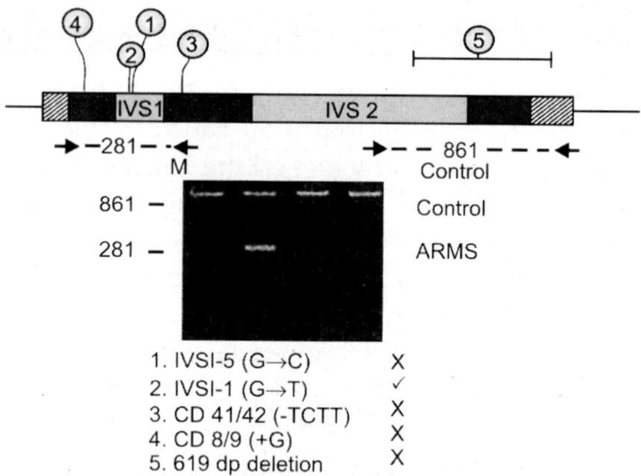

Fig. 19.1: The beta globin gene map showing some common mutations. The lower half shows agarrose gel electrophoresis of products generated using the ARMS technique.
Courtesy Dr. John Old, National Hemoglobinpathy reference Center, Oxford, UK

the problem is largely observed in India in certain communities like the Sindhis, Khatris, and Kutchis as well as in Marathas in Maharashtra. A number of teaching hospitals and NGO'S have taken up population screening, and the effect of this may be seen in the coming years. Other conditions include screening for cystic fibrosis in the Caucasian population and screening for Tay-Sach's disease is the Ashkenazi Jewish population.

Prenatal diagnosis of β-thalassemia is successfully achieved in the first trimester by chorionic villus sampling. The technique is DNA based diagnosis (Fig. 19.2).

PRESYMPTOMATIC SCREENING OF ADULTS

Presymptomatic screening of adults is carried out for family members with a history of autosomal dominant conditions with delayed onset of symptoms. Examples include screening

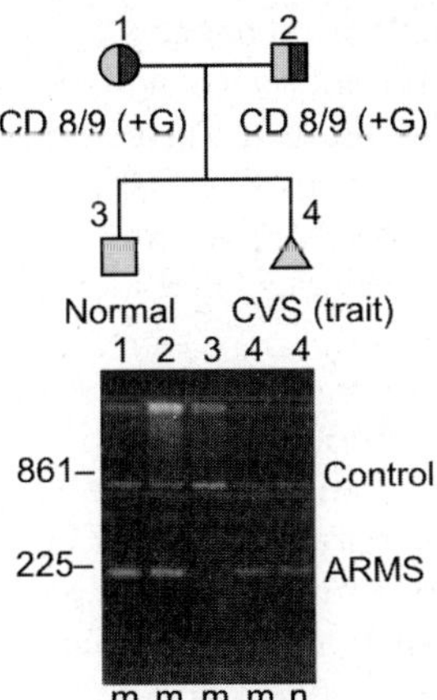

Fig. 19.2: Prenatal diagnostic evaluation for a mutation on a CVS sample. The Analysis of lane 4 using the ARMS technique shows that the fetus carries the trait and is not affected

for adult polycystic kidney disease using renal ultrasound and DNA studies, and screening for von Hippel-Lindau disease using cranial and abdominal CT scans and DNA studies. This permits genetic counseling of affected individuals and maybe necessary for effective therapy, and example of which includes early removal of tumours in Von Hippel Lindau disease or colectomy prior to the development of cancer in polyposis coli.

PREVENTION AND SCREENING FOR SOME ADULT GENETIC DISORDERS

1. Breast cancer screening is carried out using mammography and physical examination of the breast. Monthly self-examination are recommended for all women and mammograms every 2-3 years for women 40-50 years old. For patients with familial breast cancer mutation screening of the *BRCA1* and *BRCA2* genes can be carried out.

2. Screening for colorectal cancers is by testing the stool for occult blood. Endoscopy for high-risk individuals over 50, and target populations for screening include individuals with a history of colitis, familial polyposis or adenomas, and familial cancer of the colon. The screening test for such individuals includes sigmoidoscopy, ophthalmoscopy and DNA studies.
3. Screening for cervical cancer is using the Pap smear to detect cervical abnormalities every 1-3 years beginning with when the woman first becomes sexually active.
4. Screening for prostrate cancer is by digital palpation of the rectum and serum acid phosphatase concentration. The target population includes men aged 65 and above.

Principles of Population Screening for Cancer

The purpose of population screening is to divide eligible subjects into 2 groups. Those with a low risk of having cancer, and those with a sufficiently high risk to warrant further diagnostic examination. Screen is applied to asymptomatic individual and the goal is to identify individuals whose disease is at preclinical stages so it can be effectively treated.

An ideal carrier screening program will have the following attributes:

- The cancer will be a major health problem
- The cancer will be more treatable if detectable earlier
- The test should be inexpensive, cost effective as of acceptable to individuals
- The test should have a high sensitivity and specificity
- Screening will have been shown to reduce mortality.

Performance of a screening test will have no effect on disease unless individuals with abnormal results are adequately investigated and treated therefore screening programs must include follow up of abnormal results, and monitoring and tracking to measure follow up.

CHAPTER 20

PRENATAL DIAGNOSIS

INTRODUCTION

Genetic and environmental factors have an influence on various stages of development in the zygote, the preembryo, embryo, the fetus and the neonate. With the growth of genetic technology and development of high resolution ultrasound in recent years, it has become possible to detect more than 5,000 defects of hereditary and non-hereditary origin in the prenatal period. Prenatal diagnosis focuses on the diagnosis of various birth defects. Prior to development of this technology couples at risk were left with options of a risk of genetic disease or choosing other reproductive options like contraception, sterilization, or adoption. Today, these at-risk couples can make an informed choice about continuation or termination of pregnancy if a serious abnormality is detected, or think about early effective management to improve quality of life for their child. Another advantage of prenatal diagnosis is, that with normal test results, at risk couple is reassured.

Various invasive and non-invasive techniques are now available for prenatal diagnosis. The current commonly used and reliable methods of prenatal diagnosis are ultrasound, amniocentesis and chorionic villus biopsy. Maternal serum screening test at 14-16 weeks is added to these tests to pick up high-risk pregnancies for Down syndrome, and other trisomies and neural tube defects. Ultrasound is the most important tool in the detection of morphological defects of the fetus and for needle guidance in interventional techniques. For defects of genetic origin fetal tissue sampling is necessary. These tissues are used for diagnosis of chromosomal, metabolic and molecular genetic diseases.

INDICATIONS FOR PRENATAL DIAGNOSIS

Advanced Maternal Age

The most common indication for prenatal diagnosis is advanced maternal age. There is sufficient data to prove that there is an increased association between advanced maternal age and Down syndrome (Table 20.1) although other autosomal trisomies are also reported. The cause of chromosomal error in advanced maternal age is attributed to aging of the egg, which is believed to be due to the ovum being in suspended prophase. The average advanced maternal age is considered as 35 at the time of delivery, and most women at this age are offered amniocentesis or chorionic villous sampling.

Table 20.1: Co-relation between maternal age and Down syndrome

Maternal age	*Risk of Down syndrome in live borns*
25	1 in 1500
25	1 in 400
38	1 in 180
40	1 in 100
45	1 in 40

Previous Child with a Chromosomal Disorder

A couple with a history of a chromosomal disorder in a previous child, are at an increased recurrence risk, for chromosomal disorder. The risk is increased if either of the partners have balanced chromosomal rearrangement .The risk generally varies between 2 to 15%, except in a G:G translocation, where it is 100%.

Family History of a Chromosomal Disorder

In such cases, the need for prenatal diagnosis will depend on the type of chromosomal rearrangement in an index case. The karyotype of such a couple determines their recurrence risk, and prenatal diagnosis can follow.

History of Single Gene Disorder in a Previous Child or Family

Prenatal diagnosis of many single gene disorders of biochemical or molecular origin are diagnosed in pregnancy and are discussed in chapters focused on these. To plan a precise prenatal test laboratory diagnosis of an index case is important in most cases. Physicians caring for children with birth defects must make every attempt to establish a diagnosis in an index case to provide active management of the affected child, and for prenatal planning of future pregnancies.

A Positive Triple Test

The triple test is based on the estimation in the maternal serum of certain biochemical markers present in pregnancy. These are serum alfafetoprotein beta hcg, and serum estriol. (AFP, βhCG and uE3). Low AFP and high beta hCG and low estriol are indicative of increased risk of fetal aneuploidy, specially Down syndrome. With a positive triple test, fetal chromosomal studies are indicated. High alfafetprotein levels are indicative of an open neural tube defect, although certain gastrointestinal tract anomalies also are associated with it. A good ultrasound anomaly scan is important to confirm an anomaly.

Abnormal Ultrasound Findings (Soft markers for chromosomal syndromes)

Many chromosomal abnormalities, besides leading to mental retardation, have morphological abnormalities. Some of these are gross and can be picked up on ultrasound easily, while others are called soft markers. Confirmation of a syndrome in the affected pregnancy is of immense value in ascertaining a cause, deciding the time and mode of delivery, and therapy whenever possible. Accurate genetic counseling can be offered on a confirmed diagnosis.

Infertility

Many infertile couples on assisted reproductive programs have chromosomal rearrangements as a cause of their infertility. Once pregnancy is achieved, they maybe at an increased risk for a birth defect. Prenatal diagnosis can help these couples ensure an ongoing healthy pregnancy, or if abnormal, they can make an informed choice/decision.

History of Neural Tube Defects in the Previous Child or Family

Neural tube defects are mainly inherited as multifactorial disorders. When chromosomal factors are ruled out, couples with such a history should be offered maternal serum AFP screening and a a first and second trimester ultrasound scan. A 95% pick up rate can be expected in such cases.

Maternal Illness, Maternal Genetic Disease and Bad Obstetric History

With improved neonatal and pediatric care, men and women with genetic disorders can reach adulthood and reproduce. In such parents if desired, prenatal tests can be planned.

Pregnant mothers with poorly controlled insulin dependent diabetes, or epilepsy are at risk for fetal structural defects either due to their disease, or due to the drugs used to treat it. Mothers should be counseled accordingly and should be offered fetal ultrasound for detection of possible anomalies. Women with history of repeated fetal loss due to chromosomal defects in the products of conception should be offered prenatal cytogenetic evaluation.

TECHNIQUES INVOLVED IN PRENATAL DIAGNOSIS

Current techniques involved prenatal diagnosis are divided into following groups:
1. Maternal serum screening-Triple test
2. Ultrasound evaluation.
3. Obstetric procedures of fetal tissue sampling.
4. Laboratory genetic tests.

Other Techniques

1. Fluorescent in situ hybridization (FISH)
2. Preimplantation genetic diagnosis
3. Analysis of circulating fetal cells in maternal blood.

COUNSELING AND INFORMED CONSENT

For successful prenatal diagnosis, the couple needs to be counseled. Counseling should elicit a detailed clinical and family history. The counselor should confirm the indication for requested diagnosis with reference to the detection of the abnormality in question. The patient should be made aware that the laboratory test is performed as per the indication only. The safety and efficacy of the obstetric and laboratory tests should be explained. The couple should be informed about the possibility of the need for a second sample, which may be required in case of culture failure or ambiguous results.

Informed written consent is important and should be obtained from all the patients before the procedures are undertaken.

In India, prenatal diagnosis is allowed only under a specified Act. Any physician or a geneticist who provides prenatal diagnostic services in the form of counseling, obstetric procedures of fetal tissue sampling or the laboratory testing is required to obtain a license from the respective state Government, As per the act. The Pre-natal Diagnostic Techniques (Regulation and Prevention of Misuse) Act, 1994. Amended as the Preconception and Prenatal Diagnostic Techniques (Prohibition of Sex Selection ACT 2003).

PROCEDURES

Non-invasive Techniques

The Triple Test

It was observed in the West that in spite of offering prenatal cytogenetic studies to all women of advanced maternal age, the incidence of Down syndrome was not lowered. This is because many women at a much younger age also give birth to Down syndrome babies, but are not offered the triple test and are therefore not screened.

At 16 week's gestation mothers carrying Down's babies have an alteration in the levels of certain biochemical markers as compared with normal pregnancies of the same gestational age. These markers are AFP, beta hCG, and estriol (Table 20.2). The markers are also predictive of risk for other fetal aneuploidy.

Mothers with a positive screen test are considered as high-risk for fetal chromosomal aneuploidy and should be offered amniocentesis. Factors which can affect the values are maternal age, maternal weight, diabetes and gestational age and should be taken into account. Median of the multiple values (MOM) is calculated for interpretation of the results.

Table 20.2: Maternal serum triple test risk estimates

Chromosomal disorder	MSAFP	uE3	hCG
Downs syndrome	Low	Low	Raised
Trisomy 18	Low	Low	Low

Obstetric Ultrasound

Ultrasound is a valuable non-invasive tool of prenatal diagnosis, and is used for detection of structural anomalies of the fetus as well as for needle guidance in various invasive procedures.

Fetal organ development is normally completed by 18 weeks gestation. With high resolution ultrasound it has become possible to look at most of the developmental defects of the fetus, like neural tube defects, cardiac anomalies or skeletal malformations. Growth of the fetus continues till term, hence follow up scan for head size, limb measurement and renal function needs to be considered.

Many chromosomal defects have some ultrasound markers, and usually are called as soft markers (Fig. 20.1 and Table 20.3). Once such markers are observed, amniocentesis or fetal blood sampling should be considered for confirmation of a chromosomal syndrome.

Laboratory Techniques

Laboratory techniques involved in prenatal diagnosis are based on the nature of the underlying or expected defect. Basically three types of the tests are involved. These are cytogenetic (chromosomal), biochemical (enzyme assays), or molecular (DNA diagnostic). The aim of a laboratory diagnosis should be to provide rapid and reliable results.

FETAL CHROMOSOMAL STUDIES

Fetal chromosomal studies are indicated when there is an increased risk of aneuploidy on the basis of maternal age,

Table 20.3: Major chromosomal syndromes identifiable by ultrasound

Syndromes	*Ultrasound picture*
Trisomy 21	Thickened nuchal fold / VSD / Double bubble duodenal atresia / Short femur.
Trisomy 18	Choroid plexus cyst / ASD / Omphalocele / Club foot and clenched hand, overlapping fingers.
Trisomy 13	Holoprosencephaly and facial clefts / ASD / Omphalocele / Polycystic kidney / Polydactyly.
Triploidy	IUGR / VSD / ASD / Oligohydramnios / Multicystic Kidney / Anomalies of hand and feet.
45, X	Cystic hygroma / Hydrops fetalis / Lymphoedema

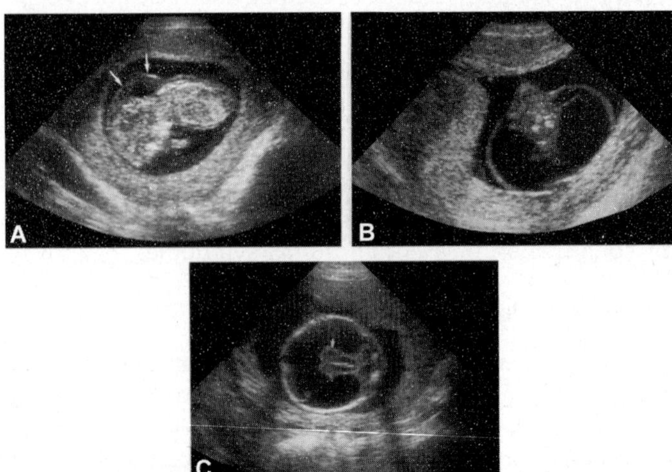

Figs 20.1A to C: Some ultrasound markers of chromosomal disease (A) Nuchal translucency in trisomy 21,45X, (B) cystic hygroma in 45X, (C) holoprosencephaly

positive triple test, previous child with chromosomal anomalies, pregnancies where one parent has a balanced structural chromosomal rearrangement, or in order to confirm fetal sex in X-linked conditions.

One of the most promising developments is interphase cytogenetics using in situ-hybridization (FISH) with non-radio active labeled probes. The results are available in 3 days. The reliability and sensitivity of the approach is being investigated in clinical practice. Karyotyping with cell culture is still recommended to confirm the finding.

FETAL ENZYME ASSAYS

Prenatal diagnosis is now possible for more than 90 inborn errors of metabolism and is indicated in all high-risk pregnancies. The amniotic fluid cells need to be grown in culture for 4-6 weeks in order to provide sufficient cells for the assay of appropriate enzymes. Currently cells from chorionic villi, direct or cultured are found to give the same results and are used when the enzymes being tested for are known to be expressed in the first trimester.

FETAL DNA DIAGNOSIS

Earlier DNA used to be extracted from amniotic cells after 3-4 weeks of culture and diagnosis was by direct demonstration of the molecular defect or by restriction fragment length polymorphisms (RFLP). Now it is possible to get sufficient amount of DNA from chorionic villi without prior culture and the test is performed earlier (9-11 weeks gestation). Chorionic villus sampling is now a preferred technique for obtaining fetal tissue for DNA analysis.

Accurate laboratory diagnosis is very important as the decision of continuation or termination of pregnancy is based on the results. Delay in results adds to anxiety leading to emotional strain. The aim of a geneticist therefore should be to provide rapid, reliable reports with a safe obstetric procedure.

FETAL TISSUE SAMPLING

Three types of tissues are predominantly used for prenatal diagnosis. The procedures are out patient, and relatively safe in expert hands. The patient has minimum discomfort with almost no complications. One of the following three techniques is commonly used for fetal tissue sampling (Table 20.4).

1. Chorionic Villous sampling (CVS) (10-12 weeks) and Late CVS (12 weeks onwards)

Table 20.4: Procedures of fetal tissue sampling

	Amniotic Fluid	*Chorionic Villi*	*Placental Villi*	*Fetal Blood*
Gestation	15-17 weeks	9-11 weeks	12 weeks +	18-20 weeks
Procedure	Simple procedure	Skilled operator required	Simple procedure	Skilled operator required
Risk of miscarriage	0.5%	1-2%	0.5%	3-4%
Reporting	12-15 days	1-15 days	1-15 days	24-72 hours
Laboratory factors	Minimum maternal cell contami-nation (MCC)	MCC, vanishing twin, placental mosaicism	Placental mosaicism	Most reliable report
Disadvantage	Delay in termination	Early termination possible	Delay in termination	Delay in termination
Patient consideration	Increased anxiety	Less emotional trauma	Increased anxiety	Apprehension

2. Amniocentesis (15-17 weeks)
3. Fetal Blood Sampling (18-20 weeks)

In case of abnormal ultrasound findings, the physician can perform amniotic fluid and cord blood sampling during the second or third trimester. Similarly, late CVS or placental biopsy is possible in the second or third trimester. Placental biopsy is useful in cases of reduced amniotic fluid volume or abnormal ultrasound findings.

Amniotic Fluid Studies

Amniocentesis was the first technique introduced in prenatal diagnosis. The use of amniocentesis for genetic diagnosis was started in 1950, when fetal sex was determined by X-chromatin studies of amniotic fluid cells. Amniotic fluid cells were first cultured in 1966 to obtain a chromosomal pattern of the fetus. In 1967, the first prenatal diagnosis of Down's syndrome (a balanced D/D translocation) was made.

With reliable reports and an ultrasound-guided procedure, amniocentesis has become a safe procedure. It has a low risk (0.5 to 1%) of miscarriage, thus has become integral part of modern obstetric care.

Amniocentesis is an outpatient procedure and is ideally performed between 15-17 menstrual week (Fig. 20.2). At this time, the ratio of viable to nonviable cells is highest. A complete ultrasound examination of the gravid uterus is made for number of fetuses and fetal viability, estimation of fetal weight by fetal biometry and placental localization. An anomaly scan for fetal malformations is done at this stage. Amniocentesis can also be done as early as 11-14 weeks (early amniocentesis), however this is not used routinely as there is an increased risk of miscarriage, and poor culture yield is likely. Amniotic fluid can be aspirated even at a later period but risk of culture failure is more likely as the ratio of viable to nonviable cells is greatly reduced after 21 weeks.

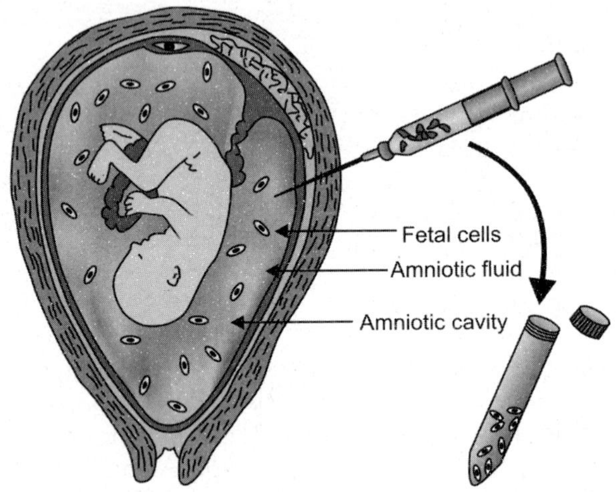

Fig. 20.2: Amniocentesis

Chorionic Villus Sampling

First trimester fetal tissue analysis by chorionic villi has been used routinely for the last 10 years. The greatest advantage of the technique is that a genetic diagnosis is possible in the first trimester.

In 1972, spontaneous divisions were first utilized for studying chromosome preparations. In 1986, first trimester fetal karyotyping from chorionic villi (9-11 weeks) was carried out. The cells from the chorionic villi were also successfully used for biochemical and DNA analysis.

The chorion consists of an outer layer of trophoblast, and an inner layer of syncitiotrophoblast with a mesenchymal core containing blood vessels. The chorion frondosum or the future placenta is selected for aspiration. This relatively simple obstetric technique is done under ultrasound guidance as an outpatient procedure. An ideal time for chorion villus sampling is 9-11 weeks and is done by the abdominal or the transcervical route. Procedure prior to 9 weeks gestation is not recommended, as up to 8 weeks gestation, there is a phase of rapid embryonic development and organogenesis. Any intervention at this stage should be strictly avoided. 15-20 mgs of fetal material can be easily obtained for analysis from a single aspiration and is sufficient for diagnosis. Cytogenetic analysis from direct cultures is available as early as 24 hours and cultured tissues take up to two weeks for the results. In experienced hands the procedure has only a 1-2% risk of fetal loss. The only associated complication of chorionic villus sampling reported was limb reduction defects.

Advantages of Chorionic Villus Sampling

1. Fetal cells are available at 9-11 weeks of gestation for chromosomal analysis, DNA analysis and enzyme assay
2. Cells from the chorionic villi are rapidly dividing and are therefore extremely suitable for chromosomal analysis
3. Sufficient fetal material can be taken as a small sample.
4. The results can be given in days or even hours.
5. It is a relatively simple obstetric technique that does not require penetration of the peritoneum or the amniotic sac.
6. If termination is decided upon, it can be carried out in the early stages of pregnancy.

FETAL TISSUE SAMPLING IN MULTIPLE GESTATIONS

Amniotic Fluid Aspiration

Cytogenetic analysis is based entirely on the samples received in the laboratory. In case of multiple gestations, it should be ensured that samples are precisely obtained from individual sacs or placentae. This is possible with good ultrasound monitoring.

Chorionic Villus Sampling (CVS) in Multiple Gestations

The incidence of CVS in multiple pregnancies is on the rise due to *in vitro* fertilization resulting in multiple pregnancies. Often such patients need prenatal diagnosis due to advanced maternal age or other genetic reasons. It is also challenging for an obstetrician if fetal reduction of an abnormal fetus is required (Figs 20.3A and B).

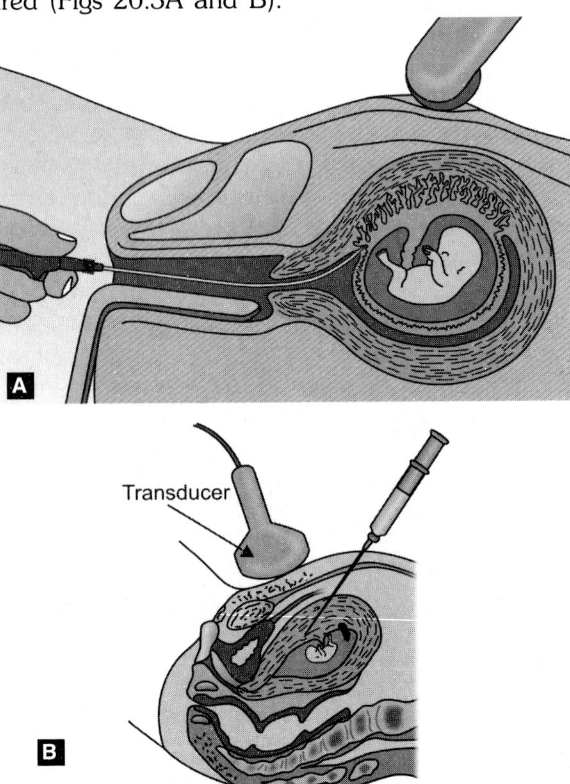

Figs 20.3A and B: Chorionic villous sampling. (A) Transcervical route, (B) Transabdominal route

In monozygotic twins, laboratory results will show the same genotype for both the twins. In dizygotic or multiple pregnancies, ultrasound examination must be concentrated on locating the septa and placentae. Separate devices are used for sampling from each sac to avoid contamination.

Fetal Blood Sampling (FBS)

Fetal blood sampling is the preferred test for rapid fetal karyotyping in advanced pregnancies or for confirming mosaicism observed in amniotic fluid cells or chorionic villi. Fetal nucleated blood cells can be cultured similar to short-term lymphocyte cultures for 24-72 hours. FBS is also used for evaluation of fetal hematological disorders, DNA diagnosis and treatment of fetal anemia by transfusion. This out patient procedure is carried out at 18 –20 weeks gestation, or later under ultrasound guidance. Fetal viability, placental localization and umbilical cord insertion is confirmed before sampling (Fig. 20.4).

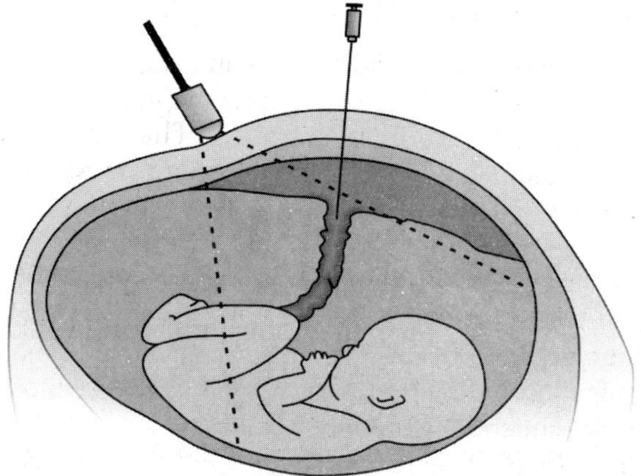

Fig. 20.4: Foetal blood sampling (Cordocentesis)

1-2 ml of fetal blood is aspirated. The sample is confirmed for its source, maternal or fetal. 0.5 to 2 ml of fetal blood is sufficient for cytogenetic diagnosis. There is a 3% fetal loss risk in the procedure. Maternal complications rare, but amnionitis and transplacental hemorrhage have been reported.

Fetoscopy, Fetal Skin Biopsy and Fetal Liver Biopsy

Fetoscopy is the endoscopic visualization of the fetus. The optimal time for this procedure is 18-20 weeks gestation. Because of the size of the instruments, only a limited field of view is possible and entire fetal visualization is not practicable. The procedure carries a fetal loss rate of about 3%. Some serious skin disorders can be diagnosed by a fetal skin biopsy taken via fetoscope. For some metabolic disorders, a fetal liver biopsy maybe necessary for diagnosis.

NEWER TECHNIQUES

Preimplantation Genetic Diagnosis (PGD)

Preimplantation genetic diagnosis is an extension of prenatal diagnosis, and the field emerged after the increasing success of *in vitro* fertilization techniques. The advantage of preimplantation diagnosis for the patient, is to have her pregnancy screened before implantation with no physical or mental stress of termination in case of abnormal results.

The first sexing of the human embryo (for an X-linked disease) was done in 1990. This was of immense value, as there are about 200 sex-linked disorders where prenatal sex determination would be useful. In the initial diagnosis, the Y specific sequence was amplified by using Polymerase Chain Reaction (PCR). Following this, in 1992 the first successful preimplantation genetic diagnosis of cystic fibrosis and Tay Sach's disease was made.

With the use of fluorescent *in situ* hybridization (FISH), the diagnosis of the most common fetal aneuploidies (X, Y, 13, 18, 21 and 16) can be carried out. The technique involves IVF procedures even in fertile patients, as several embryos are required to be screened. In addition it is recommended that PGD be followed by postimplantation genetic diagnosis.

Problems in Preimplantation Chromosomal Diagnosis

1. All cycles have to produce eggs and the procedure cannot be carried out if insufficient eggs are produced.
2. Eggs may be present but they may not be fertile.
3. All the embryos may have some chromosomal defect.
4. Due to chromosomal mosaicism, a single cell biopsy may not reflect status of the embryo.
5. The test is specific to a chromosome, and therefore the involvement of other chromosomes may not be detected.
6. It is a relatively new procedure, hence follow up with prenatal diagnosis is necessary.

Techniques of Biopsy

Polar Body Biopsy

In this technique the polar body is used for analysis. It is thus non-invasive for the embryo. This method is ideal for screening aneuploidy, as a large majority of trisomies occur during the 1st Meiotic division. However, trisomy 18 occurs after meiosis II, and therefore a 2nd Polar body analysis may be required. Only maternal defects can be analyzed by this technique and the an error in diagnosis is at times higher, due to frequent crossing over.

Cleavage Stage Biopsy

This is carried out at (6-8 Cells) on post insemination Day 3. Removal of 2 cells is possible (as single cell analysis can miss a mosaic embryo).

Blastocyst Biopsy

Multiple cells are available for analysis, resulting in a reliable diagnosis. A 1% error is possible due to confined placental mosaicism (Fig. 20.5).

Uterine Lavage

The embryo floats freely before implantation, and flushing is possible. However, all embryos may not be obtained.

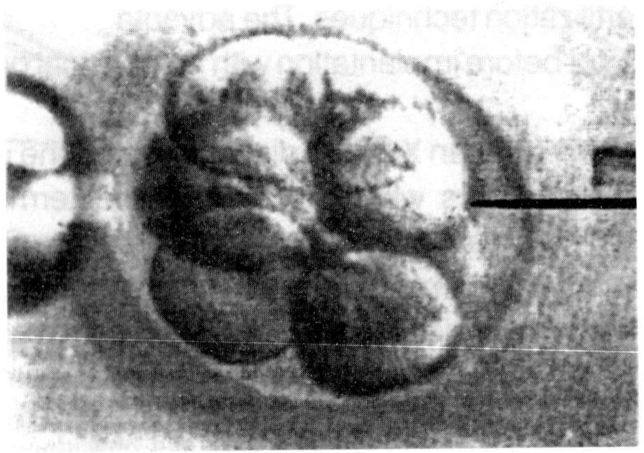

Fig. 20.5: Blastocyst biopsy for preimplantation genetic diagnosis

Fetal Cells in Maternal Blood

The possibility of recovering fetal cells from maternal blood was raised initially when XY metaphases in were demonstrated in maternal blood of pregnant women carrying a male fetus. In another technique, maternal blood was subjected to antibodies against paternal HLA alleles not present in the mother. Following flow sorting, fetal cells could be separated from maternal cells. Since then, newer techniques have demonstrated that fetal cells or at least fetal DNA exists in the maternal DNA. PCR for Y sequences on unsorted blood from pregnant women showed that women carrying a male fetus are far more likely to show a hybridization signal than those carrying a female fetus. A diagnosis of a fetus with trisomy 21, using flow sorted fetal erythroblasts obtained from maternal blood by using the FISH technique has been recently reported.

PROBLEMS IN PRENATAL DIAGNOSIS

Problems in prenatal diagnosis can arise with inadequate sample, failure in culture growth, or during interpretation of results in abnormal findings. The first two problems can be resolved by a repeat sample. Interpretation of the results is the most crucial phase in prenatal diagnosis, as pregnancy management and recurrence risk estimation is entirely based on various classical or non-classical chromosomal analysis in prenatal sample.

Recommendations in Abnormal Prenatal Cytogenetic Results

Maternal Cell Contamination

In chorionic villus cytogenetic preparations, maternal cell contamination and mosaicism is known to occur more commonly than in amniotic fluid and fetal blood sampling. When such a finding is observed it is important to assess whether the results indicate a true chromosomal abnormality in the fetus, or whether this is a confined placental abnormality with a normal fetus.

Maternal cell contamination is lowest in direct preparations and short-term cultures. In long-term cultures, it can be as high as 10-14% but with proper selection of tissue and more experience in cleaning the maternal decidua, this has been reduced. Known confined placental abnormalities are 45X, trisomy 22 and trisomy 16. The latter two can lead to placental insufficiency and IUGR. However if the chromosomal abnormality is 45X, this can be either of placental origin or the fetus may have Turner's syndrome, in which case, confirmation with amniotic fluid studies is recommended.

Mosaicism

Mosaicism can result in a major chromosome abnormality, where two or more cell lines with different karyotypes are present. True chromosomal mosaicism is one where different cell lines have originated during early post zygotic development, and are seen in the fetus. Major chromosomal trisomies, sex chromosome anomalies, chromosomal rearrangement and polyploidies can occur in the mosaic form. Post zygotic non-dysjunction is restricted to the trophoblast and extra embryonic membranes. Contamination with maternal tissue will show a mosaic cell line for fetal and maternal cells and is called confined placental mosaicism. Mosaicism can be resolved by short and long-term cultures. Mosaicism in recognized syndromes needs careful follow up by amniotic fluid studies or fetal blood sampling.

Vanishing Twin

About 7.6% pregnancies are conceived as twin pregnancies of which 6% vanish leading to one healthy twin and the other with an empty sac or remnant of the tissue. If the pregnancy is not scanned early after the missed period, the presence of one of the twins, which is going to vanish can be missed. In such a pregnancy if prenatal diagnosis is carried out by chorionic villus sampling, one can get a mixed cell line, one of which will be from persistence of trophoblast of the vanished twin, and the other from the trophoblast of the existing fetus. On some occasions, the sample may have been obtained only from the persistent trophoblast of the vanished twin. In vanishing twin cases where one fetus is healthy and the second one shows only an empty sac, patient needs to be counseled for the situation as well the need for follow up explained.

Autosomal Trisomies

Autosomal trisomies are divided into two groups. Group one, where they are associated with a clinically significant syndrome seen postnatally (Figs 20.6 and 20.7). They have a severe impact on the physical and mental development of a child, for example Trisomy 13, 18, 21. The clinical features of these syndromes are described in the chapter on chromosomal syndromes.

Group two trisomies are the ones where there is a high risk of Pseudomosaicism. In this, mosaicism is restricted only to the trophoblast and extra embryonic cells and it is not present in the fetus. Such trisomies are usually seen in chromosome number 2, 3,14, 15, 16, 20 and 22.

Trisomies of chromosome 3, 14, 16 and 22 are of placental origin hence seen more often in CVS samples, while trisomies for chromosome 2 and 20 occur frequently in amniotic fluid

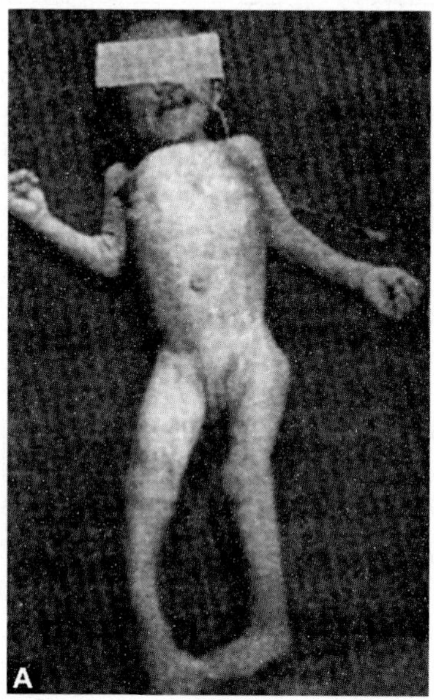

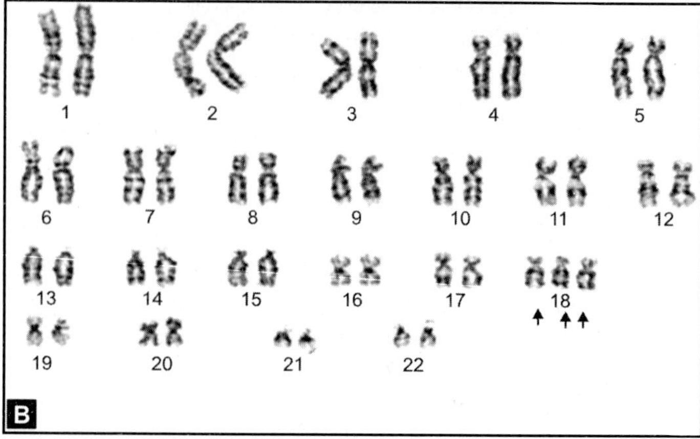

Figs 20.6A and B: (A) Fetus with trisomy 18. (B) Karyotype of the same fetus showing trisomy 18

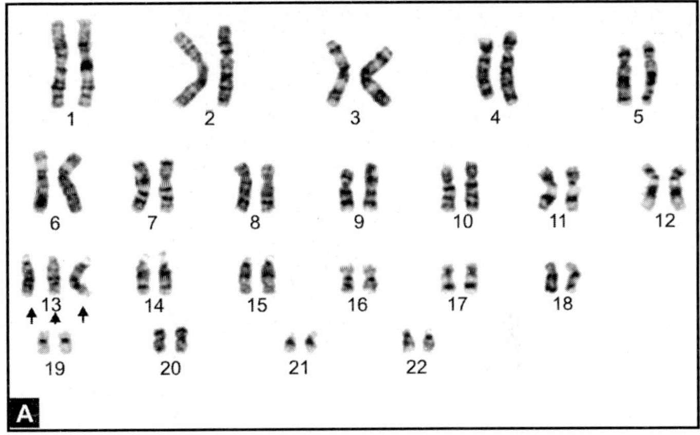

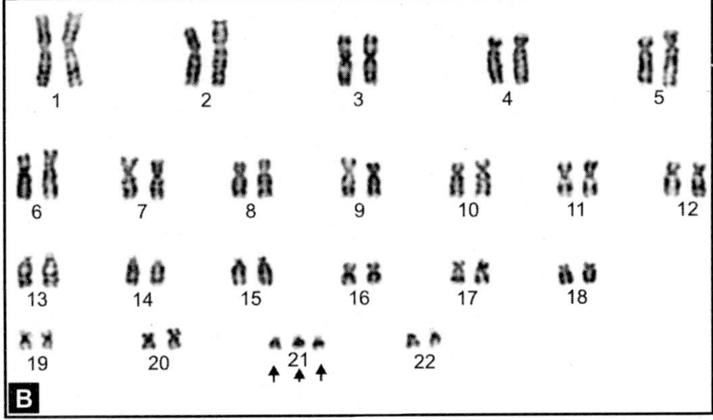

Figs 20.7A and B: Prenatal karyotypes generated by culture of amniotic fluid. (A) Trisomy 21, (B) trisomy 13

cultures. A fetus with trisomy 20 mosaicism may have a normal phenotype. Trisomy for chromosome 20 may be detected in specific fetal tissues such as kidney, rectum, oesophagus and placenta. It suggests that Trisomy 20 is confined to specific fetal tissues.

Trisomy in the Clinically Recognized Syndromes

Trisomies in the clinically recognized syndromes can also present as mosaicism, and the risk to the fetus is high. Pseudomosaicism has been demonstrated in trisomy 13, 18 and mosaic trisomies of chromosomes 7, 8, 9, 13, 18, 21. Follow up by amniocentesis or fetal blood sampling is recommended in such cases (Figs 20.8A to E).

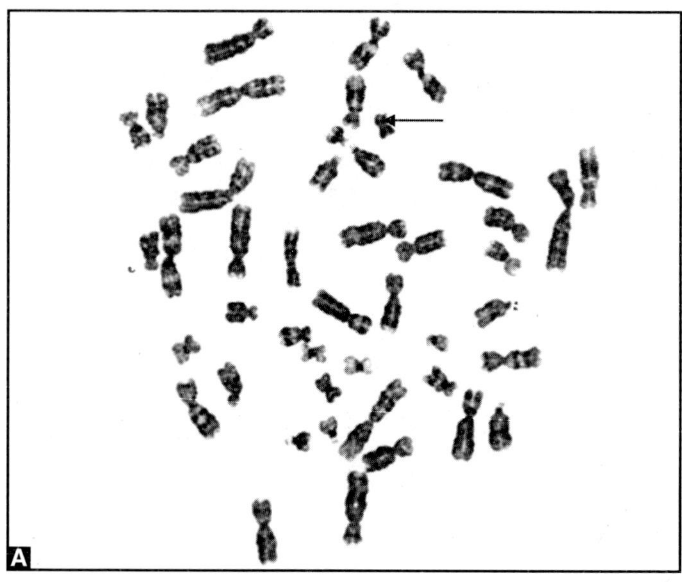

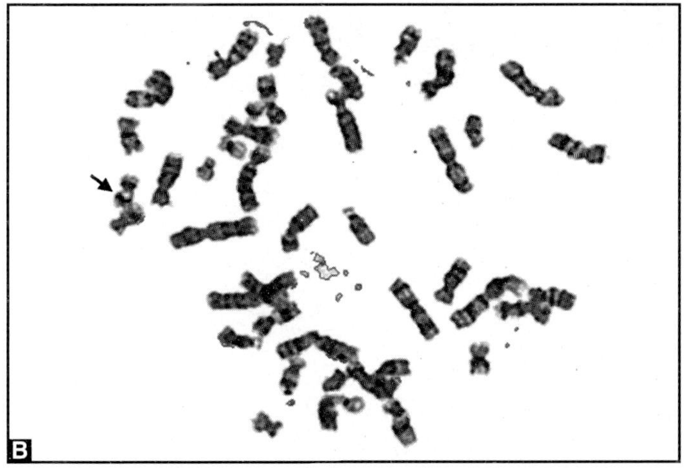
B

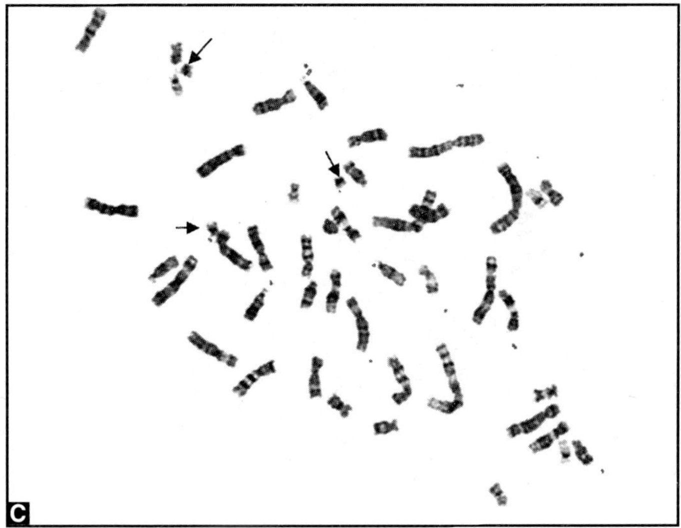
C

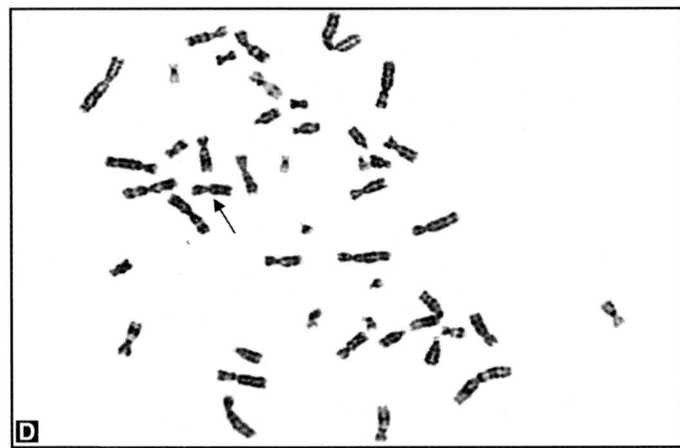

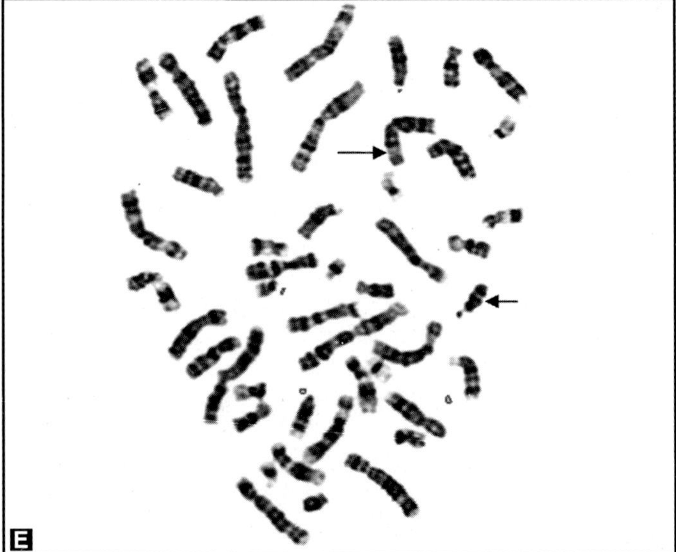

Figs 20.8A to E: Chromosomal abnormalities observed in fetal samples (A) Inversion Y (cord blood), (B) translocation t (14;21) cord blood, (C) trisomy21-(amniotic fluid) (D) 45XO-(chorionic villous sampling), (E) translocation t 8;15-(chorionic villous sampling)

Sex Chromosome Mosaicism

Sex chromosomal trisomies are compatible with life and symptoms vary from mild to severe hypogonadism. The clinical features are described in chromosomal syndromes (See chapter 18 page 296). They can be seen in mosaic forms.

True mosaicism for sex chromosomes exists in patients with sex chromosome abnormalities, leading to abnormalities of genitalia or secondary sexual development. In some CVS samples this can occur due to maternal cell contamination. It is recommended that the finding be confirmed by amniotic fluid culture or fetal blood sampling. The common sex chromosome abnormalities seen are intersex states, pseudohermaphroditism or Turner's syndrome. A brief summary of these is included in the chapter on chromosomal syndromes.

Chromosome Rearrangement

0.5% of population is known to have a chromosomal rearrangement, where the total genetic material is normal but rearranged. Types of rearrangements include translocations, pericentric and paracentric inversions and ring chromosomes. Unfortunately, phenotypes may vary from normal to severely handicapped. Hence prognosis in each individual case varies, and careful consideration is required while counseling the individual.

If such a karyotype is observed in fetal tissue, following steps are recommended:

1. Confirm parental karyotype and check for familial origin of rearrangement (maternal or paternal origin). If similar pattern is seen, and parents are normal, the risk to the fetus is low.
2. Literature survey for mental retardation or dysmorphology syndromes for correlation with the chromosome rearrangement.

3. Confirmation of the rearrangement with amniocentesis or fetal blood sampling using high-resolution banding or molecular cytogenetic techniques.

Supernumerary or Marker Chromosome

In supernumerary or marker chromosomes, assessing the prognosis is difficult. This will depend on the size of the marker chromosomes and heterochromatin involvement. The consequences can be mild to serious. Fluorescent in situ hybridization can be used to identify the segment involved. When a marker chromosome is observed, the following points need to be considered:

1. Is the marker de novo or of familial origin
2. The percentage of cells with marker chromosomes in the fetus and the parents
3. The relative size of the chromosome compared to the 'G' group of chromosomes
4. Confirmation of composition by AgNOR staining

Literature survey for risks arising from the presence of a marker chromosome.

Polyploidy

Postzygotic error can lead to diploid/triploid mosaicism and is seen in the vanishing twin syndrome. Triploidy is seen commonly in 1st trimester abortions and in pregnancy up to the second trimester. A heteroploid cell can arise due to endo reduplication ie. chromosomal replication without subsequent cell division and is mostly a cultural artifact.

Abnormal ultrasound findings are a common indication where rapid karyotyping is requested for management. If the fetus has abnormalities of classical syndromes, for example IUGR, choroid plexus cysts, renal or cardiac malformations suggestive of trisomy 18 on ultrasound scanning, and on placental biopsy the karyotype report is normal, this could be a false negative result. In this case, fetal tissue (amniotic fluid or fetal blood) should be done to confirm the karyotypic pattern.

At any time if a chromosomal rearrangement is detected in a prenatal diagnostic sample, parental karyotype should be done as soon as possible. For further pregnancy management in case of all fetal tissue samples which show an abnormal chromosomal pattern, parental karyotyping should be considered to detect the sporadic or familial origin of the same.

CHAPTER 21

TREATMENT OF GENETIC DISEASES AND HUMAN GENE THERAPY

TREATMENT OF GENETIC DISEASES

Genetic diseases occur due to deficiency of an enzyme or protein. A major motivation for gene therapy has been the need to develop novel treatments for diseases for which there is no effective conventional treatment. The goal of treatment is to modify the phenotype. Methods of treatment include:

Replacement of Deficient Enzyme/Protein

Examples of replacement of deficient enzyme/protein include treatment of SCID with blood transfusions, treatment of mucopolysaccharidoses with bone marrow transplants, treatment of Hemophilia A with cryoprecipitate/Factor VIII, treatment of Gaucher's disease with α-glucosidase, replacement of vitamin B_6 in homocystinuria, replacement of vitamin B_{12} in methylmalonicacidemia, replacement of vitamin D in vitamin D resistant rickets, thyroxine in congenital hypothyroidism and cortisone in congenital adrenal hyperplasia.

Restriction of Toxic Substrates

Examples of restriction of toxic substrates include reduction of galactose in galactosaemia, reduction of cholesterol in familial hypercholesterolemia, restriction of phenylalanine in PKU, and reduction of protein in urea cycle disorders.

Therapy of Genetic Disorders with Drugs

Therapy of genetic disorders with drugs includes treatment of Wilson's disease with penicillamine and treatment of malignant hyperthermia with dantrolene.

Surgical Approaches Such as Removal of Tissues or Organ Replacement

Removal of tissues includes colectomy in polyposis coli and organ replacement includes kidney transplants in adult polycystic kidney disease.

The term gene therapy describes any procedure intended to treat or alleviate disease by genetically modifying the genetic material of living cells to fight disease. One of the goals of gene therapy is to supply cells with copies of missing or altered genes, in an attempt to correct the disorder by altering the genetic makeup of some of the patient's cells. Gene therapy can also be used to change how a cell functions, for example by stimulating the immune system cells to attack cancer cells, or by introducing resistance to human HIV.

Cell Therapy

Cell therapy has emerged as a treatment for many diseases, and involves placement of characterized cells or embryonic stem cells in a target organ in sufficient numbers to restore the function of damaged tissue or organs. Differentiated cells may be replaced by regenerated cells or cycling stem cells, and these include hepatocytes, skeletal muscle and endothelial cells. The donor cell may be genetically engineered to synthesize and to secrete a missing entity. Examples of cell therapy also include the use of pancreatic cells and delivery of factor VIII cells engineered to secrete neurotropic factors.

The principle sources of hematopoietic stem cells for clinical transplantation include bone marrow. More recently, umbilical cord blood has been used as an alternative source of hematopoietic support. Bone marrow transplantation involves the replacement of enzymatically deficient cells with enzymatically normal cells. Allogenic bone marrow transplantation has been used to treat blood dyscrasias, hematological malignancies, and immunodeficiency states. Transplantation of haematopoietic stem cells alters course of some lysosomal and peroxisomal disorders. Hematopoietic stem-cell transplantation using bone marrow or umbilical cord blood has been the only effective long-term treatment for Hurler syndrome.

Somatic Gene Therapy

The range of disorders that might be considered amenable to this type of therapy has expanded from single-gene disorders to include cancer, AIDS, other infectious diseases, and atherosclerosis. In addition recombinant protein therapies with insulin, erythropoietin, or clotting factor could be converted for *in vivo* production via somatic gene therapy. During the past years than 300 clinical protocols and over 3000 patients have been subjected to somatic gene therapy. There are three approaches to somatic cell gene therapy: (1) *ex vivo*, where cells are removed from the body and incubated with a vector, and the gene-engineered cells are then returned to the body; (2) *in situ*, where the vector is placed directly into the affected tissues; and (3) *in vivo*, where a vector would be injected directly into the bloodstream.

Gene Therapy Strategies

For somatic gene therapy, at least three strategies for regulation of expression of the therapeutic DNA can be distinguished.

(1) A cDNA under the control of a foreign promoter can be utilized so that the product is synthesized at high levels, but without normal regulation. (2) Alternatively, genomic DNA including the sequences necessary for proper regulation of the level and tissue specificity of expression of the therapeutic gene can be used. (3) Lastly, artificial minigenes that link genomic regulatory regions with cDNA encoding the entire open reading frame, provide constructs that are of manageable size and are properly regulated. All of these strategies would typically involve random insertion of DNA sequences into the genome of the recipient. An alternative strategy would be to use site-specific recombination so that the region of a gene containing the mutation would be replaced by the normal DNA sequence. The choice of strategy will vary depending on the expression requirements of the disorder to be treated. In the case of enzyme or other protein deficiencies, where a modest increment in function may result in much improved homeostasis, any of the three nonhomologous approaches might suffice. In the case of haemoglobin disorders, the relative accessibility of bone marrow stem cells and the advantages of maintaining all the normal regulatory mechanisms make homologous recombination an extremely attractive goal. Several single-gene disorders are now candidates for gene therapy and a number of phase I clinical trials are in process. Life threatening, recessive diseases involving marrow-derived cells (e.g., adenosine deaminase deficiency, chronic granulomatous disease, and leukocyte adhesion deficiency) are considered the preferred targets for somatic gene therapy, as are disorders in which extracellular products such a hormones, clotting factors, or other serum proteins might be produced by transfected cells.

THE STRATEGIES FOR GENE THERAPY

1. *Gene augmentation therapy:* Addition of functional alleles used to treat inherited disorders caused by genetic deficiency of a gene product
2. *Targeted killing of specific cells:* Using genes encoding toxic compounds (suicide genes) or prodrugs (reagents which confer sensitivity to subsequent treatment with a drug)
3. *Targeted inhibition of gene expression:* In treatment of infectious disease
4. *Targeted mutation correction:* Using homologous recombination, antisense oligonucleotides and TFOs (triplex forming oligonucleotides)

As seen above, the genetic material may be transfused directly into cells within a patient (*in vivo* gene therapy) or cells may be removed from the patient and the genetic material inserted into the cells *in vitro*, and the modified cells transplanted back into the patient (*ex vivo* gene therapy). *Ex vivo* gene transfer involves the transfer of cloned genes into cells grown in culture. The cells that have been transformed are selected, expanded in cell culture in vitro and then introduced into the patient. In *in vivo* gene transfer, cloned genes are transferred into the tissues of the patient, and liposomes and viral vectors are used for this purpose.

PRINCIPLES OF GENE TRANSFER

Classical gene therapy required efficient transfer of cloned genes into disease cells so that introduced genes are expressed at suitably high levels. The sizes of the DNA fragment to be transferred are limited, and therefore an artificial minigene may be used, which is a cDNA sequence containing the complete coding DNA sequence, flanked by appropriate regulatory sequences to ensure a high level of expression.

Following gene transfer, the inserted genes may integrate into the chromosomes of the cell or remain as extra chromosomal genetic elements (episomes). Gene integration into chromosomes allows perpetuation by chromosomal replication following cell division. As the progeny cells contain the introduced genes, long-term stable expression may be obtained. Stem cells are an immortal population of undifferentiated precursor cells, which give rise to mature differentiated cells and are very efficient cells to target. Because normally insertion occurs randomly, the disadvantages of chromosomal integration may be that the location of the inserted genes may result in death of the host cell due to insertion into and inactivation of a gene. Aletrnatively, inserted genes may not be expressed due to integration into a highly condensed heterochromatic region, or an inserted gene may cause activation of an oncogene or inactivate a tumor suppressor gene and cause cancer.

METHODS OF GENE DELIVERY

In order to modify a specific cell type or tissue, the therapeutic gene must be efficiently delivered to the cell, in such a way that the gene can be expressed at the appropriate level and for a sufficient duration. The gene replacement used in gene therapy is delivered to the cell using a carrier vector. Two broad approaches have been used to deliver DNA to cells, namely viral vectors and non-viral vectors, which have different advantages as regards efficiency, ease of production and safety. The repertoire of delivery systems, which began with retroviral vectors, has expanded to include vectors based on adenovirus, adeno-associated virus, herpes virus, vaccinia, and other agents, and nonviral systems such as liposomes, DNA-protein conjugates, and DNA-protein-defective virus conjugates.

Viral Vectors Used for Gene Therapy

Viruses are obligate intracellular parasites, designed through the course of evolution to infect cells, often with great specificity to a particular cell type. They tend to be very efficient at transfecting their own DNA into the host cell, which is expressed to produce new viral particles. By replacing genes that are needed for the replication phase of their life cycle (the non-essential genes) with foreign genes of interest, the recombinant viral vectors can transduce the cell type it would normally infect. To produce such recombinant viral vectors the non-essential genes are provided in trans, either integrated into the genome of the packaging cell line or on a plasmid. As viruses have evolved as parasites, they all elicit a host immune system response to some extent. Mammalian virus vectors have been the preferred vehicles for gene transfer because of their high efficiency of transduction into human cells. Introduced viruses can recombine with endogenous retroviruses resulting in recombinant progeny that can undergo productive infection. Adenoviruses need repeated infections as they are non-integrating and repeated infections may provoke severe inflammatory responses (this was seen in gene therapy trials for cystic fibrosis). The most common type of vectors used in gene therapy are viruses. These viruses are genetically disabled and unable to reproduce. Mammalian virus vectors have been the preferred vehicles for gene transfer because of their high efficiency of transduction into human cells. A number of viruses have been developed, and these include retroviruses, adenoviruses, adeno-associated viruses and herpes simplex virus.

The Retroviral Systems

Retroviruses contain RNA as their genetic material instead of DNA. Retroviruses produce reverse transcriptase, which transforms their DNA into RNA. The first step in development of replication defective retroviruses involves replacement of *gag* gene (for group specific antigen), *pol* gene (encodes reverse transcriptase), and *env* gene (encodes the envelop protein) with the gene of interest. This replication-defective recombinant viral vector is transfected into a packaging cell line. Following injection, retroviruses deliver a nucleoprotein (preintegration) complex into the cytoplasm of infected cells. This complex reverse transcribes the viral genome and then integrates the resulting DNA copy into a single site in the host cell chromosomes. In absence of viral genes, the recombinant DNA or therapeutic gene is transcribed by using viral LTRs or in some cases, it is under control of the internal promoter and protein of interest is synthesized. Retroviral vectors efficiently integrate at random sites in the genome of dividing cells, permanently altering the recipient. Typically one or a few integrated copies of the recombinant vectors are found in each transduced cell. Retrovirus has a broad range of infectivity to different types of cells preferably mitotic cells. The major advantage of using retrovirus vectors is that one can determine the number of copies of gene per host cell. Retroviral vectors have several disadvantages: first, they require dividing cells as a target; second, they are difficult to produce at titers high enough for most in vivo approaches; and, third, depending on its location, retroviral integration may adversely alter the expression of a gene in the area (e.g., a proto-oncogene) and produce a transformed cellular phenotype. Currently, about 60% of approved clinical protocols for somatic gene therapy use retroviral vectors.

The Adenoviral Systems

Adenoviruses have been extensively studied, especially the Ad2 and Ad5 serotypes. The protein encoded by E1 gene is very important for viral replication. DNA up to 3.2 kb in size can replace the E1 gene to produce a replication defective recombinant vector. DNA up to 7.5 kb in size can be inserted into the genome of the adenovirus by deleting other non-essential genes. This virus has a natural tropism for respiratory epithelium. Therefore, this became a model vector for developing gene therapy in respiratory disorders. In contrast to retroviruses, adenoviruses can infect mitotic as well as post-mitotic cells. Adenovirus vectors, in contrast to retroviral vectors, offer a high titre and a better ability to infect large numbers of cells in vivo, but there is a concern about toxic effects on infected cells. In addition, the therapeutic effect is transient, with expression for only days or weeks.

The Adeno-associated Virus (AAV) Systems

This is a non-pathogenic human parvovirus and requires a helper virus for viral infection. In the absence of helper virus (adenovirus, cytomegalovirus, herpes virus), the virus integrates into human genome at specific site, 19q13.3-qter. The therapeutic gene is cloned between the two inverted terminal repeats. This recombinant plasmid is transfected along with another plasmid, which expressed viral structural proteins into the cells infected with a helper virus. Vectors based on adeno-associated virus have the potential to provide high titre, safety, and long-term expression. It is believed that the recombinant virus persists as an episome in these cells, reducing the risk of malignant transformation.

The Vaccinia Systems

The vaccinia virus is a double stranded DNA poxvirus. It infects vertebrates as well as some non-vertebrate cells. It replicates in the cytoplasm of cells. Because the vaccinia virus genome is very large, transfer vectors are constructed which contain the vaccinia virus DNA flanking the gene of interest and a selectable marker such as thymidine kinase (TK). Recombinant vaccinia virus is produced by recombination between transfer vector DNA and vaccinia DNA introduced into the cell by infection. Resulting viral rDNA can be selected based on their TK^- phenotypes. The major limitation of this viral system is that vaccinia vectors provide only transient expression, since they do not provide for DNA integration. Transient expression may be applicable in eliciting an altered immune response to malignant cells or treatment of an acute disease process.

NONVIRAL SYSTEMS FOR GENE THERAPY

Liposomes

Liposomes are spherical vesicles composed of lipid bilayers, which mimic the synthetic structure of biological membranes. The DNA lipid complexes are easy to prepare and there is no limit to the size of DNA that is transfected. However, the efficiency of gene transfer is low and the introduced DNA does not integrate into chromosomal DNA resulting in transient expression of the inserted genes.

Direct Injection

An example of this is intramuscular injection of a dystrophin minigene into a mouse model of DMD, mdx. There is a poor efficiency of gene transfer and a low level of stable integration of injected DNA.

Particle Bombardment (Gene Gun) Techniques

A micro projectile gene gun used to shoot DNA coated micro projectiles (tungsten or golden particles which are inert) into cells. The gun propels DNA-coated particles through the cell wall due to velocity and gets accommodated into the nucleus of the cells.

Receptor Mediated Endocytosis

The DNA is coupled to a targeting molecule that can bind to a specific cell surface receptor inducing endocytosis and transfer of DNA into cells. Coupling is achieved by covalently linking polylysine to the receptor molecule and then arranging for reversible binding of the negatively charged DNA to the positively charged polylysine component. A more generalised approach utilizes the transferring receptor, which is expressed in many cell types but is relatively enriched in proliferating cells and hematopoietic cells. This method has high gene transfer efficiency but does not allow integration of transformed genes. The protein-DNA complexes are not stable in serum and the DNA conjugates may be entrapped in endosomes and degraded in the lysosomes.

TARGETED INHIBITION OF GENE EXPRESSION IN VIVO

Selective inhibition of expression of a gene *in vivo*, without interfering with normal cell function is the approach for treating cancer, infectious disease, and some immunological disorders. Methods of blocking gene expression without mutating it can be accomplished at three levels.

a. *At the DNA level by blocking transcription:* Targeted inhibition of expression at the DNA level can be achieved using triple helix methods. A gene specific oligonucleotide is designed that will base pair with a defined double stranded DNA sequence of a target gene to inhibit transcription.
b. *At the RNA level by blocking mRNA ribosome attachment or mRNA attachment:* This includes antisense methods, which involve binding of gene specific oligonucleotides or polynucleotides to RNA.

c. *At the protein level by blocking post-translational processing* includes use of intracellular antibodies and oligonucleotides designed to bind and inactivate a selected protein.

GENE MODIFICATION

Gene modification involves correction of the defective gene without introducing new gene into the cells so that it will function normally. There are various ways to modify defective gene expression. These include Gene correction, in which only the defective portion of mutant gene is altered so that it will start functioning normally; Gene replacement, in which the mutant sequence of a gene is removed from the host genome and replaced with a normal functional gene, and Gene augmentation, in which introduction of a normal genetic sequence into host genome modifies the expression of mutant gene, and the defective host gene remains unaltered.

GENE THERAPY FOR MITOCHONDRIAL DISORDERS

Several methods are under investigation to develop effective carrier system for mitochondrial diseases. Some of these include bombardment of DNA-coated tungsten particles to the whole cells to insert the therapeutic gene into mitochondrial DNA, electroporation of exogenous plasmid DNA up to 7.2kb into the matrix compartment of mitochondria, and delivery of DNA by peptide targeting, which involves tagging a therapeutic gene with nuclear coded proteins, which are naturally imported into mitochondria. This technique of hijacking protein pathway has proved successful *in vitro.* Effective dissociation of the tagged DNA from proteins with the help of mitochondrial processing peptidase after entry into mitochondria is very essential without disturbing conformation of DNA. Other methods include introduction of engineered mitochondria into the cells using endocytosis, or receptor mediated therapy.

ANIMAL DISEASE MODELS FOR GENE THERAPY

An animal disease model is used for many human diseases to check the efficacy and safety of gene therapy. Several natural disease models have been found in nature, or have been generated by random mutagenesis, which does not take place at a predetermined locus. Some of these animal models include the Watanbe heritable hyperlipidaemic (WHHL) rabbit, which has a deletion of four codons of the *LDL-receptor* gene and as a result is hyperlipidemic and a model for human familial hypercholesterolemia, the mdx mouse which has mutations in the *dystrophin* gene and is a model for Duchenne muscular dystrophy, the Gunn rat, which shows deficiency of gene for enzyme UDP-glucuronyl transferase, the enzyme being absent in hereditary Crigler Najjar Syndrome resulting in increased bilirubin levels, the NOD mouse, which is diabetic and a model for human insulin dependant diabetes mellitus, and the hemophiliac dog, which has a missense mutation in the *factor IX* gene, and is a model for human hemophilia B.

Animal models of disease can also be generated by genetic manipulation by insertion of foreign DNA. These models can be used to study gene function, and to create animal models for human diseases. In order to create such genetically modified animals, the DNA of germline cells is modified. This DNA is heritable and therefore certain cells that have the capacity to differentiate into different cell types seen in the adult are considered optimal targets for introduction of foreign DNA. Such cells include the fertilized oocyte or embryonic stem cells, which are capable of giving rise to both somatic, and germline cells. When a foreign DNA molecule is artificially introduced into the cells of an animal, the animal is called a transgenic animal and the inserted DNA the transgene. In gene targeting, the mutation is introduced into a preselected endogenous gene within an intact cell. The mutation may result in inactivation of gene expression, termed a knockout mutation, or altered gene expression, and is useful for studying gene function. Transgenic animals have been used to analyse human genes by investigating gene expression and its regulation, by investigating gene function by targeted gene inactivation, by investigating gene function, and by investigating dosage effects and ectopic expression. Examples of transgenic or gene-targeted mouse models of human disease include models for cystic fibrosis, β-thalassaemia, hypercholesterolemia, Gaucher's disease, and fragile X-syndrome all produced by insertional inactivation by gene targeting. The ability to produce transgenic mice and gene targeting has permitted the design of many new animal models of disease. Another approach is genetic manipulation of animals using somatic cell nuclear transfer into an enucleated oocyte. In 1997, this approach allowed cloning of an adult mammal, a sheep called "Dolly". The successful cloning of an adult animal has major implications for research, medicine and society.

GENE THERAPY FOR INHERITED DISORDERS

Recessively inherited disorders, where disease results from a simple deficiency of a specific gene product can be treated by high-level expression of introduced normal alleles.

Examples of gene therapy for inherited disorders include:

1. *Alteration of T-cells and hematopoietic stem cells in ADA deficiency.* The gene therapy involves an *ex vivo* strategy using recombinant retroviruses containing the ADA gene.

2. *Alteration of liver cells in familial hypercholesterolemia* using an *ex vivo* strategy using retrovirus to deliver the LDL receptor gene.
3. *In cystic fibrosis,* the cells altered are the respiratory epithelial cells using an *in vivo* strategy using recombinant adenovirus or liposomes to deliver the CFTR gene.
4. *Alteration of hematopoietic stem cells* using an *ex vivo* strategy with retroviruses delivering the *GBA* gene in Gaucher's disease due to glucocerebrosidase deficiency.

AN EXAMPLE OF AN INHERITED DISORDER FOR WHICH GENE THERAPY HAS PROVED SUCCESSFUL

Severe Combined Immunodeficiency (SCID)

This disease is mainly caused by deficiency of housekeeping gene adenosine deaminase enzyme (ADA) that is mainly produced by T-lymphocytes. If ADA is not present in the body, enzyme kinase converts one of the metabolic by-products into a toxin, which destroys the T-lymphocytes. T-lymphocytes are important to the body's immune systems. They not only directly participate in immune responses, but controls activity of B-lymphocytes, cells that produce antibodies. Thus, deficiency of ADA will affect body's immune system. In 1990, the National Institute of Health (NIH) received the first approval for gene therapy testing for SCID disease. Here researchers isolated lymphocytes from the patient and exposed them to recombinant retroviruses carrying genes for ADA production. These engineered lymphocytes were then replaced into the patient where they started secreting ADA enzyme. The first patients of SCID reported to have been benefited from successful gene therapy in 1990 and 1991 were age 4 and age 9. The children are progressing well and essentially leading a healthy life.

GENE THERAPY FOR INFECTIOUS DISEASE

Gene therapy for infectious disorders involve strategies like provoking a specific immune response or specific killing of infected cells by insertion of a gene encoding a toxin or prodrug. Current gene therapy trials for infectious disease are aimed at treating patients with AIDS. The gene therapy strategies interfere with the HIV virus life cycle at three levels. By blocking HIV-1 infection, by inhibition at the RNA level using antisense, ribozymes/approaches or inhibition at the protein level involves designing intracellular antibodies against HIV proteins such as the envelope proteins. The main target for gene therapy is the expression of genes that can interfere with virus replication in CD4$^+$ T cells or stem cells. Potential therapeutic genes which will be either antisense version of the HIV *tar* gene or a mutated HIV *rev* gene that blocks the transport of HIV RNA from the nucleus and marker genes are introduced into CD4$^+$ T cells. These recombinant cells will be cultured and can be given to HIV positive persons. Other strategies include provoking an immune response against the HIV virus by transferring a gene that encodes an HIV-1 antigen such as the envelope protein gp120 and expressing it in a patient, or boosting the patients' immune system by transfer and expression of a gene encoding a cytokine such as an interferon using retroviral mediated methods.

GENE THERAPY FOR CANCER

Cancer therapy includes targeted killing of disease cells by inducing genes that encode toxins or by provoking enhanced immune responses. Some approaches focus on targeting single genes such as T*p53* gene augmentation therapy or antisense *K-ras* genes in lung cancer, where the translation of the mutant gene mRNA to the final oncoprotein product which is responsible for involuntary cell growth is prevented. In case of lung cancer, this strategy has been used against *K-ras* genes. In B-cell lymphomas, *bcl-2* is over expressed as a result of translocation of *bcl-2* gene to the immunoglobulin heavy-chain locus. This can be also hybridised with an antisense oligonucleotide, which is complementary to the *bcl-2* gene.

Potential applications of gene therapy for the treatment of cancer include approaches like artificial killing of cancer cells using genes encoding toxins or conferring drug sensitivity for example by insertion of the multiple drug resistance gene (*MDR1*). Another approach is insertion of genes encoding foreign antigens or cytokines to enhance immunogenicity of the tumor or increase anti-tumor activity of immune cells, induce normal tissues to produce anti-tumor substances like interleukin-2 or interferon and production of recombinant vaccines for prevention and treatment of malignancy. This approach involves the use of tumor infiltrating lymphocytes (TIL) as a vehicle to carry recombinant viruses containing human cytokine genes by infecting lymphocytes with a recombinant virus. These tumor-infiltrating lymphocytes attack cancerous cells and produce cytokines causing lysis of tumor cells. It is possible to enhance TIL response by transfecting recombinant viruses carrying genes such as interleukins (*IL*) 2,3,4,6,7 and tumor necrosis factor (*TNF*) whose product induces strong immunogenic response against tumor cells. For tumors arising from oncogene activation, inhibition of expression of oncogenes can be carried out using antisense oligonucleotides or triple helix oligonucleotides or intracellular antibodies can be used to bind to the oncoprotein. For tumors arising from inactivation of tumor suppressors, gene augmentation therapy can be used. Another strategy used in cancer therapy is suicide vector gene therapy. Here suicide viral vector has been used to infect the tumor cells. This recombinant viral vector contains suicide gene, which encodes an enzyme that converts non-toxic prodrug into cytotoxic product, which regresses tumor mass. Cells that get transfected with these suicide genes commit metabolic suicide. For example, herpes simplex virus thymidine kinase (*HSVtk*), cytosine deaminase and varicella zoster virus thymidine kinase are a few examples of suicide genes.

EXAMPLES OF CANCER GENE THERAPY TRIALS

1. Alteration of tumor cells *ex vivo* or *in vivo* to deliver the HSV-tk gene in brain tumors
2. Use of fibroblasts *ex vivo* and retroviruses to deliver the MDR1 (multiple drug resistance gene) gene in breast cancer. Retroviruses to deliver the MDR1 gene have also been used to alter tumor cells *in vivo* in colorectal cancer.
3. Use of retroviruses deliver IL2 genes to fibroblasts *ex vivo* or tumor cells *in vivo* in malignant melanoma
4. Use of retroviruses to deliver the IL4 gene to tumor cells or T cells ex vivo in myelogenous leukemia, or fibroblasts *ex vivo* in small cell lung cancer
5. Use of retroviruses to deliver the TNFA gene to tumor cells for the treatment of neuroblastoma.

CHAPTER 22

THE HUMAN GENOME PROJECT

In February 2001, two research groups, a biotechnology company and the other a publicly funded consortium published the draft sequence of the human genome. Accounting for just over 90% of the euchromatic portion of the 3 megabase haploid genome, this represents the fruits of a decade of intensive efforts to map and sequence the entire human genome, in the process dubbed the "Human Genome Project".

HISTORY

The idea of sequencing the entire human genome was first proposed in the mid-eighties at scientific meetings sponsored by the US Department of Energy. The US National Research Council in 1988 recommended a broader program including the following aims: (a) The generation of detailed genetic and physical maps of the human genome, (b) sequencing of the genomes of model organisms (bacteria, yeast, worms, flies and mouse), (c) the development of technologies to support these activities, and (d) research into the ethical, legal and social issues (ELSIs) raised by human genome research. The human genome project was launched in the US in 1990 as a joint effort of the DOE and the National Institutes of Health; the plan was to finish sequencing the human genome by 2005 with an estimated budget of 3 billion dollars. By 1991 the International Human Genome Project was underway with collaborations between various organisations in the US, UK, France, Japan, European Community, and later by Germany and Japan. The Human Genome Organisation (HUGO) was founded to coordinate this international effort. By 1995, significant progress had been made in generation of the genetic and physical maps of the human genome, and in the large-scale sequencing of the yeast and worm genomes, as well as targeted regions of the human genome. In 1998, Celera Genomics [formed by a merger of Applied Biosystems and The Institute of Genomic Research (TIGR)] announced that it would independently sequence the entire human genome over a 3-year period. In February 2001, the International Human Genome Sequencing Consortium and Celera Genomics independently published the draft version of the complete human genome sequence in the journals *Nature* (1) and *Science* (2), respectively. It is very likely that the complete, fully annotated version of the human genome sequence will be available before the initial deadline of 2005 and perhaps in time for the 50th anniversary of the discovery of the double-helical structure of DNA by Watson and Crick in 2003.

STRATEGY

DNA is sequenced in short reads of approximately 400 – 750 bp at a time. Smaller genomes such as those of bacteria and viruses have been sequenced in their entirety because of the limited challenge of piecing together "random" sequences. Larger genomes pose a special problem since randomly generated sequences (shotgun sequencing) would need "markers" to be able to assemble the complete sequence. This is analogous to a jigsaw puzzle – where the short, random sequences are the equivalent of pieces of the puzzle and the entire 3-billion bp sequence is the completed jigsaw puzzle. So to be able to piece together the entire picture, it was important to initially find "markers" across the entire genome that would subsequently allow the entire sequence of the genome to be assembled. The process of identifying these markers is referred to as the "mapping" of the genome.

The essential steps (Fig. 22.1) involved in facilitating the complete sequencing the human genome include the following: (a) genetic mapping, (b) physical mapping, (c) gene (transcript) mapping, and finally (d) shotgun sequencing.

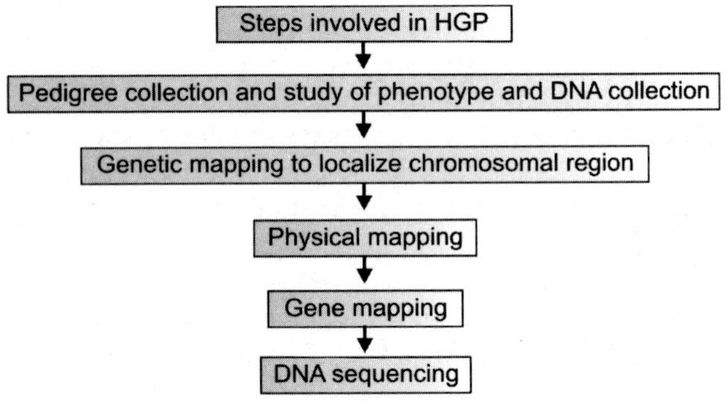

Fig. 22.1: Steps involved in human genome project

Variable sequences (i.e., polymorphisms), situated across the entire genome serve as genetic markers, and their identification constitutes the "genetic mapping" of the genome. Cutting up the genome into smaller segments, cloning them into vectors, and characterising the sequence of their ends to get small sequence tags (Sequence Tagged Sites/STS) across the genome constitutes the "physical mapping" of the genome. The vectors used for this purpose hold large DNA inserts (0.1 to 1 million bases). Using the STSs and other markers within the DNA inserts, clones spanning the entire genome were constructed and ordered.

Converting transcribed genes into their respective cDNAs by reverse transcription, and cloning and sequencing them was the basis of assembling a "gene or transcript map" of the genome. Using the latter method it was possible to sequence coding regions of a variety of unknown genes without knowing the corresponding genomic context or sequence. These sequenced genes also served the same function as STSs, and were called "Expressed Sequence Tags" (ESTs).

Having first mapped the genome using all these methods, it became possible to assemble randomly sequenced stretches of DNA into larger sequences (contigs) and subsequently to assembly the entire human genome. Genomic DNA was cut up into smaller bits using restriction enzymes and cloned into vectors that hold small inserts (2 – 50 kb) suitable for sequencing. This strategy is referred to as "shot-gun" sequencing, since essentially random bits of sequence are analysed from various clones. These sequences are then assembled by software programs using overlaps in sequence and the handles generated in the detailed mapping of the genome described above. Celera Genomics initially tried to assemble the entire genome using only sequence overlaps, but failed to do so and decided to also use the ordered markers generated by the international consortium and made freely available on the internet (GenBank).

The development of rapid and automated sequencing technologies, custom robotics, versatile sequence analysis and assembly software, and the over-whelming financial and logistical support of the public and private sectors helped bring about the spectacular success of the HGP.

SUMMARY OF THE HUMAN GENOME

- Size of the human genome: 3.2 billion bp
- Size of the euchromatic portion: 2.9 billion bp

- Total number of genes (known plus predicted): 30,000 – 40,000
- Mean size of gene: 27,000 bp
- Mean size of exon: 145 bp
- Mean number of exons per gene: 8.8
- Mean size of intron: 3,365 bp
- Mean number of amino acids encoded per gene: 447
- Protein coding sequence as a fraction of the entire genome: 1.4%
- Introns as a fraction of the genome: 36%
- Intergenic (non-gene) region of the genome: 63%
- Frequency of variation in the genome (single nucleotide polymorphisms): 1/1250 bp.

MEDICAL BENEFITS OF THE HUMAN GENOME PROJECT

Knowledge of the human genome sequence will have a profound influence in Medicine and Biology. Rather than the climax, the completion of the human genome sequence should be viewed as the beginning of the postgenomic era, a continued exploration of our molecular nature. From a medical standpoint, this knowledge will result in improved diagnosis and treatment of diseases with a genetic component.

Genes underlying inherited diseases are commonly identified by "positional cloning" i.e., using genetic linkage analysis in affected families, followed by gene hunting, and finally detection of mutations within the genes identified in the hunt. Before the advent of large-scale mapping and sequencing, this process typically took several years to accomplish. More recently, with the increasing availability of genomic sequence (released everyday over the past four years by the International Consortium), and the comprehensive mapping of the genome this process has become a lot less tedious. Consequently, at least 30 new disease genes have so far been identified that depended directly on the public release of the genomic sequence including those for breast cancer susceptibility (*BRCA2*), a form of limb girdle muscular dystrophy (*LGMD2G*), and three genes that cause non-syndromic deafness. The availability of the complete genome sequence makes it possible to comprehensively search for related genes. For example, after the identification of presenilin-1, a gene responsible for familial Alzheimer's disease, a computer search of the genome identified a closely related gene (presenilin-2), which was also shown to cause autosomal dominant Alzheimer's disease in other families.

The vast number of genes and their protein products are considered potential drug targets for the treatment of diseases. So far, a significant part of pharmaceutical research has been targeted towards the identification of such targets; however, the complete genome sequence has provided an instant treasure trove of potential targets for therapeutic strategies. Examples of these include (a) the identification of a previously unknown serotonin receptor, which is being investigated as a therapeutic target for schizophrenia, and (b) a new protease involved in the processing of beta-amyloid that is located on chromosome 21, which is being investigated as the cause of deposition of Alzheimer's disease like amyloid in the brains of patients with Down's syndrome.

With 99.999% of the genome being identical among all human beings, it is likely that the variable sequences (polymorphisms) in the genome may account for many of our individual differences. Single nucleotide polymorphisms (SNPs) occur once every 1250 bp in the human genome, and nearly 1.4 million have been identified to date. Less than 1% of these SNPs map within coding regions of genes and could potentially affect protein function. It is believed that "typing" of multiple SNPs will provide correlations with (a) susceptibility to certain disease states, especially those with a complex genetic contribution (e.g. type 2 diabetes, ischaemic heart disease, multiple sclerosis etc.), (b) differences in the response to drugs, and the incidence of side effects caused by them, and (c) disease prognosis.

Over 40% of the predicted genes have no ascribed function at this time. Their identification, without any relationship with a phenotype or function will result in accelerated research towards determining their role. Large-scale attempts to determine the function of these genes has resulted in the development of a new field called "functional genomics". With the knowledge of the entire genetic complement of the human genome, we now know all the encoded proteins; the study of these using large-scale methods, for example in the comparison of "normal" versus "disease" tissues, is called "proteomics". The availability of sequences from other organisms has also initiated the field of "comparative genomics" that is already having a major impact on the functional characterisation of the many newly identified genes.

ETHICAL LEGAL AND SOCIAL ISSUES (ELSI)

Knowledge of one's personal genetic information may be exploited by various agencies for many reasons. Insurance companies, the healthcare industry, employers, and government agencies may exploit this information. Genetic profiling could be a new basis for discrimination. It was recognized early on in the planning stages that the Human Genome Project would raise a multitude of ethical, social and legal issues. Already, the US and other European governments are in the process of drafting genetic privacy laws to prevent such information from being exploited. On the other hand, some societies do not seem to be overly concerned by this and have forged ahead forming unique relationships with the pharmaceutical industry. For example, the Icelandic government has developed collaborations with a pharmaceutical company, which will study their population for genetic variation and use it to develop new diagnostic, therapeutic and prognostic indicators.

OTHER GENOMES

Before the human nuclear genome was sequenced, genomic scientists had already sequenced genomes of the following: 599 viruses and viroids, 205 natural plasmids, 185 organelles (including the human mitochondrial genome in 1981), 31 eubacteria, 7 archaea, one fungus, two animals and one plant. With the technology in place, considerable effort is now being directed towards sequencing of other large genomes, such as the mouse, rat, zebra fish, puffer fish, and other primates. Plans are also being made to sequence other organisms that will help define key developments along the vertebrate and invertebrate lineages. Comparative genomics will then allow the characterisation of evolutionarily conserved features and the identification of genetic innovations in specific lineages.

THE FUTURE

The current draft version of the human genome sequence is expected to be fully completed by 2003. This however only represents the euchromatic portion of the genome; the heterochromatic portion is considered very difficult to sequence because it is largely composed of highly polymorphic tandem repeats. The details of all the genes and their splice forms remain to be unambiguously determined. Sequence similarity between human and mouse is likely to help identify over 95% of all exons and a significant proportion of the regulatory regions. This may not be too far off in the future since the mouse genome sequence will likely be completed within the next year. Plans are underway to clone every full-length human cDNA and have it available for the scientific community without restrictions.

Complete analysis of the polymorphic variation and its correlation with specific phenotypes holds great promise for the practice of medicine. Great advances will be made in the understanding of the molecular basis of disease which will likely lead to specific therapies. However, going from sequence to function will require a major concerted effort, perhaps larger in scale than the effort made in the Human Genome Project itself. These efforts will include the development of databases of gene expression, protein localization, protein-protein and DNA-protein interactions. New computational and technological advances will be required to fully realize the potential information embedded in the 3-billion bp of human DNA sequence now available.

CHAPTER 23

ETHICAL ISSUES IN MEDICAL GENETICS

INTRODUCTION

Ethical issues in medical practice tend to arise in every branch of medicine. They are important in medical genetics and need careful consideration, since the science of genetics was once blamed to be the practice of eugenics. The word eugenics, was first introduced by Galton. It is defined as the science of improving a race or breed by mating individuals with desired characteristics. In negative eugenics, the aim is to eliminate extreme heritable mental and physical defects. Positive eugenics is to increase the number of so called better individuals. This approach is involved in agriculture in plant and animal breeding where desirable characters can be added or removed. The application of the same principles in humans is considered to be a violation of human rights. Genetic testing and counselling was considered to be an attempt to improve the species through selective breeding. In spite of this, advancement in the field of genetics is improving the quality of life in the affected and its use in preventing life threatening and crippling diseases, is being accepted now. Genetic diagnosis concerns not only the patient, but has an effect on the immediate family as well as on the community. The results of the tests and decisions often lead to termination of a pregnancy and may stigmatise a person for not having the right genes.

Ethical issues involve moral questions and dilemmas. It is the responsibility of a geneticist to communicate all factual knowledge to the patient or family, who can on the basis of this information make a personal choice. It is essential that a counsellor at all times should offer counseling that is non-directive. What is right for one family may not be right for another, and the decision made by a family should be respected.

PRINCIPLES OF IMPARTING INFORMATION

Informed Written Consent

The informed consent should include details of the risk and technical limitations of the procedure involved in the laboratory as well as the clinical (prenatal diagnostic) procedures. The written consent protects the physician as well, as all the procedures have been thoroughly explained to the patient.

Informed Non-directive Choice

In this, the patient is given complete knowledge about all the available options and consequences of not doing the test. The patient should be given sufficient time to make a decision.

Confidentiality

Confidentiality is to be maintained in all cases and at all the costs. No information should be divulged to even the nearest relatives unless the patient so requests. All results should be discussed jointly with the couple. Failing to do this can create a misunderstanding in the members of the family, as a single member collecting all the information may not pass it on to the related members in the appropriate fashion.

Autonomy

Autonomy involves choosing a course of action as per one's decision without constraints from others.

POTENTIAL AREAS OF ETHICAL CONCERN

Certain areas in medical genetics pose ethical problems, and these include prenatal diagnosis, population screening, family screening, predictive testing and research.

Prenatal Diagnosis

Prenatal diagnosis is now available for a wide variety of structural abnormalities, which can be detected by an ultrasound examination. Other genetic disorders like biochemical, molecular and cytogenetic disorders can be detected by various laboratory tests. When the results of such tests are abnormal, patients may opt to terminate pregnancies, knowing the risk of a serious handicap in the child if the pregnancy is continued. The patient undergoing the test needs to be precisely told what to expect from the test. A laboratory test is done to rule out a specific defect only and no other defects can be ruled out. There is usually a misconception in the patient's mind as to whether the test can rule out almost any birth or genetic defect. This needs to be explained to the patient before any test is undertaken. Termination of pregnancy for the selection of the sex of an unborn child is legally prohibited in India under the prenatal diagnostic Technique (Regulation and Prevention of Misuse) Act 1994.

Population Screening

Population screening programmes for carrier detection may be carried out in certain populations with a high risk for certain autosomal recessive disorders. In autosomal recessive conditions both the partners have to be carriers in order to transmit the disease to the progeny. Carrier testing in individuals at risk for a particular disease in a population may be carried out, at the request of the individuals in question.

Screening can be carried out for thalassaemia, Tay Sach's disease and cystic fibrosis in the appropriate populations.

Newborn screening programmes when implemented are extremely important in the prevention of mental and growth retardation in some metabolic conditions.

Family Screening

During the process of genetic counseling and testing, certain genetic conditions are accidentally picked up, like a carrier of a balanced translocation or a life threatening X-linked recessive disorder where other family members are at risk. In such an event, screening tests are recommended for the family. The time for the affected individual to deal with the situation should be provided.

Predictive Testing

The developments of direct mutation analysis by various molecular techniques have opened up an opportunity to diagnose many genetic disorders of adult onset. Huntington's disease, adenomatous polyposis, and familial breast cancer are examples of such disorders. Predictive testing in a child is to be done only if requested by the parents. It is justified if it is going to help in the long-term management of a child e.g. in familial hypercholesterolaemia predictive testing can help in dietary management from an early age.

It is commonly believed that any genetic condition for which predictive testing is available but is not useful in management should not be carried out till the child attains maturity to understand it and makes an informed decision.

Another example of predictive testing is a complex one and such a situation can arise in Huntington's disease (HD). A young man may request predictive testing on the basis of his paternal grandfather being affected with HD. His test results may have the following implication: If the son is found to carry a mutation, his untested father who is not otherwise keen on knowing his status would know that he carries the mutation and has passed on the mutation to his son, since HD is an autosomal dominant disorder. These situations are difficult to handle. Here an anxious adult gets a priority over the parent and has the right to know. Confidentiality is to be strictly maintained and the status of the son should not be divulged to anyone but the patient himself.

Predictive testing leads to yet another complex situation for the purposes of Medical Insurance Companies may deny insurance on the basis of predisposition to genetic disease. The insurance companies can ask (in indicated cases) for the results of predictive testing but cannot demand the test. The companies however feel that they should either offer low sum insurances or high premiums. The issues are insoluble.

Gene Therapy

With advances in molecular biology, it possible to treat genetic diseases using gene therapy. Gene therapy has been successfully carried out for severe combined immune deficiency. In this case the patient or parents of the child with the disease are willing for any therapy, as they know there is no other cure. They are willing to participate in any programme of genetic research where there is hope. The trials in which they participate, are however uncontrolled trials where hazards or benefits are not known. The second aspect is such therapy when applied to the germ-line will be considered a eugenic approach. The current law under which gene therapy is permitted totally prevents germ line therapy. Gene therapy is also not permitted for choosing a particular character like looks, intelligence or other skills. In the United Kingdom, the committee on the ethics of Gene Therapy has recommended all gene therapy programs to be subjected to scrutiny by regional hospitals and ethical committees.

MULTIPLE CHOICE QUESTIONS AND ANSWERS

1. Which genetic disease occurs most frequently?
   (a) Autosomal dominant
   (b) Autosomal recessive
   (c) X-linked
   (d) Chromosomal abnormality
   (e) Multifactorial
2. In which part of the cell cycle are chromosomes best studied?
   (a) Interphase (b) Metaphase
   (c) Anaphase (d) Prophase
   (e) Telophase
3. Chromosomes with a central centromere are known as:
   (a) Metacentric (b) Submetacentric
   (c) Acrocentric (d) Telocentric
4. Fragile-X is diagnosed by:
   (a) G-banding
   (b) A-banding
   (c) C-banding
   (d) Folic acid deficient medium
5. What is true of the difference between gametogenesis in males and females?
   (a) Mitotic division of germ cell precursors occurs only in males
   (b) Meiosis in males begins in the fetus whereas female meiosis does not begin till puberty

(c) Dictyotene occurs during meiosis I in females but not males
(d) Oocytes do not complete meiosis II after fertilization whereas spermatocyte complete mitosis before mature sperms are formed

6. In which of the following clinical condition is a karyotype most useful?
(a) Repeated abortions
(b) Parents of a child with Down syndrome
(c) A women with H/O drugs in the 1st trimester
(d) H/o spina bifida in a previous child

7. A newborn child has hyperbilirubinemia in the neonatal period, brachycephalus, hypotonia, single palm crease, chromosome analysis will show:
(a) Trisomy 13 (b) Trisomy 18
(c) Trisomy 21 (d) XO

8. An affected male child born to normal parents can have all but one of the:
(a) Autosomal dominant
(b) Autosomal recessive
(c) Sex-linked recessive
(d) Vertical transmission
(e) Multifactorial

9. Rocker bottom feet are classically associated with:
(a) Trisomy 21 (b) Trisomy 18
(c) Trisomy 13 (d) Trisomy 9

10. Submicroscopic deletion is identified by:
(a) R-banding (b) C-banding
(c) FISH (d) G-banding

11. Which type of mutation is commonly associated with thalassemia:
(a) Insertion (b) Deletion
(c) Duplication (d) Point mutation
(e) Frame shift mutation

12. The term variable penetrance is used in connection with:
    (a) Autosomal dominant
    (b) Autosomal recessive
    (c) Multifactorial
    (d) Sex-linked recessive
13. The affected male child is hemizygous in:
    (a) Autosomal dominant
    (b) Autosomal recessive
    (c) Multifactorial
    (d) Sex-linked recessive
14. Risk of recurrence is 100% in Down syndrome when the parents have one of the following karyotype:
    (a) Trisomy 21
    (b) 14/21 translocation
    (c) Mosaic for Trisomy 21
    (d) 21/21 translocation
15. Common cardiac defect in Down syndrome is:
    (a) Mitral stenosis
    (b) AV canal defect
    (c) Fallot's tetralogy
    (d) Atrial septal defect
    (e) Transposition of great vessels
16. Folic acid prevents NTD when given to the mother
    (a) As soon as pregnancy is diagnosed
    (b) In the 1st trimester
    (c) Periconceptional period
    (d) Does not prevent NTD
17. Recurrence risk for a male child in sex-linked recessive is:
    (a) 10% (b) 25%
    (c) 50% (d) 75%
18. Vertical mode of transmission is common in:
    (a) Thalassemia (b) Polydactyly
    (c) Hemophilia (d) Spina bifida

19. Osteogenesis imperfecta is associated with one of the following:
    (a) Polydactyly
    (b) Blue Sclera
    (c) Hepatosplenomegaly
    (d) MR
20. Microcephaly on USG can be suspected at earliest at:
    (a) 1st trimester
    (b) 3rd trimester
    (c) 2nd trimester
    (d) Not diagnosed
21. Hypoglycemia is associated with:
    (a) Phenylketonurea
    (b) Galactosemia
    (c) Cystic fibrosis
    (d) Maple syrup urine disease
22. Philadelphia chromosome associated with CML is a type of:
    (a) Reciprocal translocation
    (b) Robertsonian translocation
    (c) Ring chromosome
    (d) Isochromosome
23. A balanced translocation is usually associated with:
    (a) Normal phenotype
    (b) Dysmorphic features
    (c) A genetic disease
    (d) Mental retardation
24. Evidence of an affected individual in every generation is classically associated with:
    (a) Autosomal recessive
    (b) Multifactorial
    (c) Autosomal dominent
    (d) Sex-linked recessive
    (e) Sex-linked dominant

25. A 30-year male has Lebers Hereditary Optic Neuropathy. What is the risk of recurrence in his progeny?
    (a) 25% (b) 50%
    (c) No risk (d) 75%
26. Which embryonic Hb is the precursor of Fetal Hb?
    (a) Gower 1
    (b) Gower 2
    (c) Hb Portland
27. Substitution of glutamic acid at the 6th position by valine in the beta chain results in:
    (a) Hb C disease (b) Alpha thalassemia
    (c) Sickle cell disease (d) Spherocytosis
28. Copper metabolism is affected in all but one of the following:
    (a) Indian childhood cirrhosis
    (b) Wilson's disease
    (c) Menke's Kiky Hair syndrome
    (d) Hemochromatosis
29. Congenital Rubella is associated with all but one of the congenital anomalies:
    (a) Congenital heart disease
    (b) Hydrocephalus
    (c) Cataracts
    (d) Micropthalmia
    (e) Microcephaly
30. The karyotypic abnormality in Cri-du Chat syndrome is:
    (a) 4p- (b) 5p-
    (c) 9p- (d) 18p-
31. Uniparental disomy is a feature of:
    (a) Angelman syndrome
    (b) William's syndrome
    (c) DiGeoge's syndrome
    (d) RubinsteinTaybi syndrome

32. Short stature is a classical feature of:
    (a) Klinefelter's syndrome
    (b) Turner's syndrome
    (c) Fragile X
    (d) XXY syndrome
33. What is holandric inheritance:
    (a) Inheritance from mother to offspring
    (b) Inheritance from father to offspring
    (c) Inheritance from father to his male offspring
    (d) Inheritance from mother to her male offspring
34. In a female newborn, the risk of being a carrier for a sex-linked recessive disorder, when her mother is a carrier is:
    (a) 30% of the progeny
    (b) 50% of the progeny
    (c) 50% of the female progeny
    (d) 25% of the female progeny
35. Noonan's syndrome has a phenotype akin to:
    (a) Turner's syndrome
    (b) Fragile X
    (c) Klinefelter's Syndrome
    (d) XXY syndrome
36. The chromosomal pattern in Testicular Feminisation syndrome is:
    (a) XX (b) XXY
    (c) XY (d) XO
37. Female Pseudohermaphroditism can be due to all but one of the following conditions:
    (a) Congenital adrenal hyperplasia
    (b) Progesterone administration to mother
    (c) Maternal virilising tumors
    (q) Administration of steroids to mother

38. Fetal alcohol syndrome is associated with all but one of the following:
    (a) Characteristic facies
    (b) Skeletal defects
    (c) Heart defects
    (d) Congenital cataracts
39. Potter's syndrome is associated with all but one of the following:
    (a) Renal agenesis
    (b) Hypoplastic lungs
    (c) Oligohydramnios
    (d) Polyhydramnios
40. Deformations are caused by:
    (a) Chromosomal aberrations
    (b) Single gene defect
    (c) Mechanical factors
    (d) Developmental defect during embryogenesis
41. Hypoplastic mandible is a feature of:
    (a) Treacher Collins syndrome
    (b) Pierre Robin syndrome
    (c) Aperts syndrome
    (d) Crouzon's disease
42. What is the risk recurrence in future pregnancies when the abortus is chromosomally abnormal:
    (a) Increased (b) Decreased
    (c) Unchanged
43. An adult male has no signs of Marfan's syndrome, but two of his progeny are affected. How would you assess the genotype of the father?
    (a) Variable expressivity
    (b) Non-penetrance
    (c) e Allelic heterogenicity

44. All but one of the following are true of multifactorial traits:
    (a) Recurrence risk is the same for all 1st degree relatives
    (b) Recurrence risk drops as the relationship to the affected individual becomes more remote
    (c) Recurrence risk does not depend upon sex
    (d) Recurrence risk is higher in relatives of severely affected probands
45. A newborn child birth Down syndrome:
    (a) Is likely to have a close relative with Down syndrome
    (b) Will show Barr bodies in the buccal smear
    (c) Is more probable with a mother over the age of 35
46. Match the congenital anomaly with the type of malformation:

(a) Deformation	(1) Amniotic band syndrome
(b) Disruption	(2) Club foot in a twin pregnancy
(c) Dysplasia	(3) Potter's syndrome
(d) Malformation	(4) Cleft lip and palate
(e) Sequence	(5) Thanatophoric Dwarfism

47. An individual is XXXXY Give the correct combination of active and inactive genes:
    (a) Active and three inactive X chromosomes
    (b) 2 active and 2 inactive X chromosomes
    (c) 3 active and 1 inactive X chromosomes
    (d) None of the above
48. A newborn infant is diagnosed to have Down syndrome. How would you proceed with the counseling?
    (a) Counsel mother first
    (b) Counsel father first
    (c) Counsel both separately
    (d) Counsel both together
49. Fanconi/ Bloom syndrome is associated with:
    (a) Triploidy
    (b) Trisomy
    (c) Monosomy
    (d) Chromosome breakages
    (e) Fragile sites

50. The human haploid genome has approximately:
    (a) 3 billion base pairs of DNA
    (b) 3 million base pairs of DNA
    (c) 70,000 base pairs of DNA
51. Where would you advise prenatal diagnosis for Neural tube defects:
    (a) A woman with long-standing IDDM
    (b) H/o Rubella in the first trimester
    (c) Exposure to X-rays in the first trimester
52. Which of these is the specific test for NTD?
    (a) Maternal Serum Triple Test
    (b) USG in the first trimester
    (c) Amniocentesis at 15 weeks with beta hCG estimation
53. What parameters in the Triple test suggest Down's syndrome:
    (a) High AFP with low beta HCG
    (b) Low AFP with high beta HCG
    (c) Isolated high AFP
    (d) Isolated high beta HCG
54. At what period of pregnancy is amniocentesis advisable?
    (a) 9-11 weeks (b) 15-17 weeks
    (c) 22-24 weeks
55. Select the specific prenatal diagnostic test for a woman with 20 weeks of pregnancy. The fetus is found on USG to have duodenal atresia and nuchal edema:
    (a) CVS sampling
    (b) MSAFP
    (c) Amniocentesis
    (d) Fetal blood sampling
56. Which prenatal test is applicable in a woman who is a heterozygote for DMD?
    (a) CVS (b) Amniocentesis
    (c) USG (d) Serum creatine

57. A 36-year-old woman with 15 'weeks pregnancy wants to know the risk for Down's. Which test would you suggest:
    (a) CVS (b) MSAFP
    (c) Amniocentesis (d) USG
58. Foetal karyotyping is indicated in all but one of the following conditions
    (a) A 40-year-old primi
    (b) H/o Downs in a previous child
    (c) Maternal karyotype shows" 14/21 translocation
    (d) H/o polydactyly in the family
59. Which of the following infectious agents are potentially teratogenic:
    (a) Rubella virus (b) Toxoplasmosis
    (c) Herpes simplex (d) Varicellae
    (e) Cytomegalovirus (f) All of above
60. Prenatal genetic counselling is indicated when the mother is on:
    (a) Antiepileptics
    (b) Occasional antihistaminics
    (c) Folic acid
    (d) Insulin
61. Which of these statements about genetic polymorphisms is true:
    (a) Can be demonstrated by cytogenetic analysis
    (b) Seen on clinical examination
    (c) Reflect alteration of DNA sequences
    (d) Can be used to distinguish twins
62. Tick of the correct statement about multifactorial anomalies:
    (a) They are a group of embryologically unrelated malformations
    (b) They are isolated anomalies
    (c) The recurrence risk in the same generation varies
    (d) Recurrence risk is not sex related

63. Genetic disease is commonly treated by:
    (a) Somatic gene therapy
    (b) Amelioration of metabolic abnormalities
    (c) Amelioration of clinical phenotype
64. X inactivation in females is best described by one of the following statements:
    (a) It occurs in postnatal life
    (b) It is associated with demethylation
    (c) It is a part of Turner's syndrome
    (d) It produces dosage compensation for the X linked gene
65. Most of the nuclear DNA consists of:
    (a) Introns
    (b) Exons
    (c) Repetitive sequences like SINES and LINES
    (d) Unique sequences that function as genes
66. All the following are microdeletion syndromes *except:*
    (a) Angelman syndrome
    (b) Cri du chat syndrome
    (c) Miller Dieker syndrome
    (d) Prader Willi syndrome
67. A proto-oncogene may be activated by any of the following *except*:
    (a) Chromosomal rearrangement
    (b) Deletion
    (c) Point mutation
    (d) Amplification
68. The Hardy Weinberg Law is based on all the following *except*:
    (a) Genes involved are autosomal dominant
    (b) Random mating within a population
    (c) No migration of population
    (d) No mutation occurring at the locus

69. High resolution banding is useful because:
    (a) It allows individual single copy genes to be identified
    (b) It uses chromosomes in the mid metaphase stage
    (c) It is used to identify fragile sites
    (d) It can demonstrate small alterations of chromosomal structure
70. Genomic imprinting:
    (a) Is responsible for parent of origin effect in the expression of some genes
    (b) Randomly turns off genes from either parent
    (c) Occurs normally only in makes
    (d) Occurs in normal females
71. Congenital Adrenal Hyperplasia in a newborn female is manifested by:
    (a) Ambiguous genitalia
    (b) Breast development
    (c) Cubitus valgus
    (d) Webbing of neck
72. Cystic Fibrosis is suspected when a child presents with:
    (a) Recurrent respiratory infections
    (b) Immune deficiency
    (c) Lactose intolerance
    (d) PUG
73. VATER Association has all except one of these:
    (a) Anal atresia
    (b) TO fistula
    (c) Duodenal atresia
    (d) Cardiac anomaly
    (e) Hydrocephalus
74. Miller Dieker syndrome is:
    (a) Multifactorial
    (b) Microdeletion
    (c) Trisomy
    (d) Normal karyotype

75. William's syndrome has all the following characteristics *except*:
    (a) Hypocalcemia.
    (b) Constipation
    (c) Aortic Stenosis
    (d) Pulmonary stenosis
76. Deafness is associated with all but one of the following:
    (a) Treacher Collins syndrome
    (b) Waardenberg's syndrome
    (c) Pendred's syndrome
    (d) Turner's syndrome
77. X linked dominant mode of transmission is seen in:
    (a) Rett syndrome
    (b) Hemophilia A
    (c) Fragile X syndrome
    (d) DiGeoges syndrome
78. Hydrocephalus is a finding in all except one of the following:
    (a) Dandy Walker syndrome
    (b) Arnold Chiari malformation
    (c) VATER Association
    (d) Macrocephaly.
79. Obesity is associated with all but one of the following:
    (a) Laurence Biedl Moon syndrome
    (b) Beckwith Wiedemann syndrome
    (c) Prader Willi syndrome
    (d) Angelman syndrome
80. Primary Amenorrhea is associated with:
    (a) Turner's syndrome
    (b) XXX syndrome
    (c) Klinefelter's syndrome
    (d) Arnold Chiari malformation

81. Match the urine odor with the Inborn error of Metabolism:

(a) PKU	1. Sweaty urine
(b) Tyrosinemia	2. Cabbage odor
(c) Isovaleric academia	3. Tomcat urine
(d) Multiple carboxylase deficiency	4. Mousy urine
(e) Methionine malabsorbtion malabsorbtion	5. Rancid or fishy

82. Non-ketotic acidosis is diagnostic of:
    (a) Methylmalonic academia
    (b) Propionic academia
    (c) Multiple carboxyl deficiency
    (d) MCAD medium chain acytyl Co-A dehydrogenase. deficiency
83. Cherry red spot on the retina is found in all except one of the following:
    (a) Tay-Sachs disease
    (b) Niemann Pick disease
    (c) Sandhof disease
    (d) Krabbe's disease
84. Hepatosplenomegaly is found in all except one of the following:
    (a) Tay Sachs disease
    (b) GM1 Gangliosidosis
    (c) Gaucher's disease
    (d) Niemann Pick disease
85. Sphingomyelinase deficiency is responsible *for:*
    (a) Mucolipidosis
    (b) Krabbe's disease
    (c) Niemann Pick disease
    (d) Sandhof disease
86. Neonatal hyperbilirubinemia occurs in one of the following:
    (a) Phenylketonuria (b) Tyrosinemia
    (c) Galactosemia (d) Organic acidemias

87. Mucopolysaccharidosis type 1 is due to deficiency of:
    (a) Hexosaminidase
    (b) Alpha-1-iduronidase
    (c) Phenyl alanine hydroxylase
    (d) Glucose 1:6 transferase
88. All but one indicate an inborn error of metabolism:
    (a) A healthy infant with no dysmorphic features suffers vascular collapse on day 2 of life
    (b) An infant, initially bright has regression of milestones and shows no interest in the outside world.
    (c) Child born to consanguinous parents
    (d) A child with mental retardation with slanting eyes and single palmar crease
89. Hereditary spherocytosis is due to:
    (a) Structural protein abnormality
    (b) Abnormality of membrane transport.
    (c) Altered cellular receptor
    (d) Enzyme deficiency
90. Match the following diseases with the mutation induced protein alteration:

(a) Galactosemia	1. Alteration of major collagen or connective tissue
(b) Osteogenesis imperfecta	2. Dysfunction of a sugar converting enzyme
(c) Tay Sachs	3. Expansion of a segment - trinucleotide repeats
(d) Huntington's disease	4. Dysfunction of an enzyme in removing sugar side chains from long chain lipids

91. Which one of these is a cytogenetic abnormality seen in chronic myeloid leukemia:
    (a) Interstitial deletion in 13q
    (b) Translocation between chromosome 15 & 17 t(15;17)

(c) Translocation between chromosome 9 & 22 t(9;22)
(d) Multiple chromosomal breaks

92. Presymptomatic testing for hereditary cancers is possible in:
(a) Familial breast and ovarian cancer
(b) Leukemias
(c) Retinoblastoma
(d) Osteosarcoma

93. Oocyte completes its meiosis II division in the fetus:
(a) At puberty (b) Before ovulation
(c) During ovulation (d) After fertilization

94. The most common genetic change occurring in the development of tumor is:
(a) Activation of c-myc gene due to chromosomal rearrangement
(b) Activation of c-myc by somatic mutation
(c) Inactivation or loss of P53 gene/by somatic mutation
(d) Mutation in the ras group of oncogenes

95. Any ideal genetic screening program has all the following features *except*:
(a) The cost of having a program is less than not having one
(b) Management option are better when patients are screened and found positive
(c) The disease to be screened is lethal or has serious consequences
(d) The disease is curable after diagnosis

96. All the following are correct *except:*
(a) Gene therapy is useful when a genetic disease to diagnosed before bull
(b) It is useful when the genetic disease is diagnosed after birth
(c) It is useful in genetic and non-genetic disorder
(d) Give therapy is a prophylactic form of treatment

97. Match the terminology in ethical principles:

(a) Justice	1 Not allowing harm to the patient
(b) Autonomy	2 Respect patients decision against treatment
(c) Fidelity	3 To keep the commitment
(d) Beneficence	4 To equal treatment to all cases
(e) Rights	5 Do no harm

98. On which of the following tissues is cytogenetic analysis performed:
    (a) Formalin preserved tissues
    (b) Paraffin blocks of tissues
    (c) Serum
    (d) Dried blood spots
    (e) Lymphocytes
99. Pharmacogenetics deals with:
    (a) Study of drugs
    (b) Effect of drugs on human body
    (c) Genetic susceptibility of an individual on drug metabolism
    (d) Teratogenetic effect of the drug
100. All of following is true except one for couples having special interest in knowing the zygosity of twins:
    (a) General interest
    (b) To confirm if they are identical
    (c) To assess if they will have twins again
    (d) Paternity assessment

ANSWERS

1. (e) Multifactorial diseases occur due to the additive results of genes plus environmental factors. Most of the adult onset diseases are multifactorial. Examples of these include hypertension, type II diabetes and coronary heart disease.
2. (b) Somatic cells undergo cell division to produce generally identical daughter cells. In germ cells, mitosis takes place after reduction division. The cell cycle is divided into four stages—prophase, metaphase, anaphase and telophase. In metaphase, the chromosomes contract and move to the centre of the cell. Due to their elongated morphology, they are ideal for studying chromosomal defects.
3. (a) Chromosomes can be classified according to the centromere position. When the centromere is in the middle of a chromosome, it is called metacentric, when slightly above the centre, submetacentric, at the end of the chromosome, acrocentric and at the tip, telocentric.
4. (d) Fragile X is an X-linked disorder where affected males have delayed and mental retardation, The incidence is 1:1500 males. The molecular defect is a CGG repeat or a triplet repeat expansion. Cytogenetically, the fragile site involves the FMR-1 gene on Xq27. This fragile site becomes visible only under special culture techniques using folate deficient medium. Recently, molecular genetic techniques to identify the expansion have been used for the diagnosis of this condition.
5. (d) Meiosis I takes place in the oogonia before birth where as Meiosis II occurs only after fertilization.

6. (b) Down syndrome is associated with presence of extra chromosome 21. Others do not show abnormal chromosome patterns.
7. (c) Trisomy 21. Trisomy 21 means the presence of an extra chromosome 21. This is the commonest chromosomal anomaly seen in the population. Incidence of trisomy 21 increases with advancing maternal age.
8. (d) Vertical transmission denotes the inheritance of the abnormality from either of the parents to the progeny. The parents also have to have a recognizable abnormality, and cannot be normal. An exception is the rare event of germ cell mosaicism where the affected genes are expressed only in the parental germ cells and not the somatic cells, and therefore the parents have a normal phenotype.
9. (b) Trisomy 18.
10. (c) These group of disorders are called contiguous gene or microdeletion sydromes, and cannot be identified using normal banding techniques. Using fluorescent in situ hybridisation, specific probes are used for hybridisation and analysed using special filters.
11. (d) The word point mutation means that a single base is substituted by another in the DNA. Various types of mutations are seen in thalassemia. There are about 500 different mutations in the Indian population.
12. (a) Autosomal dominant disorders are transmitted from an affected parent to a child. It is often noted that in a known dominant disorder, the affected members show a variable phenotype. This can be due to variable penetrance. This means multiple members of the family affected with the same mutation show varying clinical features.

13. (d) Sex linked recessive. The affected males are hemizyous. The gene located on the X chromosome is sufficient to manifest the disease, since males have only one copy of the X chromosome.
14. (d) In Down syndrome, there are three copies of chromosome 21. Down syndrome can occur due to error at meiosis leading to a disomic gamete which is fertilized by a normal gamete. In translocation 21/21, it is certain that always a 21/21 chromosome will be transmitted, as both chromosome 21s are involved. Thus after fertilization with the normal 21 chromosome from the other partner the gamete always will be trisomic for 21. For the remaining 21 /centric fusion translocations, the empiric recurrence risk is less than 2% if the father is a carrier and 15% if the mother is a carrier.
15. (b) About 40% of children with Down syndrome have structural lesions such as atrioventricular septal defects, isolated ventricular septal defects, patent ductus arteriosus, or anomalous origin of the subclavian arteries. All newborns with Down syndrome should undergo cardiac evaluation.
16. (c) The ectoderm of the neural plate, called neuroectoderm gives rise to the central nervous system, consisting of the brain and spinal cord. By the end of the third week, neural folds begin to move together fuse and neural tube is formed. By the time a woman knows she is pregnant these events take place. Folic acid is important and necessary for the development of the neural tube, and its deficiency may contribute to neural tube defects. Maintaining these levels in the preconception period is therefore important.

17. (c) The risk for transmission from a female carrier to male child is 50%. The male has only one sex chromosome, and the mother with her two X chromosomes has a 50% chance of passing on an affected chromosome.
18. (b) Most skeletal dysplasias are transmitted in the autosomal dominant fashion. This means either of the parent is affected. However, characteristic of autosomal dominant conditions, is non penetrance, where there is an absence of a trait or a disease in the parent or variation in the symptoms due to reduced expressivity.
19. (b) Blue sclerae are characteristic of osteogenesis imperfecta (OI). Four genetic OI syndromes are recognised Type I and Type IV are autosomal dominant and Type II and III are autosomal recessive.
20. (c) Microcephaly results due to an abnormality of the central nervous system, in which the brain and consequently, the skull fails to grow. Children are mentally retarded. The face is of normal size. The cause of microcephaly is often uncertain and could be due to genetic abnormalities or infectious due to the TORCH group of infections. Diagnosis of microcephaly requires successive ultrasound scans during the second trimester and confirmed in the third trimester.
21. (b) Hypoglycemia is associated with galactosemia. This is an inborn error of carbohydrate metabolism and is due to deficiency of the enzyme galactose 1 phosphate uridyl transferase, an essential enzyme in the metabolism of the galactose. Newborns present with vomiting, lethargy, failure to thrive and jaundice.

The symptoms appear in second week of life. If untreated mental retardation can occur. The complications are avoided by early diagnosis by checking reducing substances in the urine. Treatment consists of feeding infants milk substitutes which do not contain galactose or lactose, the sugars present in the milk.

22. (a) Philadelphia chromosome is a type of reciprocal translocation between the long arms of chromosomes 9 and 22. Its presence in a case of CML indicates good prognosis. Aim of cytotoxic therapy in CML is to destroy all cells with Philadelphia chromosome so that it is not detectable after therapy.

23. (a) There are two types of translocations, Robertsonian and reciprocal. Robertsonian translocations occur when two acrocentric chromosomes join together. In balanced translocations, carriers have 45 chromosomes but no loss of chromosomal material, and are healthy. In unbalanced translocations the chromosome number is 46, with trisomy for one of the chromosomes involved in the translocation, leading to spontaneous abortion, or a liveborn infant with trisomy. Robertsonian translocations arise spontaneously, or are inherited from a parent carrying a balanced translocation. In reciprocal translocations, there is exchange of chromosomal material between two different chromosomes due to breakage and rejoining. Balanced translocations occur in healthy individuals, but there is a risk of mental retardation in individuals with denovo translocations, as a small loss of DNA material may not be visualised by routine microscopy, and the missing material causes disease.

24. (c) An autosomal dominant disease can manifest in the heterozygous state in both the sexes, therefore appearance of the trait in every generation is expected. 50% of the progeny is will carry the trait as a parent can transmit either a chromosome which is completely normal or with a trait.
25. (c) Leber's hereditary optic neuropathy is a disorder which occurs due to mitochondrial mutations, either sporadic or inherited. The transmission is maternal as only the egg contributes to the cytoplasm and mitochondria in the zygote. Progeny of a carrier mother will receive the mutation but an offspring of a carrier father will be normal. The pedigree pattern may be difficult to recognize, as carrier individuals are asymptomatic.
26. (b) Fetal haemoglobin (alpha2 gamma2) forms less than 2% of the fraction of total haemoglobin. These consist of 2 alpha chains identical to those found in HbA and 2 gamma chains. The gamma chains are members of the beta globin family. Hb F in fetal life accounts for 60% of the total haemoglobin. A few weeks after conception, embryonic haemoglobin (delta2 epsilon2). Hb Gower 1 is synthesised by the embryonic yolk sac.
27. (c) Sickle cell disease is a hereditary disease, where the mutation in the globin gene changes the amino acid glutamine to valine by changing the codon GAG to GTG.
28. (d) Disorders of copper metabolism are associated with a high copper level in the liver and raised serum levels of copper and ceruloplasmin. These are Menke's disease, an X-linked disorder and Wilson's disease, an autosomal recessive disorder. Indian childhood cirrhosis is believed to be multifactorial

in origin. Neurological symptoms appear in early life and are common to all three disorders. Hemochromatosis is an autosomal recessive disorder caused by accumulation of toxic quantities of iron in different organs. The diagnosis is based on increased serum ferritin and iron. If untreated, the disease results in premature death due to cirrhosis, diabetes and cardiac failure.

29. (b) Maternal rubella infection, also known as German measles occurs when the mother is affected with the rubella virus in pregnancy, leading to congenital rubella infection, Clinically it manifests as rash and fever and the diagnosis is confirmed by rubella titre. The infection is transmitted transplacentally. The symptoms of rubella embryopathy include fetal growth retardation, hepatosplenomegaly, congenital cataracts, deafness and mental retardation. In hydrocephalus there is an enlargement of ventricular system of the brain which occurs due to an imbalance in the production and absorption of cerebrospinal fluid. Hydrocephalus is not seen as apart of rubella embryopathy.

30. (b) The name cri-du-chat syndrome is associated with this syndrome, as the cry of the newborn child is high pitched, shrill and cat like. This was the first autosomal deletion syndrome to be described. The infants are severely mentally retarded and may have cardiac defects (30%). Most children have denovo defect, but about 15% result from a chromosomal imbalance inherited from a normal carrier parent, and tend to be more severe.

31. (a) In uniparental disomy, there is inheritance of both copies of the same chromosome from a single parent rather than a single copy from each parent. The

phenotype is associated due to lack of imprinting of certain genes. If there is paternal uniparental disomy of chromosome 15, the associated disorder is known as Angelman syndrome and if maternal the it is known as Prader Willi syndrome. This is called genomic imprinting, which is differential expression of a gene, depending on whether it is inherited from the father or the mother.

32. (b) Turner syndrome is a sex chromosomal disorder which occurs due to absence of the second X chromosome (45x) or due to a structural abnormality of one X chromosome. The average height in Turner syndrome is 145 cm, as there may be a loss of genes responsible for height in the regions of the missing X chromosome.

33. (c) Holandric inheritance or 'Y' linked inheritance suggests that only males are affected. In this condition affected males transmit to all his sons and to none of his daughters like family surname. Certain 'Y' linked traits like hairy pinna and baldness are Y linked. It has been recently reported that H-Y histocompatibility genes responsible for spermatogenesis are located on the Y chromosomes and should be considered as having holandric inheritance.

34. (c) X-linked recessive traits are determined by a gene located on the X chromosome and is manifests in males The diseases inherited as autosomal disorders are transmitted by heterozygous females who are healthy and pass on to 50% of their sons. A female will pass only one of her X to her daughters which could be normal or affected there is 50% chance that they will have an affected gene. The affected sons will transmit diseased gene to their daughters

but they being heterozygous are not affected and are carriers.

35. (a) Noonan's syndrome has phenotype akin to Turner syndrome. The affected individuals are short statured, have webbed neck cardiac anomaly and wide spaced nipple. The gene is inherited as autosomal dominant and is located on chromosome 12q.

36. (c) Testicular feminization syndrome is associated with 46XY karyotype. In this condition phenotype of a person is female there is breast development at puberty. The testes are present in the inguinal canal. There is absence of uterus and vagina may be small pouch like. Patients can present for the first-time as a case of primary amenorrhea. Though testes produce androgen there is absence of androgen sensitive receptors. Female shave female psychic sex. The testes can turn malignant hence should be removed at puberty. Oestrogen is recommended to prevent osteoporosis.

37. (d) An individual having pseudohermaphroditism is has female karyotype and the external genitalia are virilised thus resembling that of a male or are ambiguous. The main cause is congenital adrenal hyperplasia. Which occurs due to reduced cortisol production leading to increased ACTH secretion causing adrenal hyperplasia. Maternal virilizing tumors like arrhenoblastoma also leads to pseudohermaphroditism.

38. (d) Fetal alcohol syndrome shows characteristic facial features like short palpebral fissures, maxillary hypoplasia, micropthalmus, thin upper lips, growth retardation and sometimes limb deformities. The infants at birth show alcohol withdrawal symptoms.

39. (d) Potter's syndrome is a birth defect classified as sequence. The condition occurs as a sequence of malformation due to renal agenesis leading to absence of urine production leading to reduced amniotic fluid volume giving secondary deformation and pulmonary hypoplasia.
40. (c) The deformations are caused by abnormal intrauterine moulding of structures which are otherwise structurally normal. Involvement of musculoskeletal system is common and occurs in fetuses with congenital neuromuscular problems like congenital myotonic dystrophy or as in spina bifida due to positional deformities of the legs. The deformation also occurs in the second trimester due to small sized uterus, fibroids, multiple gestation.
41. (b) Pierre Robin syndrome is a syndrome of maldevelopment of the first branchial arch results in various congenital malformations of the eyes, ears, palate and mandible. Hypoplasia of the mandible is a classical feature of this syndrome.
42 (b) 60% of the abortuses show a chromosomal error usually numerical anomalies. Subsequent karyotyping of the parent in these show only 0.5% having a chromosomal carrier defect. Thus cause of previous errors is due to error at meiosis I or II leading to non-disjunction which can be a chance occurrence.
43. (b) Marfan's syndrome is inherited as an autosomal dominant condition. Ideally it is transmitted from parent to his child. If parent is unaffected it may fall into a characteristic seen in autosomal condition as non-penetrance. It can also be seen where paternity can be considered.
44. (c)

45. (c) Is more probable with a mother over the age of thirty five years.

46. Match the congenital anomaly with the type of malformation

(a) Deformation	(1) Amniotic band syndrome
(b) Disruption	(2) Club foot in a twin pregnancy
(c) Dysplasia	(3) Potter's syndrome
(d) Malformation	(4) Cleft lip and palate
(e) Sequence	(5) Thanatophoric dwarfism

Ans. (1b, 2a, 3e, 4d, 5c)

47. (a) In the somatic cells of the female mammals out of two X chromosomes only one X chromosome is active while the second is inactive. This in active chromosome is seen lying at the periphery of the nucleus attached to a nuclear membrane and is termed Barr body. The inactive chromosome is either paternal or maternal and in different cells of a same person. This inactivation is random but fixed so daughter cells of these cells carry the same inactive chromosome. If a female or a male is carrying more than one X chromosome the number of X chromosomes get inactivated and are seen as Barr bodies in the interphase cell. The inactivation occurs as early as 15-16 days of gestation. Inactivation begins in the region Xq13 and spreads along the chromosome.

48. (d) Genetic counselling is a process of communication where an advice is given about the condition in question as regards confirmation of the clinical diagnosis, prognosis, management as well as prenatal diagnosis for future pregnancies. When an infant is diagnosed to have a genetic condition, both the parents should be counselled together. This helps them to understand the condition better as well as gives mutual emotional support.

49. (d) Fanconi's syndrome patient's have pancytopenia, radial aplasia, patchy pigmentation of the skin. Congenital heart disease and renal anomalies are also noted. Cytogenetic preparations from the lymphocytes show chromosomal breakages. Bloom syndrome patients clinically show small cutaneous telangiectases. Their chromosomes show breakages and rearrangement.

50. (a) Human genome consists of 3 billion basepairs. These encode our genetic information. All amino acids are coded by three base pairs. Any missing link can lead to disease.

51. (a) The children of women with insulin dependent diabetes mellitus have risk of congenital anomalies that is two to , three folds greater than that of general population. The most common malformation observed is congenital heart disease and neural tube defects.

52. (a) Maternal serum Triple test involves study of three analyses (HCG, alfafetoprotein and serum estriol. The alfafetoprotein is the main plasmaprotein in fetal life and is slowly replaced by albumin. It is possible to measure these levels in the fetal blood, amniotic fluid and maternal serum. In neural tube defects and abdominal wall defects the this fetal protein is leaked into the amniotic fluid and circulated in maternal blood raised s.AFP along with ultrasonography between 15-17 weeks can diagnose about 90% of neural tube defects.

53. (b) Down syndrome fetuses are biochemically immature and show low levels of serum AFR (Ref. Ans. 52). Human chorionic gonadotropin originates from the placenta. Its level falls sharply between 10-20 weeks. These are markedly high in Down syndrome

screening. Along with serum estriol these are used as marker for predicting risk for Down, Edward syndrome Tri 18. Since there can be false positives and negatives tests should be interpreted and assessed correctly. The ideal time for Down's screening is 14-16 weeks.

54. (b) Amniocentesis is usually done between 15-17 weeks gestation when viable (80%) to non-viable (20%) cells is highest. The volume of amniotic fluid is about 200 ml of which 15-20 ml is aspirated under ultrasound guidance. Amniocentesis at earlier gestation has few viable cells and there is increased procedure related risk of miscarriage. Around 24 weeks gestation ,the viable cells are only 10 to 12%.

55. (d) With abnormal ultrasound findings at 20 weeks the most preferred test is fetal blood sampling Duodenal atresia and nuchal oedema are ultrasound markers of Down syndrome. Rapid karyotyping is of great value and is possible with fetal blood which can give results within 48 hr to 72 hr with amniotic fluid karyotyping takes minimum 12-15 days.

56. (a) Male fetus of a woman who IS heterozygote for DMD is at risk for a disease. It is possible to do dystrophin gene analysis where a deletion in the gene is responsible for DMD, from DNA extracted from a CVS sample. Since this is a sex linked disorder fetal sexing is done first and if male the sample is subjected for dystrophin gene analysis.

57. (c) A 36-year-old woman has an increased risk of Down syndrome due to her age. Non-invasive tests like USG markers or Triple test are used as screening tests for mothers who are less than 35 at the time of delivery. Amniocentesis is performed between 15-17 weeks gestation (Ref ti Ans. 54). And is ideal for diagnosis of Down syndrome.

Here are the answers for 33-57
please delete questions 22 and 45
please check the answer for 37. b does not seem to be the correct answer.

58. (d) Isolated polydactyly can be inherited as an autosomal dominant disorder. Fetal chromosomal studies will not identify this and it is therefore not justified since it will not alter the management of the pregnancy. The diagnosis of polydactyly could be made during a fetal anomaly scan, if careful examination of the fetal hand is made.

59. (f) All of the above. Congenital rubella manifests with central diffuse cataracts, congenital heart disease, salt and pepper retinitis, jaundice, hepatomegaly, myocarditis, blueberry muffin rash and sensorineural deafness. The major sites of Involvement in congenital toxoplasmosis are the CNS, retina, choroid, and muscles. Severely affected infants are hydrocephalic or microcephalic, have hepato-splenomegaly, ventricular dilatation and diffuse calcifications. Infants congenitally infected with herpes simplex may die in utero or may be born with jaundice, skin lesions, chorioretinitis, and signs of systemic infection. Congenital varicella zoster Infection leads to microphthalmia, cataracts, chorioretinitis, and cutaneous and bony aplasia or hypoplasia. Infants with congenital CMV present with sepsis, intrauterine growth retardation, chorioretinitis microcephaly, hepatosplenomegaly, anemia, thrombocytopenia and periventricular calcifications.

60. (a) Epileptic women on anticonvulsant drugs have an increased risk of congenital malformations in the fetus. If multiple drugs are used, the risk is increased.

Whether the risk is due to the disease or the drugs or a combination of both is uncertain. Drugs like valproic acid, phenytoin, and carbamazepine are known to cause neural tube defects. Pre and perinatal folic acid and prenatal diagnosis by AFP estimation is indicated for the possibility of neural tube defects.

61. (c) DNA polymorphisms are due to an alterations in the DNA sequence, and do not cause disease. The techniques used include RFLP analysis using Southern blotting or PCR.
62. (b) Most multifactorial anomalies are isolated anomalies and involvement of other body parts is as part of a sequence of events.
63. (c) Genetic disease is commonly treated by amelioration of the clinical phenotype, as yet there is very little specific treatment available. However, the success in the treatment of severe combined immuno-deficiency caused by deficiency of adenosine deaminase, cystic fibrosis and the Haemophilus has been shown. Several gene therapy trials using various vectors for several diseases are currently underway.
64. (d) In somatic cells of female mammals, one of the 2 X chromosomes is inactivated. In males there is only one X chromosome. In spite of having a double dose of genes on the X chromosome in females, the gene product is the same as males. This is because one X chromosome undergoes inactivation, and this is called dosage compensation.
65. (c) Interspersed repeats are repeated DNA sequences located at dispersed regions in the genome. Most of these elements namely the LINES (long interspersed nuclear elements) and SINES (short

interspersed nuclear elements) are located in gastrogenic regions, but some of them are located in introns. The most common LINE element in humans is the L 1 element and the most common SINE is the Alu family of repeats.

66. (b) 5p-syndrome, also known as cri-du-chat syndrome is a chromosomal syndrome in which the clinical diagnosis is confirmed by chromosome analysis using Giemsa trypsin banding. Microdeletion syndromes are not seen using the above technique as the size of the deletion is too small, and a special technique called fluorescent in situ hybridisation is required for the visualisation of the underlying chromosomal aberration.

67. (b) Human cellular genes that regulate normal cell growth and that are homologous to the genetic material of transforming ANA tumour viruses (retroviruses) are called protooncogenes. Mutagenesis may be initiated by insertional mutagenesis but more commonly the tumorigenesis results from unregulated activation of the related endogenous oncogene by chromosomal translocation.

68. (b) The Hardy Weinberg law is based on the assumption that mating within the population is totally random, there is migration of the population, there is no occurrence of mutation at the locus being studied, and there is no selection for a particular genotype at the said locus.

69. (d) For high resolution banding the chromosomes are selected in prophase and prometaphase, where they are elongated, as they are less condensed than metaphase chromosomes. To attain this, partial synchronisation of mitosis in the culture is aimed,

by arresting DNA synthesis. The cells are then released from the arrest and many mitotic cells are obtained. The staining procedure is same as that of Giemsa trypsin banding, but due to elongation of the chromosomes many sub-bands are visualised and a banding level of 850 can be achieved.

70. (a) The sex of the parent contributing a specific chromosome may affect the expression of some of the genes on the chromosome. Imprinting is a strong parental chromosomal influence on the expression of a particular gene. An example of genomic imprinting is the Angelman and Prader-Wilii syndromes, both resulting from a deletion of 15q11-13. In Angelman syndrome, the maternal region is deleted, while in Prader-Willi syndrome, the paternal region is deleted.

71. (a) Congenital adrenal hyperplasia is due to deficiency of 21-hydroxylase, which is an enzyme in the pathway of progesterone metabolism, and synthesis of steroids. In the severe salt-wasting form there is deficiency of mineralocorticoids, and ambiguous genitalia in female children. In the milder form there is simply virilization of the female external genitalia.

72. (a) Cystic fibrosis is the most common autosomal recessive disorder occurring in northern Europeans with a carrier frequency of about 1 in 20. The disease affects exocrine gland function, resulting in chronic lung disease and malabsorption. The gene for cystic fibrosis and several mutations are known, making carrier detection and prenatal diagnosis possible. Many carriers (heterozygotes) with one mutant CF gene have been shown to have abnormalities in the vas deferens, and therefore this is an investigation that should be carried out in cases of male infertility.

73. (d) The VATER association is a group of congenital anomalies occurring as a dysmorphic syndrome, with no specific pattern of inheritance. The acronym VATER stands for vertebral anomalies, anal atresia, tracheoesophageal fistula, and renal and radial anomalies. Another group of anomalies VACTERYL includes in addition to VATER, cardiac anomalies and hydrocephalus.

74. (b) Miller Dieker syndrome is a microdeletion syndrome, involving a microdeletion of the chromosomal region on 17p 13.3. It is characterised by microcephaly, lissencephaly, seizures and growth and mental retardation.

75. (a) In William's syndrome there is microdeletion of 7q23. Patients present with elfin facies, supravalvular aortic stenosis and hypercalcemia, not hypocalcemia.

76 (d) Turner syndrome occurs due to absence or structural defect of the one of the X chromosomes. It presents with short stature, weobed neck, shield chest with widely spaced nipples and ovarian streak gonads, and coarctation of the aorta. Deafness is not known to be associated with Turner's syndrome, but is known to be associated with Treacher Collins, Waardenburg's and Pendred syndrome.

77. (a) Rett syndrome is an X-linked dominant condition, and is caused by mutations in the MEPC gene on the X chromosome. X linked dominant conditions are rare. Both the males and females are affected, but the condition is lethal in males. Fragile X syndrome and hemophilia A and B are X-linked recessive conditions with affected males and female carriers. DiGeorge syndrome is caused by a deletion of chromosome 22q.

78. (c) Hydrocephalus is a condition where there is an accumulation of cerebrospinal fluid leading to dilation of the ventricles due to blockage in the CSF circulation. There is thinning of the cortex and increase in the size of the head. Prenatal diagnosis by ultrasound examination can detect this, however sometimes hydrocephalus may not appear until birth. The VATER association is sometimes associated with cardiac defects and hydrocephalus and it is termed the VACTERYL association. All cases of macrocephaly are not associated with hydrocephalus, but hydrocephalus may be a cause of microcephaly.

79. (d) Angelman syndrome is associated with a maternal deletion of chromosome 15q11-13. It is called the "happy Puppet syndrome", and presents with mental retardation, microcephly, ataxia, epilepsy and absent speech. Prader Willi syndrome is caused by a paternal deletion of chromosome 15q11-13, and both these disorders occur due to genomic imprinting. Prader Willi syndrome, Beckwith Weidemann syndrome and Laurence Moon Biedl syndrome are all associated with obesity.

80. (a) One of the clinical manifestations of Turner syndrome is sexual infantilism and streak ovaries. Most females with Turners do not produce estrogens, and therefore have high levels of gonadotropins and ovarian failure, leading to primary amenorrhea.

81.

(a)	PKU	1. Sweaty urine
(b)	Tyrosinemia	2. Cabbageodor
(c)	Isovaleric academia	3. Tomcat urine
(d)	Multiple carboxylase deficiency	4. Mousy urine
(e)	Methionine malabsorption	5. Rancid or fishy

Ans. (1c, 2e, 3d, 4a, 5b)

82. (d) MCAD deficiency (medium-chain acyl-CoA dehydrogenase) deficiency is a disorder of ketogenesis or fatty acid oxidation. It is the most common and least severe disorder compared with short chain and long chain deficiencies, occurring at 1 in 9-15,000 live births. Patients are well in infancy and present with the first episode of hypoglycemia at 2 yr of age, due to prolonged fasting or intercurrent illness. Ketone concentrations are low or undetected.
83. (d) Cherry red spot is seen in Niemann Pick A, Tay Sach's, infantile GM1, Farber's and Sialidosis, which are all lysosomal storage diseases. Krabbe's disease is due to galactocerebrosidase B-galactosidase deficiency and is associated with optic atrophy.
84. (a) Tay Sachs disease (GM2 gangliosidosis) has a clinical onset by 3-6 months and is characterised by profound loss of central nervous system function, and is due to deficiency of hexosaminidase A. There is no hepatosplenomegaly in Tay Sachs. GM1 gangliosidosis (generalized or infantile form), Gaucher's disease and Niemann Pick A, B and C all have hepatosplenomegaly.
85. (c) Sphingomyelinase deficiency is responsible for Niemann Pick disease. The deficiency manifests in the first month of life and is associated with failure to thrive, hepatosplenomegaly cherry red spot in the macula (50% in Niemann Pick A) and by foam cells in the marrow. Death occurs due to sphingomyelin accumulation by the age of 4.
86. (c) Hyperbilirubinemia characteristically occurs in the newbons on the 3rd day of life and is termed physiologic jaundice. Jaundice on the first day of life is always pathologic and could be due to

hemolytic disease of the newborn. The hyperbilirubinemia in galactosemia appears after first week of life, after established feeding. The neonate manifests with liver failure (bilirubinemia, coagulation defects hypoglycemia) and frequently cataracts. The disoder occurs due to deficiency of an enzyme galactose 1 phosphate uridyl transferase, which is necessary for metabolism of galactose.

87. (b) The mucopolysaccharidoses are a group of lysosomal storage disorders where a deficiency of a specific lysosomal enzyme responsible for degradation of complex macromolecules lead to its accumulation. The affected children are mostly normal at birth, have coarse facial features and develop involvement of the skeletal, vascular and central nervous system. Based on the clinical and genetic differences, six different types of MPS are recognised. Type I MPS also known as Hurler's syndrome is due to deficiency of alpha 1 iduronidase, and is characterised by dysostosis multiplex, cloudy cornea, hepatosplenomegaly, CNS dysfunction kyphosis and Alder-Reilly bodies in the WBC.

88. (d) These are classical signs of Down syndrome, a chromosomal disorder associated with presence of an extra chromosome 21.

89. (a) Hereditary spherocytosis is an autosomal dominant disorder due to a defect in the protein lattice (spectrin, ankyrin, protein 4.2) which determines red cell shape. It varies in clinical severity and may manifest as a severe hemolytic anemia with growth failure and splenomegaly to a well compensated mild hemolytic anemia. An osmotic fragility test confirms the presence of spherocytes, which are also seen on a peripheral blood smear.

90. Match the following:

(a) Galactosemia tissue	1. Alteration of major collagen or connective
(b) Osteogenesis Imperfecta	2. Dysfunction of a sugar converting enzyme
(c) Tay Sachs	3. Expansion ot a segment - trinucleotide repeats
(d) Huntington's disease	4. Dysfunction of an enzyme in removing sugar side chains from long chain lipids

Ans. (1b, 2a, 3d, 4c)

91. (c) 85% of patients with chronic myeloid leukaemia show a translocation between the distal portions of the chromosome 9 and 22, also known as the Philadelphia chromosome. Patients with this chromosomal rearrangement have a better prognosis.
92. (a) A proportion of the heritable type of breast and ovarian cancer is caused by mutations in the BRCA 1 locus on 17q or the BRCA2 locus on chromosome 22. Mutation analysis in the affected individual can be carried out.
93. (d) Primary oocytes are produced after the third month in a female fetus. Initiation of meosis starts in the female fetus. The primary oocytes are arrested at the dictyotene stage of prophase. At puberty, oocytes are released from miotic arrest and start maturing. Meiosis I is completed, and miotic II begins around ovulation and completed only after fertilization. The ovum is thus said to be in suspended prophase.
94. (c) A wide variety of malignancies show inactivation of the p53 tumor suppressor gene, by loss or somatic

mutation, and is the underlying cause of pathogenesis in many cancers. Germ line mutation of p53 is also known, in a rare dominantly inherited tumor predisposing syndrome the Li-Fraumeni syndrome.

95. (d) Genetic screening is the most important tool in controlling genetic disease. By identifying carriers the disease can be controlled by choosing various reproductive options like prenatal diagnosis and selective termination, adoption or conception with egg or donor sperms. Identification of a genetic disorder does not mean that it can be cured, unlike some metabolic disorders like PKU and galactosemia which can be very well controlled with dietary restrictions.

96. (d) Gene therapy can be applied at 2 levels somatic and germ line somatic gene therapy is used prenatally and postnatally it is also an accepted mode of treatment for non-genetics disorder. Germ line therapy is yet no accepted due to ethical considerations

97. Match the terminology in ethical principles.

a	Justice	1	Not allowing harm to the patient
b	Autonomy	2	Respect patients decision against treatment
c	Fidelity	3	To keep the commitment
d	Beneficence	4	To give equal treatment to all cases
e	Rights	5	Do no harm

Ans. (1b, 2a, 3d ,4e, 5d)

98. (e) Cytogenetic studies need cells which can divide either naturally or by stimulants. Therefore they must be live cells. A variety of tissues like blood, bone marrow, chorionic villi, or amniotic fluid cells can be used.

99. (c) The term pharmacogenetics refers to the effect of genes on the response to drug therapy. The response may be in the form of altered metabolism of the drug, leading to the necessity of increased a decreased drug dosing, side effects of the drugs, and factors causing drug resistance.

100. (d) Zygosity determination of twins means finding out whether twins are identical. Monozygotic, arising from one egg and one or dizygotic or fraternal, arising from two fertilized eggs. In one-third of the cases children are of different sexes hence dizygosity is confirmed. In twins of the same sex the zygosity is clear by physical appearance by the age of two. Most monozygotic twins have the same blood group and their DNA pattern is the same. It is only in disputed paternity that paternity assessment is sought.

Index

A

B

C

D

E